T0249578

Interventional Procedures in Hepatobiliary Diseases

Editors

ANDRÉS CÁRDENAS
PAUL J. THULUVATH

CLINICS IN LIVER DISEASE

www.liver.theclinics.com

Consulting Editor
NORMAN GITLIN

November 2014 • Volume 18 • Number 4

ELSEVIER

1600 John F. Kennedy Boulevard • Suite 1800 • Philadelphia, Pennsylvania, 19103-2899

http://www.theclinics.com

CLINICS IN LIVER DISEASE Volume 18, Number 4
November 2014 ISSN 1089-3261, ISBN-13: 978-0-323-32658-2

Editor: Kerry Holland
Developmental Editor: Casey Jackson

Clinics in Liver Disease (ISSN 1089-3261) is published quarterly by Elsevier Inc., 360 Park Avenue South, New York, NY 10010-1710. Months of issue are February, May, August, and November. Business and Editorial Offices: 1600 John F. Kennedy Blvd., Ste. 1800, Philadelphia, PA 19103-2899. Customer Service Office: 3251 Riverport Lane, Maryland Heights, MO 63043. Periodicals postage paid at New York, NY and additional mailing offices. Subscription prices are $295.00 per year (U.S. individuals), $145.00 per year (U.S. student/resident), $401.00 per year (U.S. institutions), $395.00 per year (foreign individuals), $200.00 per year (foreign student/ resident), $498.00 per year (foreign institutions), $340.00 per year (Canadian individuals), $200.00 per year (Canadian student/resident), and $498.00 per year (Canadian institutions). Foreign air speed delivery is included in all *Clinics* subscription prices. All prices are subject to change without notice. **POSTMASTER:** Send address changes to *Clinics in Liver Disease*, Elsevier Health Sciences Division, Subscription Customer Service, 3251 Riverport Lane, Maryland Heights, MO 63043. **Customer Service: Telephone: 1-800-654-2452 (U.S. and Canada); 314-447-8871 (outside U.S. and Canada). Fax: 314-447-8029. E-mail: journalscustomer service-usa@elsevier.com (for print support); journalsonlinesupport-usa@elsevier.com (for online support).**

Reprints. For copies of 100 or more of articles in this publication, please contact the Commercial Reprints Department, Elsevier Inc., 360 Park Avenue South, New York, NY 10010-1710. Tel.: 212-633-3874; Fax: 212-633-3820; E-mail: reprints@elsevier.com.

Clinics in Liver Disease is covered in *MEDLINE/PubMed (Index Medicus)*, Science Citation Index Expanded, Journal Citation Reports/Science Edition, and Current Contents/Clinical Medicine.

Contributors

CONSULTING EDITOR

NORMAN GITLIN, MD, FRCP (LONDON), FRCPE (EDINBURGH), FACG, FACP
Formerly, Professor of Medicine, Chief of Hepatology, Emory University; Currently, Consultant, Atlanta Gastroenterology Associates, Atlanta, Georgia

EDITORS

ANDRÉS CÁRDENAS, MD, MMSc, AGAF
GI/Endoscopy Unit, Institut de Malalties Digestives i Metaboliques, University of Barcelona, Hospital Clinic, Barcelona, Spain

PAUL J. THULUVATH, MD, FRCP
Medical Director, The Institute for Digestive Health and Liver Disease, Mercy Medical Center; Professor of Medicine and Surgery, University of Maryland School of Medicine, Baltimore, Maryland

AUTHORS

JUAN G. ABRALDES, MD, MMSc
Associate Professor of Medicine, Cirrhosis Care Clinic, Liver Unit, Division of Gastroenterology, University of Alberta, Edmonton, Alberta, Canada

RAFAEL BAÑARES, MD, PhD
Professor of Medicine, Scientific Director of IiSGM, Gastroenterology and Hepatology Department, Hospital General Universitario Gregorio Marañón, IiSGM; School of Medicine, Universidad Complutense de Madrid (UCM), Madrid, Spain; Centro de investigación en red de enfermedades hepáticas y digestivas (CIBEREHD), Barcelona, Spain

SUBHAS BANERJEE, MD
Associate Professor; Chief of Endoscopy, Division of Gastroenterology and Hepatology, Stanford University School of Medicine, Stanford, California

TODD H. BARON, MD
Professor of Medicine, Director of Advanced Therapeutic Endoscopy, University of North Carolina, Chapel Hill, North Carolina

MICHEL BLE, MD
Barcelona Hepatic Hemodynamic Laboratory, Liver Unit, Hospital Clínic, IDIBAPS (Institut d'Investigacions Biomèdiques August Pi i Sunyer, University of Barcelona), Barcelona, Spain

BRIAN C. BRAUER, MD, FASGE
Associate Professor of Medicine, University of Colorado Anschutz Medical Campus, Aurora, Colorado

ANDRÉS CÁRDENAS, MD, MMSc, AGAF
GI/Endoscopy Unit, Institut de Malalties Digestives i Metaboliques, Hospital Clinic, University of Barcelona, Barcelona, Spain

MARÍA-VEGA CATALINA, MD
Medical Staff, Gastroenterology and Hepatology Department, Hospital General Universitario Gregorio Marañón, IiSGM, Madrid, Spain; Centro de investigación en red de enfermedades hepáticas y digestivas (CIBEREHD), Barcelona, Spain

ALVARO DÍAZ-GONZALEZ, MD
GI/Endoscopy Unit, Institut de Malalties Digestives i Metaboliques, Hospital Clinic, University of Barcelona, Barcelona, Spain

ANGELS ESCORCELL, MD, PhD
Liver Unit, Institut de Malalties Digestives i Metaboliques, Hospital Clinic, University of Barcelona, Barcelona, Spain

ALEJANDRO FERNÁNDEZ-SIMON, MD
GI/Endoscopy Unit, Institut de Malalties Digestives i Metaboliques, Hospital Clinic, University of Barcelona, Barcelona, Spain

JUAN CARLOS GARCÍA-PAGÁN, MD
Head of the Hepatic Hemodynamic Unit, Barcelona Hepatic Hemodynamic Laboratory, Liver Unit, Hospital Clínic, IDIBAPS (Institut d'Investigacions Biomèdiques August Pi i Sunyer, University of Barcelona); CIBERehd (Centro de Investigación Biomédica en Red de Enfermedades Hepáticas y Digestivas); University in Barcelona, Barcelona, Spain

VIRGINIA HERNANDEZ-GEA, MD
Barcelona Hepatic Hemodynamic Laboratory, Liver Unit, Hospital Clínic, IDIBAPS (Institut d'Investigacions Biomèdiques August Pi i Sunyer, University of Barcelona); CIBERehd (Centro de Investigación Biomédica en Red de Enfermedades Hepáticas y Digestivas); University in Barcelona, Barcelona, Spain

AWINASH KUMAR, MD
Department of Hepatology, Institute of Liver and Biliary Sciences, New Delhi, India

ROBERT J. LEWANDOWSKI, MD
Associate Professor, Section of Interventional Radiology, Department of Radiology, Robert H. Lurie Comprehensive Cancer Center, Northwestern Memorial Hospital, Chicago, Illinois

JEET MINOCHA, MD
Assistant Professor, Division of Interventional Radiology, Department of Radiology, University of Illinois Hospital and Health Sciences System, Chicago, Illinois

ROSA MIQUEL, MD
Pathology Department, Hospital Clinic, Institut d'Investigacions Biomediques August Pi i Sunyer (IDIBAPS); University in Barcelona, Barcelona, Spain

KAVISH R. PATIDAR, DO
Resident Physician, Department of Internal Medicine, Virginia Commonwealth University Hospital, Richmond, Virginia

BOGDAN PROCOPET, MD
Barcelona Hepatic Hemodynamic Laboratory, Liver Unit, Hospital Clínic, IDIBAPS (Institut d'Investigacions Biomèdiques August Pi i Sunyer, University of Barcelona), Barcelona, Spain; Gastroenterology Department, 3rd Medical Clinic, University of Medicine and Pharmacy "Iuliu Hatieganu"; Gastroenterology Department, Regional Institute of Gastroenterology and Hepatology "O. Fodor", Cluj-Napoca, Romania

WAEL E. SAAD, MD, FSIR
Professor & Division Director of Vascular & Interventional Radiology, Department of Radiology, University of Michigan, University of Michigan, Ann Arbor, Michigan

RIAD SALEM, MD, MBA
Professor, Section of Interventional Radiology, Department of Radiology, Robert H. Lurie Comprehensive Cancer Center, Northwestern Memorial Hospital, Chicago, Illinois

ARUN J. SANYAL, MD
Professor of Medicine, Physiology and Molecular Pathology; Associate Professor, Division of Gastroenterology, Department of Internal Medicine, Virginia Commonwealth University School of Medicine, Richmond, Virginia

SHIV K. SARIN, MD, DM, FNA, DSc
Senior Professor and Head, Department of Hepatology, and Director, Institute of Liver and Biliary Sciences, New Delhi, India

PHILIPPE SARLIEVE, MD
Assistant Clinical Professor, Department of Radiology, University of Alberta, Edmonton, Alberta, Canada

RAJ J. SHAH, MD, FASGE, AGAF
Associate Professor of Medicine, University of Colorado Anschutz Medical Campus, Aurora, Colorado

M. SHADAB SIDDIQUI, MD
Assistant Professor of Medicine, Section of Hepatology, Hume-Lee Transplant Center, Virginia Commonwealth University, Richmond, Virginia

R. TODD STRAVITZ, MD
Professor of Medicine, Section of Hepatology, Hume-Lee Transplant Center, Virginia Commonwealth University, Richmond, Virginia

MALCOLM SYDNOR, MD
Associate Professor, Radiology and Surgery; Director, Vascular Interventional Radiology, Virginia Commonwealth University Hospital, Richmond, Virginia

PUNEETA TANDON, MD, FRCPC
Associate Professor of Medicine, Cirrhosis Care Clinic, Liver Unit, Division of Gastroenterology, University of Alberta, Edmonton, Alberta, Canada

NIRAV THOSANI, MD
Instructor, Division of Gastroenterology and Hepatology, Stanford University School of Medicine, Stanford, California

PAUL J. THULUVATH, MD, FRCP
Medical Director, The Institute for Digestive Health and Liver Disease, Mercy Medical Center; Professor of Medicine and Surgery, University of Maryland School of Medicine, Baltimore, Maryland

JAVIER VAQUERO, MD, PhD
Researcher, Gastroenterology and Hepatology Department, Hospital General Universitario Gregorio Marañón, IiSGM, Madrid, Spain; Centro de investigación en red de enfermedades hepáticas y digestivas (CIBEREHD), Barcelona, Spain

Contents

Preface: Interventional Procedures in Hepatobiliary Diseases xiii

Andrés Cárdenas and Paul J. Thuluvath

Transjugular Liver Biopsy 767

Michel Ble, Bogdan Procopet, Rosa Miquel, Virginia Hernandez-Gea, and Juan Carlos García-Pagán

Liver biopsy is still the gold standard for evaluation of acute and chronic liver diseases, despite achievements regarding noninvasive diagnosis and staging in liver diseases. Transjugular liver biopsy (TJLB) has proved a good option when ascites and/or significant coagulopathy precludes a percutaneous approach. Because diagnostic hemodynamic procedures can be performed during the same session, it is useful in many clinical settings, regardless of the absence of percuteaneous contraindications. TJLB is a safe technique able to provide good-quality specimens with a low rate of complications. This article presents an overview of TJLB that discusses the technique, applicability, indications, contraindications, complications, and diagnostic accuracy.

Measurement of Portal Pressure 779

Juan G. Abraldes, Philippe Sarlieve, and Puneeta Tandon

Portal pressure is estimated through measuring the hepatic venous pressure gradient (HVPG). The main clinical applications of HVPG measurements include diagnosis, classification, and monitoring of portal hypertension, risk stratification, identification of candidates for liver resection, and monitoring efficacy of β-adrenergic blockers. Clinically significant portal hypertension is defined as an HVPG of 10 mm Hg or greater. Patients who experience a reduction in the HVPG of 20% or greater or to lower than 12 mm Hg in response to β-blocker therapy have a markedly decreased risk of bleeding (or rebleeding), ascites, and spontaneous bacterial peritonitis, resulting in improved survival rates.

Endoscopic Band Ligation and Esophageal Stents for Acute Variceal Bleeding 793

Andrés Cárdenas, Alejandro Fernández-Simon, and Angels Escorcell

 Video of endoscopic band ligation technique accompanies this article

Patients with portal hypertension and esophageal varices are at risk of bleeding due to a progressive increase in portal pressure that may rupture the variceal wall. Appropriate treatment with initial general measures such as resuscitation, a restrictive transfusion policy, antibiotic prophylaxis, pharmacologic therapy with vasoconstrictors, and endoscopic therapy with endoscopic band ligation are mandatory. However, 10% to 15% of patients fail initial endoscopic therapy, and, thus rescue therapies are needed. This article reviews the current endoscopic strategies with band ligation and esophageal stents for patients with acute variceal bleeding.

Endoscopic Treatment of Gastric Varices   809

Shiv K. Sarin and Awinash Kumar

Gastric varices (GV) are present in one in 5 patients with portal hypertension and variceal bleeding. GV bleeds tend to be more severe with higher mortality. High index of suspicion, early detection and proper locational diagnosis are important. An algorithmic approach to the management of GV bleeding prevents rebleeds and improves survival. Vasoactive drugs should be started with in 30 minutes (door to needle time) and early endotherapy be done. Cyanoacrylate injection in experienced hands achieves hemostasis in >90% patients. A repeat session is sometimes needed for complete obturation of GV. Transjugular intrahepatic portosystemic shunt and balloon retrograde transvenous obliteration are effective rescue options. Secondary prophylaxis of GV bleeding is done with beta-blocker and endotherapy.

Endovascular Management of Gastric Varices   829

Wael E. Saad

Bleeding from gastric varices is a major complication of portal hypertension. Although less common than bleeding associated with esophageal varices, gastric variceal bleeding has a higher mortality. From an endovascular perspective, transjugular intrahepatic portosystemic shunts (TIPS) to decompress the portal circulation and/or balloon-occluded retrograde transvenous obliteration (BRTO) are utilized to address bleeding gastric varices. Until recently, there was a clear medical cultural divide between the strategy of decompressing the portal circulation (TIPS creation, for example) and transvenous obliteration for the management of gastric varices. However, the practice of BRTO is gaining acceptance in the United States and its practice is spreading rapidly. Recently, the American College of Radiology has identified BRTO to be a viable alternative to TIPS in particular anatomical and clinical scenarios. However, the anatomical and clinical applications of BRTO were not defined beyond the conservative approach of resorting to BRTO in non-TIPS candidates. The article discusses the outcomes of BRTO and TIPS for the management of gastric varices individually or in combination. Definitions, endovascular technical concepts, and contemporary vascular classifications of gastric variceal systems are described in order to help grasp the complexity of the hemodynamic pathology and hopefully help define the pathology better for future reporting and lay the ground for more defined stratification of patients not only based on comorbidity and hepatic reserve but on anatomy and hemodynamic classifications.

Transjugular Intrahepatic Portosystemic Shunt   853

Kavish R. Patidar, Malcolm Sydnor, and Arun J. Sanyal

Transjugular intrahepatic portosystemic shunt (TIPS) is an established procedure for the complications of portal hypertension. The largest body of evidence for its use has been supported for recurrent or refractory variceal bleeding and refractory ascites. Its use has also been advocated for acute variceal bleed, hepatic hydrothorax, and hepatorenal syndrome. With the replacement of bare metal stents with polytetrafluoroethylene-covered stents, shunt patency has improved dramatically, thus, improving outcomes. Therefore, reassessment of its utility, management of its complications, and understanding of various TIPS techniques is important.

Transarterial Chemoembolization and Yittrium-90 for Liver Cancer and Other Lesions 877

Jeet Minocha, Riad Salem, and Robert J. Lewandowski

> Transarterial chemoembolization (TACE) is the recommended treatment of intermediate stage hepatocellular carcinoma (HCC). Radioembolization with yttrium 90 has overcome the shortcomings of external beam radiation in the treatment of liver cancer. TACE and radioembolization have led to encouraging response, survival, and quality of life outcomes, with reduced toxicity profiles. This result has led to the use of these therapies in patients with hepatic metastases, most commonly from colorectal cancer. This article reviews the current state of the practice of TACE and radioembolization and presents recent scientific data that support their role in the treatment of HCC and hepatic metastatic disease.

Endoscopic Retrograde Cholangiopancreatography for Cholangiocarcinoma 891

Todd H. Baron

> Cholangiocarcinoma is an increasingly common malignancy. Patients usually present with biliary obstruction. The role of endoscopic retrograde cholangiopancreatography (ERCP) is almost exclusively for drainage of the biliary tree, although diagnostic ERCP is still performed at the time of drainage to obtain a tissue diagnosis using brush cytology and intraductal biopsies. Peroral cholangioscopy may facilitate tissue diagnosis by allowing for directed biopsies. Biliary drainage is achieved by endoscopic stent placement. Careful preprocedural planning is necessary to select the ideal areas for drainage and to minimize contrast injection and subsequent cholangitis in hilar lesions.

Endoscopic Retrograde Cholangiopancreatography for Primary Sclerosing Cholangitis 899

Nirav Thosani and Subhas Banerjee

> Although there are no randomized, controlled trials evaluating the efficacy of endoscopic retrograde cholangiography (ERC) in primary sclerosing cholangitis (PSC) patients, substantial indirect evidence supports the effectiveness of ERC in symptomatic PSC patients with a dominant stricture. Currently cumulative evidence supports the role of ERC with endoscopic dilation with or without additional short-term stent placement for symptomatic PSC patients with a dominant stricture. Differentiating benign dominant strictures from cholangiocarcinoma (CCA) remains difficult; however, newer endoscopic techniques and advanced cytologic techniques are likely to improve sensitivity for the diagnosis of CCA over that achieved by traditional cytology brushing alone.

Endoscopic Retrograde Cholangiography for Biliary Anastomotic Strictures After Liver Transplantation 913

Alejandro Fernández-Simon, Alvaro Díaz-Gonzalez, Paul J. Thuluvath, and Andrés Cárdenas

> Biliary complications after liver transplantation (LT) are an important cause of morbidity and mortality. In most cases, an anastomosis of the bile duct is performed as a duct-to-duct reconstruction, which makes endoscopic

therapy with endoscopic retrograde cholangiography (ERC) feasible. Biliary anastomotic strictures (AS) are the most common cause of biliary complications. The early detection of an AS, which can sometimes be challenging given that its clinical presentation is often subtle, is of key importance to obtain high treatment success. In this review, we focus on the management of AS after LT with a special emphasis on ERC.

Cholangioscopy in Liver Disease

927

Brian C. Brauer and Raj J. Shah

Since its introduction, cholangioscopy has been used diagnostically and therapeutically. The working channel size has increased, permitting direct visualization for tissue sampling and to guide application of lithotripsy for difficult stones. Cholangioscopy utilizes endoscope and catheter-based systems. The application of slim gastroscopes for direct cholangioscopy provides better image resolution than conventional systems. Cholangioscopy has proven effective in the management of large biliary stones and for the diagnosis and exclusion of biliary tumors. Commercially available cholangioscopes are fiberoptic; those with digital video technology remain in a prototype development phase. This review covers available cholangioscope technologies, indications, technique, efficacy, and complications.

Molecular Adsorbent Recirculating System and Bioartificial Devices for Liver Failure

945

Rafael Bañares, María-Vega Catalina, and Javier Vaquero

Acute liver failure and acute-on-chronic liver failure remain clinical problems with unacceptable morbidity and mortality. The development of extracorporeal liver support systems that replace the detoxification, synthetic, and regulatory functions of the native liver represent a long-sought potential solution, but all the devices currently available are still far from ideal. In general, artificial (cell-free) and bioartificial liver support devices have shown their ability to decrease some circulating toxins, to ameliorate hepatic encephalopathy and other intermediate variables, and to be relatively safe. Their effects on the survival of patients with ALF or ACLF, however, have not been conclusively shown.

Intensive Care Unit Management of Patients with Liver Failure

957

M. Shadab Siddiqui and R. Todd Stravitz

Acute liver failure (ALF) and acute-on-chronic liver failure (ACLF) usually mandate management within an intensive care unit (ICU). Even though the conditions bear some similarities, precipitating causes, and systemic complications management practices differ. Although early identification of ALF and ACLF, improvements in ICU management, and the widespread availability of liver transplantation have improved mortality, optimal management practices have not been defined. This article summarizes current ICU management practices and identifies areas of management that require further study.

Index

979

CLINICS IN LIVER DISEASE

FORTHCOMING ISSUES

February 2015
Consultations in Liver Disease
Steven L. Flamm, *Editor*

May 2015
Hepatic Encephalopathy
Robert S. Brown Jr, *Editor*

August 2015
Hepatocellular Carcinoma
Adrian Reuben, *Editor*

RECENT ISSUES

August 2014
Liver Transplantation: Update of Concepts and Practice
Kalyan Ram Bhamidimarri and Paul Martin, *Editors*

May 2014
Portal Hypertension
Jorge L. Herrera, *Editor*

February 2014
The Impact of Obesity and Nutrition on Chronic Liver Diseases
Zobair M. Younossi, *Editor*

Preface

Interventional Procedures in Hepatobiliary Diseases

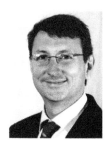 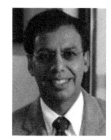

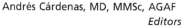

Andrés Cárdenas, MD, MMSc, AGAF   Paul J. Thuluvath, MD, FRCP
Editors

Hepatology has progressed enormously as a specialty in the past two decades. It has evolved from a purely clinical specialty to a field where multiple interventional procedures take a lead role in the management of patients. The incorporation of new therapeutic interventions for patients with liver disease as well as for liver transplant recipients has exponentially grown and subspecialty fields have emerged within the liver disease arena. Interventional procedures play a critical role in the management of patients with hepatobiliary diseases because they offer diagnostic and definite treatment options for an array of conditions. Interventions include those that directly measure portal pressure, perform transjugular liver biopsy, and place transjugular intrahepatic portsosystemic shunts as therapy for complications of portal hypertension. Another commonly performed intervention is digestive and hepatobiliary endoscopy, which offers not only diagnostic but also therapeutic choices in various areas such as portal hypertension and hepatobiliary disease. Endoscopy plays a fundamental role in the management of patients with almost all types of liver disease. In addition, both hepatology and endoscopy have become very specialized and thus a thorough knowledge of the indications, findings, therapeutic possibilities, and complications that arise from endoscopic interventions is a must for the practicing clinician. The rising incidence of liver cancer has also placed radiofrequency ablation and chemoembolization of liver lesions at the forefront of interventional therapies for hepatocellular carcinoma. Finally, the management of acute liver failure has certainly evolved with new therapeutic options, such as liver assist devices, that can help manage these patients in the intensive care unit. It is for this reason that we consider this issue of *Clinics in Liver Disease* devoted to "Interventional Procedures in Hepatobiliary Diseases" a timely and unique one. In this issue, we have invited an outstanding group of experts in the above-mentioned fields who share their vast experience and critically appraise important developments in interventional procedures of patients with hepatobiliary diseases.

Clin Liver Dis 18 (2014) xiii–xiv
http://dx.doi.org/10.1016/j.cld.2014.08.001
liver.theclinics.com

We sincerely hope that this issue has succeeded in summarizing the current status of interventional procedures in the management of hepatobiliary diseases. We express our gratitude to all the authors for their exceptional contributions. Finally, we thank Dr Norman Gitlin for inviting us as guest editors, as well as Casey Jackson and Kerry Holland, for their editorial support and assistance.

Andrés Cárdenas, MD, MMSc, AGAF
Institut de Malalties Digestives i Metaboliques
University of Barcelona
Hospital Clinic–Villarroel 170, Esc 3-2
08036 Barcelona, Spain

Paul J. Thuluvath, MD, FRCP
The Institute for Digestive Health & Liver Disease
Mercy Medical Center
301 St Paul Place
Baltimore, MD 21202, USA

E-mail addresses:
acardena@clinic.ub.es, acv69@hotmail.com (A. Cárdenas)
thuluvath@gmail.com (P.J. Thuluvath)

Transjugular Liver Biopsy

Michel Ble, MD[a], Bogdan Procopet, MD[a,b,c], Rosa Miquel, MD[d,e],
Virginia Hernandez-Gea, MD[a,e,f], Juan Carlos García-Pagán, MD[a,e,f],*

KEYWORDS

- Transjugular liver biopsy • Tru-Cut needle • Menghini needle • Tissue sample quality
- Liver specimen • Ultrasound guidance • HVPG • Cirrhosis stage

KEY POINTS

- Transjugular liver biopsy (TJLB) is a safe procedure able to obtain diagnostic liver specimens from patients with diffuse liver disease. Concomitant measurement of the hepatic venous pressure gradient (HVPG) provides relevant information to assess the risk of decompensation, esophageal varices formation and efficacy of portal hypertension treatment.
- Usually, under local anesthesia, the right-sided transjugular approach is used but the femoral veins, left internal jugular vein (LIJV) or external jugular veins could be alternatives routes. Ultrasound guidance makes the jugular puncture easier and safer.
- A 20 mm length specimen containing 11 complete portal tracts is the minimum requirement for a good quality sample. In comparison with percutaneous liver biopsy (PLB), TJLB is definitely not an inferior technique because this goal may be achieved with multiple passes without increasing the risk of bleeding.
- In chronic fibrotic disorders, the use of Tru-cut needle provides longer and and more compact samples than with Menghini technique.
- Major complications (hepatic hematoma or intraperitoneal hemorrhage) due to the procedure are exceptional. However, minor complications (neck hematoma at the site of jugular puncture, accidental carotid puncture) may appear in up to 7%. Despite being a longer procedure than PLB, TJLB is well tolerated. Moreover, conscious sedation and systemic analgesics may increase acceptance.

Disclosures: None.
[a] Hepatic Hemodynamic Laboratory, Liver Unit, Hospital Clínic, IDIBAPS (Institut d'Investigacions Biomèdiques August Pi i Sunyer, University of Barcelona), C/ Villarroel 173, Barcelona 08036, Spain; [b] Gastroenterology Department, 3rd Medical Clinic, University of Medicine and Pharmacy "Iuliu Hatieganu", Str. Victor Babes 8, Cluj-Napoca 400012, Romania; [c] Gastroenterology Department, Regional Institute of Gastroenterology and Hepatology "O. Fodor", Strada Constanţa 5, Cluj-Napoca 400158, Romania; [d] Pathology Department, Hospital Clinic, Institut d'Investigacions Biomediques August Pi i Sunyer (IDIBAPS), C/ Villarroel 173, Barcelona 08036, Spain; [e] University in Barcelona, Gran Via de les Corts Catalanes, 585, Barcelona 08007, Spain; [f] CIBERehd (Centro de Investigación Biomédica en Red de Enfermedades Hepáticas y Digestivas), Instituto de Salud Carlos III, C/ Monforte de Lemos 3-5, Pabellón 11, Planta 0, Madrid 28029, Spain
* Corresponding author. Hepatic Hemodynamic Laboratory, Liver Unit, Hospital Clínic, Villarroel 170, Barcelona 08036, Spain.
E-mail address: jcgarcia@clinic.ub.es

INTRODUCTION: NATURE OF THE PROBLEM

Despite new advances in the noninvasive diagnosis of chronic liver disease (CLD), liver biopsy is still the gold standard for evaluation of acute and chronic liver injury.[1,2] Recently, liver biopsy has been questioned because of drawbacks, such as sampling error[3,4] and intra- and interobserver variability[5]; however, the role of liver biopsy in diagnosis of liver disease remains highly valuable. Liver biopsy remains essential for the diagnosis of some liver diseases, such as nonalcoholic steatohepatitis, abnormal liver tests from unknown origin, or autoimmune hepatitis. Moreover, TJLB is indicated particularly in patients with fulminant hepatitis or acute liver failure of unknown cause; in the setting of bone marrow transplantation, where it helps to differentiate between sinusoidal obstruction syndrome, graft-versus-host disease, recurrent malignancy, and drug toxicity[6,7]; and in patients with alcoholic hepatitis where histologic alterations have prognostic relevance.[8]

TJLB was first described in 1964 in dogs,[9] and in 1967 a transjugular catheterization of the hepatic veins was first performed in humans as an approach to the biliary tract for cholangiography.[10] TJLB is usually performed when ascites and/or a significant coagulopathy preclude a percutaneous approach due to the risk of severe hemorrhage. Given that it is possible to measure hepatic hemodynamics during the same procedure, however, TJLB is used even in the absence of contraindications for PLB. TJLB may increase the probability of obtaining a good biopsy sample by performing several passes without increasing the risk of complications. This article presents an overview of TJLB. The technique, applicability, indications, contraindications, complications, and diagnostic profitability and outcomes of the different sampling approaches are discussed.

INDICATIONS/CONTRAINDICATIONS

TJLB is an effective and safe technique for obtaining liver tissue in patients with end-stage liver disease and entails lower incidence of hemorrhagic complications than PLB.[11] As a consequence, TJLB has traditionally been indicated for conditions where there is a high risk of bleeding.[12] Other common indications of TJLB are morbid obesity, small livers, or suspicion of hepatic peliosis.[13] Patients with heart failure and cirrhosis[14] often need a careful assessment of liver function that may include HVPG assessment and TJLB[15] to evaluate the need of combined heart and liver transplantation. **Box 1** summarizes the indications of TJLB.

There is no specific contraindication for TJLB and the risk-benefit ratio should be evaluated on a case-by-case basis. TJLB should be avoided when central venous access is absent (inferior vena cava obstruction) or in cases of polycystic liver disease, suspicion of cholangitis, and uncontrolled sepsis. **Box 2** summarizes some of the relative contraindications.

TJLB is not indicated in patients with focal hepatic lesions. In special circumstances, however, when PLB is contraindicated and there is strong indication of biopsy, TJLB could be performed under external US guidance.

TECHNIQUE/PROCEDURE
Preparation

1. Patient should be informed about the technique and its risks.
2. Written informed consent should be provided.
3. Checklist
   a. Rule out contrast allergy.

Box 1
Indications of transjugular liver biopsy
Absolute
Ascites
Severe coagulopathy
Need for additional intervention (HVPG)
Relative
Morbid obesity
Small cirrhotic liver
Right pleural effusion/infection
Suspicion of hepatic peliosis
Hepatic hemangioma
Failure of PLB
Condition where TJLB could be the first choice for histologic assessment
Alcoholic hepatitis
Fulminant hepatitis
Acute liver failure from unknown etiology
Abnormal liver tests in bone marrow transplant recipients
Suspicion of cirrhosis with associated portal hypertension
Suspicion of idiopathic portal hypertension/patients with HIV
Concomitant kidney biopsy

b. Assure 6 hours fasting.
c. Check prothrombin time or international normalized ratio and platelet count.
d. Check serum creatinine.
e. Establish an adequate management in patients on anticoagulant therapy.
   i. The authors' approach is that oral anticoagulant treatment (warfarin) is switched to subcutaneous low-molecular-weight heparin at least 3 days prior to TJLB. The day of the procedure, half-dose is administered and if there are no complications, warfarin treatment is started the same afternoon.

Box 2
Contraindications to transjugular liver biopsy
Lack of central venous access (inferior vena cava obstruction; occlusion of hepatic veins)
Glenn shunt; Fontan procedure
Polycystic liver disease
Hepatic hydatid disease
Acute cholangitis
Uncontrolled sepsis
Allergy to contrast agent
Uncooperative patient

4. Electrocardiografic traces, blood pressure, and heart rate should be monitored during the procedure.
5. Insert a venous catheter into an antecubital vein to have easy intravenous access if required.
6. To increase patient comfort and relaxation and if there are no contraindications (hepatic encephalopathy, severe respiratory insufficiency, or allergy), light sedation with intravenous midazolam (0.02 mg/kg) should be used. Midazolam infusion at this low dose does not affect hepatic venous pressure measurements[16] and increases tolerability.
7. Oxygen may be administered via a nasal cannula (2 L/min).
8. Antibiotic prophylaxis
   a. There is no consensus regarding the need for antibiotic prophylaxis for TJLB.[17] Antibiotic prophylaxis should be managed on a case-by-case basis and according with local epidemiology.
   b. In selected liver transplant recipients in poor clinical condition and with proved or suspected impaired biliary drainage who undergo a liver biopsy, targeted prophylaxis depending on local epidemiology may be offered to decrease the probability of sepsis.[18]

Necessary Material

See necessary materials in **Box 3**, **Fig. 1**.

Position

1. The patient should be dressed with a hospital gown and placed in a supine position on the angiography table, under the fluoroscopy arch.
2. The head should be slightly turned in the opposite direction of the puncture site.

Box 3
Necessary material for transjugular liver biopsy

Drapes, disinfectant sponges, gauze pads, scalpel, and 10-mL Luer-lock syringes

Sterile gloves, eye protection, a gown, a surgical cap, a mask, and a full-size sterile drape

Anesthetic syringe and 2% lidocaine anesthetic solution

Midazolam

Iodinated contrast medium

18-G needle for jugular vein access

0.035-inch (0.89-mm) J-shaped, angled guide wire

9F–10F (11-cm long) introducer

Biopsy needle

- 9F Colapinto needle together with the 9F sheath
- Tru-Cut Quick-Core or FlexCore biopsy kit system

Additional material

- 5F multipurpose catheter with J tip (for difficult hepatic vein catheterization)
- Two-lumen balloon catheter and invasive pressure measurement kit (for HVPG measurement)
- Stiff guide-wire (eg, Amplatz Super Stiff)

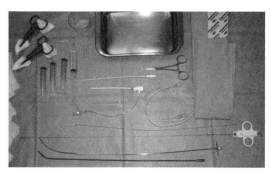

Fig. 1. Table set for TJLB: drapes, disinfectant sponges, scalpel, 10-mL Luer-lock syringes, anesthetic syringe, iodinated contrast medium, 18-G needle for jugular vein access, 9F–10F (11-cm long) introducer, 9F Colapinto needle together with the 9F sheath catheter, and the Tru-Cut needle.

Approach

1. Right internal jugular vein (RIJV) is the preferred approach[19] but the LIJV, external jugular, subclavian, or even femoral can be used.
2. When an RIJV approach is not feasible, biopsy from the LIJV can be performed but requires crossing obliquely through the mediastinum and heart with the rigid metal cannula. The LIJV approach enables very secure engagement of the right or middle hepatic vein orifice with the rigid biopsy cannula. The oblique course of the cannula through the mediastinum directs the cannula laterally and into the hepatic veins.[20]

Technique/Procedure (Detail Steps)

1. Previous US evaluation gives precise information of topographic location of the RIJV, confirms its permeability, and permits tailoring the puncture to the specific anatomy of the individual patient.[21]
2. For better venous filling and to avoid air embolism, the table can be positioned in moderate Trendelenburg position, patients can be asked to do a Valsalva maneuver, and/or the legs can be lifted with a cushion or with infusion of saline solution.
3. The doctor should perform a surgical hand scrub and wear face mask, eye protection, gown and sterile gloves.
4. The doctor should be placed at the top of the patient's head.
5. The puncture site is then disinfected with 2% chlorexidine.
6. The skin is covered with a sterile drape.
7. Subcutaneous local anesthetic (2% lidocaine) infiltration should be performed.
8. The patient's head should be minimally rotated 45° to the contralateral side of the puncture site so the common carotid artery does not lie posterior to the LIJV, thus decreasing the possibilities of its accidental puncture.[22,23]
9. Under US visualization, the RIJV is penetrated through the skin with an 18-gauge [G] needle catheter.
10. When reflux of dark venous blood is obtained in the syringe, a 0.035-in (0.89-mm) J-shaped, angled guide wire is inserted into the vein. The wire is guided under fluoroscopic control through the right side of the heart and the needle is then withdrawn.
11. A 9F–10F (11-cm long) introducer is inserted via Seldinger technique over the guide wire.

12. The 9F tetrafluoroethylene (TFE) sheath catheter with curved tip, delivered within the TJLB kit, is launched through the introducer via the superior vena cava, right atrium, inferior vena cava, and the right hepatic vein or an appropriate alternative hepatic vein (**Fig. 2**). In cases in which the hepatic veins are difficult to catheterize, a guide wire or a 5 F, J-tip multipurpose catheter may be used.
13. HVPG can be measured at this point and preferably with a 2-lumen balloon catheter, which can be introduced into the hepatic vein over the guide wire. Once HVPG is measured, the balloon catheter should be exchanged by the 9F TFE catheter.
14. To prevent cardiac arrhythmias, continuous cardiac monitoring is recommended while the catheter is passing the right atrium.
15. Biopsy performance
    a. Menghini technique: The 9F sheath catheter's position into the hepatic vein should be verified by injecting contrast agent. Then the Colapinto needle is advanced into the sheath until it reaches the hepatic vein. The needle should advance easily into the sheath and no force should be applied to avoid the sheath's perforation and accidental puncture of the cava vein or heart wall. The needle is then moved forward 1–2 cm through the wall of the hepatic vein to then puncture the liver. To perform the puncture, a syringe is attached to the edge of the needle and aspiration force should be applied while puncturing (Menghini technique) (**Fig. 3**). This practice is easier and safer when patients hold their breath. The direction of the needle tip (indicated by the arrow marker at proximal extremity of the needle) should be usually oriented anteriorly if the right hepatic vein is catheterized or posteriorly if the median vein is catheterized. Biopsy from the left hepatic vein is used less because of a higher risk extracapsular puncture due to lower left lobe dimensions. The starting point of the biopsy should be at 3–4 cm from the hepatic vein ostium because it provides a central position and decreases the risk of extracapsular puncture. This position also avoids accidentally losing the hepatic vein when pulling back the needle into the sheath.
    b. The Tru-Cut technique: After catheterization of the hepatic vein with a selective catheter, the transjugular introducer sheath is advanced with the stiffening

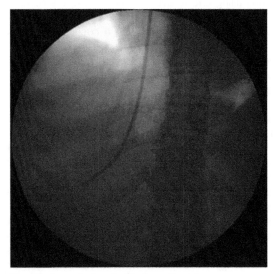

Fig. 2. The 9F sheath catheter entering in the hepatic vein.

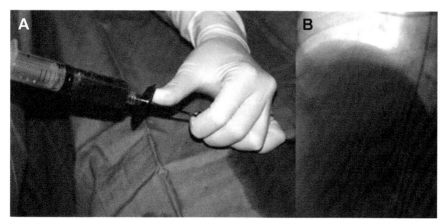

Fig. 3. Liver biopsy—Menghini technique: the direction of the needle tip (indicated by the edge of the arrow at proximal extremity of the needle) is usually oriented anteriorly if the right hepatic vein is catheterized (*A*). Under fluoroscopic guidance, the needle is then moved forward quickly 1–2 cm through the wall of the hepatic vein and punctures the liver (*B*).

cannula through a guide wire. The Tru-Cut needle is prepared by pulling back the plunger until a firm click is felt. Then, the Tru-Cut needle is advanced with the stiletto fully retracted in the hepatic vein through the stiffening cannula. The stiffening cannula gives the orientation of the puncture as in the Menghini technique. When the needle is in the appropriate position, advance the stiletto 1–2 cm into the parenchyma and than fire the cutting cannula by fully depressing the plunger with the thumb to capture tissue within the specimen notch (**Fig. 4**).

16. If the liver specimen is absent or inadequate, other attempts should be made until success is achieved.
17. Once the sample is secured, contrast medium should be injected to detect possible capsular perforation; in such cases, embolization coils can be injected via the transjugular catheter until the leak is sealed.

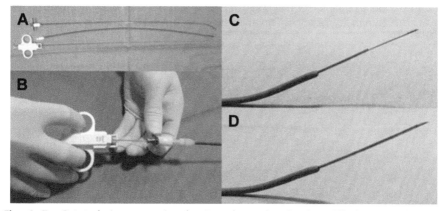

Fig. 4. Tru-Cut technique: transjugular introducer sheath, the stiffening cannula, and the Tru-Cut needle (*A*). Descend the Tru-Cut needle with the stiletto fully retracted in the hepatic vein through the stiffening cannula. The stiffening cannula (arrow edge) gives the orientation of the puncture (*B*). Tru-Cut needle in armed position—the notch is visible (*C*). Tru-Cut needle fired—the cutting cannula is covering the notch (*D*).

18. At least 3 adequate samples (at least 15 mm in length) should be obtained (**Fig. 5**).
19. The specimens are carefully placed in formalin or other solutions as required for the anatomopathologic study.

COMPLICATIONS AND MANAGEMENT

The total rate of complications was 6.7% in a systematic review of 60 adult series, which included more than 7500 patients.[13] When pain and patient tolerance are included in analysis, the reported rate increases until 29%.[24] Increased right upper quadrant pain, new onset, or worsening of previous dyspnea should raise suspicion of complicated TJLB, so appropriate explorations to detect complications should not be delayed.

The most frequent complications are related with jugular puncture and include neck pain, local hematoma, and accidental puncture of carotid artery; however, the use of US guidance substantially lowers these complications. The complications related to TJLB and the usual management are summarized in **Table 1**. In comparison with PLB, TJLB is less painful (analyzed by a visual analogic scale) and requires less analgesia. Despite that TJLB is a longer procedure and requires a less comfortable position, the overall tolerance and the acceptance are equal between the 2 techniques.[24]

Duration of TJLB varies between 30 and 60 minutes. There are no specific indications about postoperative care of these patients, which usually is based on local guidelines and expertise. The authors recommend, however, observing the patient for at least 2 hours. Pain can usually be managed with minor analgesics (eg, acetaminophen or codeine). There is no need for regular follow-up US or laboratory tests unless complications appear.

SAMPLE QUALITY AND CLINICAL IMPLICATIONS (IF PROCEDURE IS USED FOR DIAGNOSTIC PURPOSES)

TJLB procedure is technically successful in more than 96% of the cases[13] and technical failure is mostly related with the impossibility to catheterize the hepatic veins or to cannulate the jugular vein.

Sample Quality

To be considered optimal for diagnosis of diffuse liver disease, the specimens should be at least 15 mm long and contain at least 6 CPTs.[1] Reliable grading and staging of

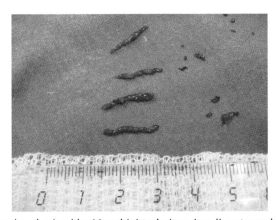

Fig. 5. Biopsy samples obtained by Menghini technique in a liver transplant recipient.

Table 1
Complications related to the TJLB

Frequent	Management
Neck pain	Self-limited; conservative
Neck hematoma	Conservative
Carotid puncture	Conservative; contralateral puncture/reschedule
Abdominal pain	Self-limited; conservative—antalgics
Supraventricular arrhythmia	Self-limited; rarely specific management
Rare	**Management**
Horner syndrome	Conservative
Pneumothorax	Conservative for small pneumothorax; aspiration
Small hepatic hematoma	Conservative
Subclinical capsular puncture	Conservative
Hemobilia	Conservative
Hepatoportal fistula	Conservative
Arteriovenous fistula	Angio CT scan; embolization
Large hepatic hematoma	Angio CT; transfusion if needed; embolization; surgery
Intraperitoneal hemorrhage	Angio CT; transfusion if needed; embolization
Biliary fistula/leak	Conservative/endoscopic retrograde cholangiopancreatography and biliary stenting
Accidental renal puncture	Conservative

liver disease require a biopsy of at least 20 mm in length and at least 11 portal tracts.[25,26] A biopsy shorter than 2 cm but containing at least 11 CPTs may still be considered suitable for grading and staging.[25] In a systematic review of 64 studies with more than 7500 biopsies, TJLB offered adequate quality samples in 96% of the cases[13] and the specimens obtained were considered adequate for histologic diagnosis in the most of them.

There is a great variability among studies, however, concerning sample quality. The quality increases with the experience of the center and number of biopsies done per year.[27,28] Nevertheless, in a systematic review of published studies, there was no difference in terms of the sample's length, fragmentation, or number of CPTs between studies with less or more than 100 TJLB.[13]

There are only a few studies that compare the 2 types of needles: the aspiration system (Menghini needle) and the semiautomatic system, Tru-Cut needle (Quick-Core and FlexCore). The automated biopsy device seems more effective than the Menghini technique in terms of sample quality and procedure time,[29–31] although other studies have not confirmed this.[32] In a systematic review using data from different studies, the Tru-Cut needle obtained significantly longer, less fragmented, and more adequate specimens for histologic diagnosis.[13] The mean length was not significantly correlated with CPT number using either Colapinto or Tru-Cut needle. Although the number of portal tracts might be considered adequate, they tend to be observed at the margin of the tissue in many of the Tru-Cut needle biopsies, probably because the tissue is much thinner than in PBL. There is also technical artifact (compression artifact), which may interfere with the optimal interpretation of liver lesions.

The 2 automated needle systems (18-G FlexCore and 18-G Quick-Core) also have been compared, and the 18-G FlexCore TJLB needle provided better liver specimens,[33] although there is only one study dedicated to this issue. Moreover, the FlexCore TJLB needle is currently not available in Europe.

In a recent study, the caudal orientation of the Tru-Cut needle notch resulted in a higher quality of samples compared with the cranial or lateral orientation.[34] Although the study's hypothesis is interesting, the validation in the human cohort lacks accuracy. In the retrospective analysis of the human cohort, in the random group, the orientation of the notch is not stated and hypothetically a majority of the biopsies could have caudal orientation also. The quality criteria used by pathologists for comparison and the number of CPTs are not detailed in the 2 compared groups. Diameter, length of the specimen, and utility for histologic studies do not depend on the size of the needle when comparing 18-G to 19-G needles, despite the higher fragmentation rate with thicker needles.

Clinical Implications

Liver biopsy remains the milestone for diagnosis of liver disease. To reduce at minimum the risk of procedure-related complications, however, a complete clinical evaluation must be done. According to the clinical question, the appropriate technique (PLB or TJLB) should be chosen. Traditionally, TJLB was considered inferior to PLB because of a lower quality of the obtained samples. More recent studies have strongly demonstrated, however, that TJLB samples are comparable with PLB[24,28] without differences regarding the impact on clinical decisions based on biopsy results.[35]

In older studies, samples obtained with TJLB proved to have great diagnostic significance and in 11% of cases were crucial for final diagnosis.[36] TJLB is comparable to PLB in terms of mean CPTs and complication rates. Moreover, TJLB offers the feasibility of multiple passes, increasing the length and the diagnostic value of the specimen without increasing the risk of complications.[37] Another advantage of TJLB is the measurement of HVPG during the same intervention, adding substantial diagnostic and prognostic information.[38] Therefore, it could be stated that TJLB offers 2 gold standards in the assessment of liver diseases.

CURRENT CONTROVERSIES/FUTURE CONSIDERATIONS

Despite being a safe technique, TJLB implies invasiveness and potential complications along with lower acceptance from patients. These reasons have contributed to the accelerated development of noninvasive techniques for the diagnosis and staging of CLD. Nevertheless, currently, none of them can fully replace liver biopsy and, therefore, it remains a key diagnostic method for several clinical scenarios. For instance, it remains the only method to differentiate between simple steatosis and steatohepatitis in patients with NAFLD. It is also crucial in the diagnosis and the management of autoimmune hepatitis and provides valuable diagnostic and prognostic information in alcoholic hepatitis.

SUMMARY

TJLB is a safe, effective, and well tolerated. The use of semiautomatic needle systems enables larger and less fragmented samples, with a fewer number of passes, and reduces procedure time. Quality of the specimen is comparable to PLB with a similar rate of complications despite the use of more passes and coagulopathy. In addition, HVPG measurements can be obtained during the procedure and offer supplemental diagnosis and prognostic information.

REFERENCES

1. Bravo AA, Sheth SG, Chopra S. Liver biopsy. N Engl J Med 2001;344:495–500.
2. Campbell M, Reddy K. Review article: the evolving role of liver biopsy. Aliment Pharmacol Ther 2004;20:249–59.
3. Bedossa P, Dargere D, Paradis V. Sampling variability of liver fibrosis in chronic hepatitis C. Hepatology 2003;38:1449–57.
4. Ratziu V, Charlotte F, Heurtier A, et al. Sampling variability of liver biopsy in nonalcoholic fatty liver disease. Gastroenterology 2005;128:1898–906.
5. Regev A, Berho M, Jeffers LJ, et al. Sampling error and intraobserver variation in liver biopsy in patients with chronic HCV infection. Am J Gastroenterol 2002;97:2614–8.
6. McDonald GB. Hepatobiliary complications of hematopoietic cell transplantation, 40 years on. Hepatology 2010;51:1450–60.
7. Nadolski G, Mondschein JI, Shlansky-Goldberg RD, et al. Diagnostic yield of transjugular liver biopsy samples to evaluate for infectious etiology of liver dysfunction in bone marrow transplant recipients. Cardiovasc Intervent Radiol 2014;37:471–5.
8. Altamirano J, Miquel R, Katoonizadeh A, et al. Histologic scoring system for prognosis of patients with alcoholic hepatitis. Gastroenterology 2014;146:1231–9.
9. Dotter CT. Catheter biopsy. Experimental technic for transvenous liver biopsy. Radiology 1964;82:312–4.
10. Hanafee W, Weiner M. Transjugular percutaneous cholangiography. Radiology 1967;88:35–9.
11. Ahmad A, Hasan F, Abdeen S, et al. Transjugular liver biopsy in patients with end-stage renal disease. J Vasc Interv Radiol 2004;15:257–60.
12. Harinath S, Srinivas S, Caldwell C, et al. Liver biopsy - evolving role in the new millennium. J Clin Gastroenterol 2005;39:603–10.
13. Kalambokis G, Manousou P, Vibhakorn S, et al. Transjugular liver biopsy–indications, adequacy, quality of specimens, and complications–a systematic review. J Hepatol 2007;47:284–94.
14. Te HS, Anderson AS, Millis JM, et al. Current state of combined heart-liver transplantation in the United States. J Heart Lung Transplant 2008;27:753–9.
15. Møller S, Bernardi M. Interactions of the heart and the liver. Eur Heart J 2013;34:2804–11.
16. Steinlauf A, Garcia-Tsao G, Zakko MF, et al. Low-dose midazolam sedation: an option for patients undergoing serial hepatic venous pressure measurements. Hepatology 1999;203:1070–3.
17. Venkatesan AM, Kundu S, Sacks D, et al. Practice guidelines for adult antibiotic prophylaxis during vascular and interventional radiology procedures. J Vasc Interv Radiol 2010;21:1611–30.
18. Lopez-Sanchez C, Len O, Gavalda J, et al. Liver biopsy – related infection in liver transplant recipients: a current matter of concern? Liver Transpl 2014;20:552–6.
19. Gamble P, Colapinto R, Stronell R, et al. Transjugular liver biopsy: a review of 461 biopsies. Radiology 1985;157:589–93.
20. Yavuz K, Geyik S, Barton RE, et al. Transjugular liver biopsy via the left internal jugular vein. J Vasc Interv Radiol 2007;18:237–41.
21. Soyer P, Lacheheb D, Levesque M. High-resolution sonographic guidance for transjugular liver biopsy. Abdom Imaging 1993;362:360–2.
22. Snoey ER, Clements RC, Price D. Effect of head rotation on vascular anatomy of the neck: an ultrasound study. J Emerg Med 2006;31:283–6.

23. Ortega R, Song M, Hansen CJ, et al. Ultrasound-guided internal jugular vein cannulation. N Engl J Med 2010;362:e57.
24. Procopet B, Bureau C, Métivier S, et al. Tolerance of liver biopsy in a tertiary care center: comparison of the percutaneous and the transvenous route in 143 prospectively followed patients. Eur J Gastroenterol Hepatol 2012;24:1209–13.
25. Colloredo G, Guido M, Sonzogni A, et al. Impact of liver biopsy size on histological evaluation of chronic viral hepatitis: the smaller the sample, the milder the disease. J Hepatol 2003;39:239–44.
26. Guido M, Guido C, Fassan M, et al. Clinical practice and ideal liver biopsy sampling standards: not just a matter of centimeters. J Hepatol 2006;44:823–4.
27. Chau T, Tong S, Li T, et al. Transjugular liver biopsy with an automated trucut-type needle: comparative study with percutaneous liver biopsy. Eur J Gastroenterol Hepatol 2001;14:19–24.
28. Cholongitas E, Quaglia A, Samonakis D, et al. Transjugular liver biopsy: how good is it for accurate histological interpretation? Gut 2006;55:1789–94.
29. Bañares R, Alonso S, Catalina M, et al. Randomized controlled trial of aspiration needle versus automated biopsy device for transjugular liver biopsy. J Vasc Interv Radiol 2001;12:583–7.
30. Choo SW, Do YS, Park KB, et al. Transjugular liver biopsy: modified ross transseptal needle versus quick-core biopsy needle. Abdom Imaging 2000;25:483–5.
31. McAfee J, Keeffe E, Lee R, et al. Transjugular liver biopsy. Hepatology 1992;15: 726–32.
32. Papatheodoridis GV, Patch D, Watkinson A, et al. Transjugular liver biopsy in the 1990s: a 2-year audit. Aliment Pharmacol Ther 1999;13:603–8.
33. Behrens G, Ferral H, Giusto D, et al. Transjugular liver biopsy: comparison of sample adequacy with the use of two automated needle systems. J Vasc Interv Radiol 2011;22:341–5.
34. Clark TW, McCann JW, Salsamendi J, et al. Optimizing needle direction during transjugular liver biopsy provides superior biopsy specimens. Cardiovasc Intervent Radiol 2013. http://dx.doi.org/10.1007/s00270–013–0819–4.
35. Beckmann M, Bahr MJ, Hadem J, et al. Clinical relevance of transjugular liver biopsy in comparison with percutaneous and laparoscopic liver biopsy. Gastroenterol Res Pract 2009. http://dx.doi.org/10.1155/2009/947014.
36. Trejo R, Alvarez W, Garcia-Pagan JC, et al. The applicability and diagnostic cost-efectiveness of transjugular liver biopsy. Med Clin 1996;107:521–3.
37. Cholongitas E, Senzolo M, Standish R, et al. A systematic review of the quality of liver biopsy specimens. Am J Clin Pathol 2006;125:710–21.
38. Bosch J, Abraldes JG, Berzigotti A, et al. The clinical use of HVPG measurements in chronic liver disease. Nat Rev Gastroenterol Hepatol 2009;6:573–82.

Measurement of Portal Pressure

Juan G. Abraldes, MD, MMSc[a],*, Philippe Sarlieve, MD[b],
Puneeta Tandon, MD, FRCPC[a]

KEYWORDS

- Portal hypertension • Cirrhosis • HVPG • β-blockers • Catheterization

KEY POINTS

- Measurement of the hepatic venous pressure gradient (HVPG) is the gold standard technique used to quantify the degree portal hypertension in liver disease.
- In patients with cirrhosis, HVPG measurement provides independent prognostic information on survival and the risk of decompensation.
- The HVPG response to pharmacologic therapy for portal hypertension identifies which patients benefit most from treatment.
- Measurement of HVPG helps assess the risk of liver failure and death after liver resection in patients with compensated chronic liver disease and hepatocellular carcinoma.

INTRODUCTION

Portal hypertension, a frequently presenting clinical syndrome, is defined as a pathologic increase in portal venous pressure. This increase causes the pressure gradient between the portal vein and the inferior vena cava (the so-called portal perfusion pressure of the liver or portal pressure gradient) to increase greater than the normal range of values (1–5 mm Hg). When the portal pressure gradient increases to greater than 10 to 12 mm Hg, complications of portal hypertension can arise; these complications include formation of portosystemic collaterals and varices, upper gastrointestinal bleeding resulting from ruptured gastroesophageal varices and portal hypertensive gastropathy, ascites, renal dysfunction, hepatic encephalopathy, arterial hypoxemia, disorders in the metabolism of drugs or endogenous substances that are normally eliminated by the liver, bacteremia, and hypersplenism.[1] The importance of portal hypertension is underscored by the high incidence and severity of these complications.

The authors declare that they have no conflicts of interest.
[a] Cirrhosis Care Clinic, Liver Unit, Division of Gastroenterology, University of Alberta, Edmonton, Alberta T6E 4X8, Canada; [b] Department of Radiology, University of Alberta, 2A2.41 WC Mackenzie Health Science Centre, Edmonton, Alberta T6G 2R7, Canada
* Corresponding author. University of Alberta, 1-51 Zeidler Ledcor Center, Edmonton, Alberta T6E 2X8, Canada.
E-mail address: Juan.g.abraldes@ualberta.ca

Clin Liver Dis 18 (2014) 779–792
http://dx.doi.org/10.1016/j.cld.2014.07.002

liver.theclinics.com

The main cause of this syndrome in Western countries is cirrhosis of the liver, a disease that affects mainly adults and that represents the third to fifth leading cause of death in men older than 50 years in Europe and the United States.

HEPATIC VENOUS PRESSURE GRADIENT
Rationale

Hepatic vein catheterization with measurement of the hepatic venous pressure gradient (HVPG) is currently the gold standard technique for determining portal pressure. It is calculated as the difference between the wedged hepatic venous pressure (WHVP) and the free hepatic venous pressure (FHVP).[2] The WHVP is measured by occluding a main hepatic vein; stopping the blood flow causes the static column of blood to transmit the pressure that is present in the preceding vascular territory—in this case, the hepatic sinusoids. This measurement, in the absence of presinusoidal obstruction, reflects portal pressure.[3] The hepatic vein can be occluded through either wedging the catheter into a small branch of a hepatic vein or inflating a balloon at the tip of the catheter.[3] Occlusion of the hepatic vein through inflating a balloon is preferred, because the volume of the liver circulation transmitting portal pressure is much larger than that attained through wedging the catheter (**Fig. 1**),[4] which reduces the variability of the measurements.[5] Studies have shown that the WHVP provides an accurate estimate of portal pressure in alcoholic and viral cirrhosis.[6] The FHVP, as the name suggests, is a measure of the pressure of unoccluded hepatic vein. Free hepatic venous pressure, and not right atrial pressure, should be used to calculate the hepatic venous pressure gradient, because HVPG calculated with right atrial pressure shows a worse correlation with clinical outcomes.[7] Liver catheterization allows a transjugular liver biopsy to be performed during the same procedure.

Because HVPG reflects portal pressure, changes in this measurement indicate alterations in the factors that determine portal pressure, namely hepatic vascular resistance, collateral resistance or portal blood flow inflow, or their combination.[4] Changes in hepatic resistance can be caused by changes in fibrosis, regenerative nodules, appearance of thrombosis (mechanical factors), or a change in hepatic vascular tone (dynamic factors). In this sense, HVPG can be a reliable surrogate of

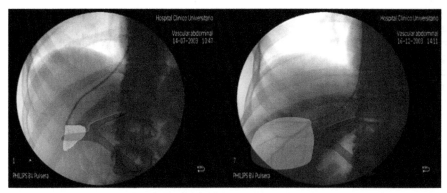

Fig. 1. Hepatic venous pressure gradient measurement with the wedged end-hole catheter (*left panel*) and the balloon catheter (*right panel*). After occluding the hepatic vein, the static column of blood transmits the pressure of the preceding vascular territory: the hepatic sinusoids. In the absence of a presinusoidal obstruction, this reflects the pressure of the portal vein. The volume of liver-transmitting pressure is much larger (and thus less prone to artifacts) with the balloon catheter.

the degree of liver fibrosis, but it also integrates many other pathogenic aspects occurring in liver diseases.

The Procedure

Guidelines for reliable HVPG measurements were recently published by hepatologists interested in the procedure[2,8] but still lack widespread standardization across radiology units. **Box 1** provides a technical summary of the procedure.

Catheterization of the hepatic vein can be performed under light sedation (midazolam, up to 0.02 mg/kg).[9] Higher doses of midazolam or deep sedation significantly alter pressure measurements.[10] The technique to obtain HVPG values is straightforward; however, achieving accurate measurements requires specialist training.

Complications

Measuring the HVPG is a safe procedure. Major complications are infrequent and include local injury at the puncture site (femoral, jugular, or antecubital veins), such as bleeding, hematoma, and, more rarely, arteriovenous fistulae or Horner syndrome (in the case of jugular puncture). Ultrasonographic guidance should be always used when available, because it considerably reduces the risk of complications of the procedure. Passage of the catheter through the right atrium might cause supraventricular arrhythmias (most commonly ectopic beats, but in the authors' experience these are self-limited in more than 90% of occasions).

Contraindications

A history of allergic reaction to iodinated radiologic contrast medium is not a contraindication to hepatic vein catheterization, because carbon dioxide (CO_2) can be used as a contrast agent. Although coagulation disorders are common in patients with cirrhosis, commonly used tests have low predictive value for the actual risk of bleeding.[11] Only cases of severe thrombocytopenia (platelet levels $<20 \times 10^9$/L) or very prolonged international normalized ratio values (>3) call for the replacement of platelets or transfusion of fresh frozen plasma.

Associated Procedures

In addition to pressure measurements, other procedures can also be performed during hepatic vein catheterization, including hepatic blood flow (using indicator dilution techniques), transjugular liver biopsy (discussed elsewhere in this issue), and retrograde CO_2 portography. Furthermore, performing right heart catheterization through the same venous access prolongs the procedure only by 5 minutes, with a minimal incremental risk. Right heart catheterization allows the measurement of pulmonary artery pressure, pulmonary wedged pressure, and cardiac output, which can be very useful in the investigation of cardiopulmonary complications of cirrhosis and for pretransplant evaluation.

Reporting

Box 2 shows a list of items that should be included in a report of HVPG measurements.

Follow-up

The procedure can be performed on a day-hospital or ambulatory basis (provided that a recovery room is available). Patient can normally be discharged 1 hour after the procedure. If femoral access is used, the patient requires a 24-hour period of complete bedrest. Transjugular liver biopsy requires special consideration (reviewed elsewhere in this issue).

Box 1
Hepatic venous pressure gradient procedure

1. The procedure should be performed in fasting conditions.

2. Sedation: midazolam, up to 0.02 mg/kg, does not alter HVPG measurements. Higher doses or the use of deep sedation (propofol/remifentanil) alter pressure measurements. Sedation might be intensified after completing the HVPG measurements, before the biopsy procedure.

3. Monitoring: continuous electrocardiography, arterial blood pressure, and pulse oximetry.

4. Calibration: most transducers are now precalibrated. If not precalibrated, the transducer should be calibrated against known external pressures before starting measurements (eg, 13.6 cm H_2O should read 10 mm Hg, 27.2 cm H_2O should read 20 mm Hg, and 40.8 cm H_2O should read 30 mm Hg).

5. Zeroing: place the transducer at the level of the right atrium (midaxillary line). With transducer open to air (zero pressure), adjust the recorder to read zero.

6. Pressure tracings: permanent records should be obtained either through hard copy or electronically for subsequent review (**Fig. 2**).

7. Scale: use an appropriate scale for venous pressure measurements (full range up to 50 mm Hg).

8. Venous access: under local anesthesia, the right jugular vein is catheterized, a venous introducer is placed, and the catheter is advanced under fluoroscopic control into the inferior vena cava and a hepatic vein. Real-time ultrasound facilitates venous access. Hepatic venous pressure gradient can be performed from the left jugular vein or a femoral vein, but these are second choices.

9. Free hepatic venous pressure: the FHVP is measured by maintaining the tip of the catheter "free" in the hepatic vein, at 2 to 4 cm from its opening into the inferior vena cava. The FHVP should be close to inferior vena cava pressure; if the difference between these pressure values is greater than 2 mm Hg, the catheter is likely inadequately placed or a hepatic vein obstruction is likely present. In these cases, inferior vena cava pressure should be used for calculating HVPG. Hepatic venous pressure gradient should not be calculated with the atrial pressure.

10. Wedged hepatic venous pressure: the WHVP is measured by occluding the hepatic vein, either by wedging the catheter into a small branch of a hepatic vein or by inflating a balloon at the tip of the catheter. Adequate occlusion of the hepatic vein is confirmed by slowly injecting 5 mL of contrast dye into the vein with the balloon inflated. No reflux of the dye or washout through communications with other hepatic veins should be observed. Otherwise, WHVP might be underestimating portal pressure. No need exists to obtain measurements in different veins.

11. Balloon versus end-hole occlusion: occluding the hepatic vein through inflating a balloon is preferred, because the volume of the liver circulation transmitting portal pressure is much larger than that attained through wedging the catheter. This technique reduces the variability of the measurements. If an end-hole catheter is used, measurements should be taken from at least 2 different sites and averaged. Catheters with side holes should not be used.

12. Duration of measurements: the WHVP should be measured until the value remains stable (usually >40 seconds). A 15-second stabilization is enough for FHVP.

13. All measurements should be taken at least in duplicate (or triplicate if differences of >1 mm Hg are recorded). The final value is calculated as the mean of these measurements.

14. Any event that might cause an artifact, such as coughing, moving, or talking, should be noted.

15. If large pressure oscillations are noted with the respiratory cycle (as may occur in obese patients or patients with tense ascites or encephalopathy), values at end-expiration should be used.

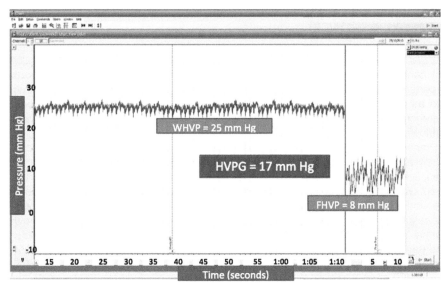

Fig. 2. A typical tracing of a HVPG. Equilibration of WHVP requires more than 20 seconds. The HVPG is calculated as the difference between WHVP and FHVP.

APPLICATIONS OF HVPG MEASUREMENT
Diagnosis of Portal Hypertension

Hepatic venous pressure gradient is rarely used for diagnostic purposes. Portal hypertension is usually diagnosed on clinical grounds (from the presence of its complications) or based on results of imaging studies. A particular setting in which HVPG might be of diagnostic utility is in investigating ascites that is not obviously caused by portal hypertension. The HVPG can assist with differentiating between a cardiac origin (increase in both FHVP and WHVP, with normal HVPG), tumoral ascites (normal

---

Box 2
Items to be included in a report of a hepatic vein catheterization with HVPG measurements

1. Access route (jugular vs femoral vs forearm), including laterality

2. Type of catheter/s used for accessing the hepatic vein and for pressure measurements (balloon vs end-hole catheter)

3. Hepatic veins used for pressure measurements (right vs middle vs left)

4. FHVP

5. WHVP

6. HVPG

7. Inferior vena cava pressure

8. Right atrial pressure (if measured)

9. Limitations (if any) of the measurements

10. Complications

11. Associated procedures

FHVP, WHVP, and HVPG), or ascites from portal hypertension in the setting of cirrhosis (increased HVPG).

Classification of Portal Hypertension

Any condition that interferes with blood flow within the portal system can cause portal hypertension, and therefore this condition is classified according to the site of obstruction as prehepatic (involving the splenic, mesenteric, or portal veins), intrahepatic (parenchymal liver diseases), and posthepatic (diseases involving the hepatic venous outflow).

Prehepatic portal hypertension is most frequently caused by portal vein thrombosis. Intrahepatic causes of portal hypertension are the most common. In Western countries, liver cirrhosis is responsible for approximately 90% of cases of portal hypertension, whereas schistosomiasis disease is the leading cause in some areas of the world. Intrahepatic portal hypertension can be further subclassified according to the results of hepatic vein catheterization. Presinusoidal portal hypertension shows normal WHVP and FHVP values, as is the case for noncirrhotic portal hypertension and hepatic granulomatosis (which occurs during the early stages of primary biliary cirrhosis and schistosomiasis, sarcoidosis, tuberculosis). Sinusoidal portal hypertension gives rise to increased WHVP and normal FHVP and is found in most chronic liver diseases, except for primary biliary cirrhosis. In postsinusoidal portal hypertension, both the WHVP and FHVP are increased, as seen in Budd-Chiari syndrome (hepatic vein thrombosis). Causes of posthepatic portal hypertension include heart failure, constrictive pericarditis, or occlusion of the suprahepatic vena cava.[2]

Assessment of Disease Severity and Prognosis in Cirrhosis

The use of the HVPG for the measurement of portal pressure is "as close as we have come to a validated surrogate outcome measure in hepatology."[12] This assertion is based on consistent observational data showing that improvements in the HVPG (either medication-induced or related to treatment of the cause of cirrhosis, such as abstinence from alcohol) are associated with improvements in clinical outcomes.

Risk prediction in cirrhosis

The HVPG is a strong and independent predictor of outcomes in compensated and decompensated cirrhosis. Cross-sectional studies addressing clinical-hemodynamic correlations have shown that an HVPG of 10 mm Hg or greater is necessary for gastroesophageal varices to form.[13,14] The importance of this HVPG threshold has been confirmed in a large observational study nested in a randomized trial evaluating patients with compensated cirrhosis.[14] An HVPG of 10 mm Hg or greater was associated with an increased risk of developing varices, hepatic decompensation (40% at 4 years),[15] and hepatocellular carcinoma on follow-up.[16] As a result of its prognostic utility, the HVPG threshold of 10 mm Hg or greater is termed *clinically significant portal hypertension*. The HVPG is also relevant in patients with decompensated cirrhosis, for whom it provides information about the risk of death during follow-up.[17–19] In this setting, 16 mm Hg is considered the optimum cutoff value.[17,20,21] In the setting of acute variceal hemorrhage, an HVPG of greater than 20 mm Hg is an independent predictor of rebleeding and of mortality.[22–24] Based on these clinical-hemodynamic links, recent guidelines support the recommendation that the HVPG be used to risk-stratify patients, particularly in the research setting.[25,26] For example, trials evaluating therapies for the prevention of varices should ideally focus on patients with a baseline HVPG of 10 mm Hg or greater. Moreover, investigators have suggested that trials evaluating pharmacologic therapy for primary and secondary prophylaxis should ideally include HVPG measurements,[27] although this can be logistically challenging. In the authors' view, in trials studying secondary prophylaxis, in which the rate of events is high, there is no need to use surrogate end points such as HVPG measurements. In trials targeting patients with early chronic liver disease, in which the rate of events is very low, HVPG could be used as a surrogate of efficacy. However, further validation of HVPG response as a surrogate with new drug classes (other than β-blockers) would be desirable.

Risk prediction in viral hepatitis

The HVPG has utility in the setting of chronic viral hepatitis. Through assessing the liver as a whole, including the potential functional changes in the hepatic microvasculature, it has the potential to provide supplemental information to histology.[28] The correlation of the HVPG with histologic fibrosis has been established in both hepatitis B[29] and C[6] virus–related chronic hepatitis. From these data, most patients with significant fibrosis ($\geq$F2 according to the METAVIR scoring system) have an HVPG greater than 5 mm Hg.[29] Antiviral therapy–related changes in the HVPG are a good way to evaluate disease progression and regression in cases of advanced chronic hepatitis C. Several studies have compared HVPG measurements taken before and after antiviral therapy in patients with chronic hepatitis C. These studies have shown a significant HVPG reduction in patients with advanced-stage fibrosis (F3 and F4) after treatment of chronic hepatitis C, particularly in the presence of a sustained viral response.[30,31] In patients with compensated cirrhosis without obvious clinically significant portal hypertension (eg, without esophageal varices), the HVPG is useful to predict the response to antiviral therapy. Reiberger and colleagues[32] showed that an HVPG cutoff of 10 mm Hg or greater was an independent predictor of response to combination pegylated interferon and ribavirin therapy (sustained virologic response of 14% vs 51% in those with HVPG <10 mm Hg). The development of thrombocytopenia was also more pronounced in patients with the higher HVPG. Although promising as a tool to select patients, with the advent of novel hepatitis C therapies, the predictive power of an HVPG of 10 mm Hg or greater will require complete reevaluation.[33]

Alcoholic hepatitis

Acute alcoholic hepatitis (AAH) is a severe condition with a high mortality rate. Compared with patients with viral or alcohol-related cirrhosis, AAH is associated with higher HVPG values. This finding is likely related to the activation of inflammatory vasoactive mediators and the subsequent increases in both portal blood inflow and functional vascular resistance to portal flow.[34,35] In a study of 60 patients with severe AAH (Maddrey discriminant function value of >32), multivariate analysis revealed that an HVPG of greater than 22 mm Hg (measured within 8 days of admission), a Model for End-Stage Liver Disease (MELD) score of greater than 25 points, and encephalopathy were independent predictors of in-hospital mortality. Forty-eight percent of patients had an HVPG greater than 22 mm Hg. The in-hospital mortality rate in these patients was 66% compared with 13%, suggesting that this variable could be a valuable tool to risk-stratify patients with severe AAH.[36] More recent data, however, suggest that HVPG does not significantly add to the predictive value of histology.[37]

HVPG and liver transplantation

In a retrospective study of patients with cirrhosis awaiting liver transplantation, Ripoll and colleagues[19] found that the HVPG provides prognostic value regarding survival, independent of both the MELD score and age. Each 1-mm Hg increase in the HVPG predicted a 3% increase in risk of death. These findings have not been translated into practice, because although the calibration (the ability to predict survival in an individual patient) of MELD improved with the addition of HVPG, the discrimination (the ability to rank patients according to prognosis) did not.

As in the pretransplant setting, the HVPG has a role in the selection and treatment of patients with posttransplant hepatitis C. In patients transplanted for hepatitis C virus–related cirrhosis, a 1-year posttransplant HVPG (area under the curve [AUC], 0.96) was more accurate than liver biopsy (AUC, 0.80) in identifying those patients at highest risk of clinical decompensation from hepatitis C recurrence.[38] In this setting, the improved sensitivity of HVPG for detecting a compromised liver has been attributed to the atypical pattern of perisinusoidal fibrosis deposition that occurs posttransplantation. In addition, HVPG might better reflect the non–fibrosis-related pathophysiologic events that contribute to disease progression, such as liver microvascular dysfunction.[4] Portal hypertension (an HVPG of $\geq$6 mm Hg) was, for example, detected in 5%, 16%, and 60% of patients with stage 0, 1, and 2 fibrosis, respectively. At 1-year posttransplantation, an HVPG of 6 mm Hg or greater was associated with clinical decompensation (ascites, hepatic encephalopathy) in 67% versus 2% of patients with an HVPG of less than 6 mm Hg.[38] In other studies, cutoffs of 6 mm Hg or greater and 10 mm Hg or greater have predicted posttransplantation hepatitis C virus–related decompensation and even death.[39] Given its superior accuracy to biopsy, HVPG is likely the optimal investigation for the assessment of chronic viral hepatitis recurrence after liver transplantation.[38–41] Again, the availability of new treatments, much more effective and with less side effects, will markedly change current patient selection strategies. Consistent with the nontransplant setting, serial HVPG measurements may also have a role once posttransplant antiviral therapy has commenced, with this measurement improving the most in patients achieving a sustained virologic response to antiviral therapy.[42]

HVPG and hepatocellular carcinoma

In patients with compensated cirrhosis, Ripoll and colleagues[16] reported that the HVPG, together with assessment of albumin levels and viral origin, was an independent predictor of the risk of developing HCC. This risk was 6 times higher in patients with clinically significant portal hypertension (HVPG $\geq$10 mm Hg) than in patients with cirrhosis and HVPG values less than 10 mm Hg.

The HVPG also plays an important role in the HCC treatment algorithm.[43] In patients with well-compensated cirrhosis and resectable HCC, the presence of clinically significant portal hypertension markedly increases the risk of unresolved hepatic decompensation occurring within 3 months of hepatic resection.[44,45] Surgical resection for HCC should therefore be restricted to patients without clinically significant portal hypertension.[46,47]

Assessment of the response to pharmacologic therapy to decrease portal pressure

Variceal bleeding and ascites occur when HVPG values reach at least 12 mm Hg.[13,48] Longitudinal studies have shown that if the HVPG decreases to less than 12 mm Hg, either through drug therapy[49,50] or spontaneously (owing to an improvement in liver disease),[18] variceal bleeding is totally prevented and varices decrease in size. However, even if this target is not achieved, a decrease in HVPG of at least 20%[50] from baseline levels offers almost total protection from variceal bleeding in the long term. In patients surviving a bleeding episode, achievement of these targets (decrease in HVPG to <12 mm Hg or $\geq$20% from baseline) constitutes the strongest independent predictor of protection from subsequent variceal bleeding, reduces the risk of other portal hypertension–related complications (eg, ascites, spontaneous bacterial peritonitis), and is associated with an improved survival (**Fig. 3**).[51–53] This survival benefit

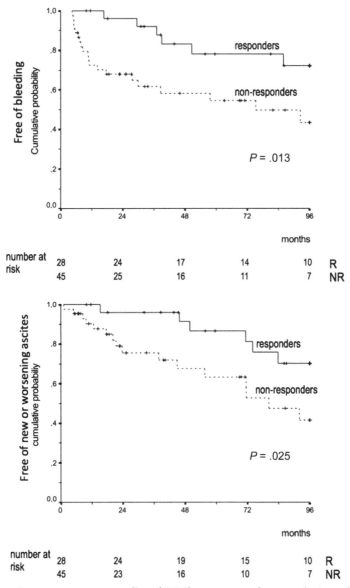

Fig. 3. Hepatic venous pressure gradient (HVPG) response and prognosis. In patients with cirrhosis who have recovered from an episode of acute variceal bleeding, and subsequently treated with β-blockers, an HVPG decrease greater than 20% or to less than 12 mm Hg (responders) is associated with a long-term decrease in the risk of variceal bleeding and ascites. (*From* Abraldes JG, Tarantino I, Turnes J, et al. Hemodynamic response to pharmacologic treatment of portal hypertension and long-term prognosis of cirrhosis. Hepatology 2003;37(4):902–8; with permission.)

was not attributed to an improvement in liver function.[54] These studies are of enormous conceptual importance, because they indicate that the overall prognosis in patients with cirrhosis who survive a variceal bleeding episode can be improved by decreasing portal pressure. The HVPG threshold of 12 mm Hg is less precise for predicting bleeding from fundal gastric varices, and occasionally bleeding may occur in those who have measurements less than this threshold.[55]

The clinical application of the prognostic value of HVPG changes is hampered by the need for repeated measurements of HVPG, and by the fact that a significant number of patients might bleed before a second HVPG measurement is taken.[56] Two studies have shown that evaluation of the acute HVPG response to intravenous propranolol therapy is a useful tool in predicting the efficacy of nonselective β-blockers in preventing first bleeding or rebleeding.[57,58] The acute HVPG response to propranolol was independently associated with survival in these patients.[57] Importantly, the threshold decrease in HVPG that defined a good response (associated with decreased bleeding and mortality) in these studies was 10% to 12% from baseline, rather than the 20% decrease that applies with the chronic response.

A relevant question is whether monitoring pharmacologic therapy for portal hypertension in day-to-day practice has any benefit. The benefits of β-blockers in preventing first bleeding and rebleeding were demonstrated in trials in which treatment was not HVPG-guided; that is, β-blockers were given empirically, either without assessment of HVPG response or, if it was assessed, it was not a factor in guiding therapy.[59] To date, an HVPG-guided treatment strategy has not yet been associated with improved clinical outcomes,[60,61] largely because the therapy that should be offered to nonresponders remains unclear.[56,60] Given the invasive nature of the HVPG measurement and the lack of standardization across centers, HVPG-guided therapy is likely to remain limited to the setting of clinical research until further data are available.

Another important issue is whether the classification of a person as a hemodynamic responder can be maintained over the long term.[62] To do this, annual HVPG measurements were taken in 40 hemodynamic responders (in the setting of secondary prophylaxis) for a mean follow-up of 48 months. Although all patients with alcoholic cirrhosis who remained abstinent retained hemodynamic responsiveness, only 36% of patients with alcoholic cirrhosis who did not remain abstinent and 50% of patients with viral cirrhosis did so. The loss of hemodynamic response was associated with an increased risk of rebleeding, death, and liver transplantation.

Assessment of new therapeutic agents

The first step in the assessment of a potential new agent for treating portal hypertension should involve testing its capacity to modify portal pressure (evaluated as HVPG). However, the demonstration of a portal hypertensive effect for a new drug might not translate into objective clinical benefit. The association between pharmacologic reduction in portal pressure and improved outcomes has been consistently demonstrated only for β-blocker–based therapies.

SUMMARY

Measurement of HVPG remains one of the most useful techniques in hepatology. Hepatic venous pressure gradient is close to the best surrogate marker in chronic liver diseases: it reflects disease severity and has strong prognostic value with regard to survival and decompensation in patients with compensated cirrhosis, during acute bleeding and before liver resection. Furthermore, repeat measurements of HVPG provide unique information on the response to the medical treatment of portal hypertension and represent an invaluable tool for developing new drugs for this disease. Moreover, because changes in HVPG also correlate with the extent of structural changes in the liver, this measurement is increasingly used to assess the effects of antiviral therapy in hepatitis B– and C–related cirrhosis and in assessing the effect of antifibrotic agents. Because of the wide range of applications of this measurement, hepatologists should be familiar with the procedure for assessing HVPG and interpretation of the results.

ACKNOWLEDGMENTS

The authors wish to thank R. Borowski and R. Thomlison for their expert secretarial support.

REFERENCES

1. Groszmann RJ, Abraldes JG. Portal hypertension: from bedside to bench. J Clin Gastroenterol 2005;39(4 Suppl):S215.
2. Bosch J, Abraldes JG, Berzigotti A, et al. The clinical use of HVPG measurements in chronic liver disease. Nat Rev Gastroenterol Hepatol 2009;6:576–82.
3. Groszmann RJ, Glickman M, Blei AT, et al. Wedged and free hepatic venous pressure measured with a balloon catheter. Gastroenterology 1979;76(2):253–8.
4. Abraldes JG, Araujo IK, Turon F, et al. Diagnosing and monitoring cirrhosis: liver biopsy, hepatic venous pressure gradient and elastography. Gastroenterol Hepatol 2012;35(7):488–95.
5. Zipprich A, Winkler M, Seufferlein T, et al. Comparison of balloon vs. straight catheter for the measurement of portal hypertension. Aliment Pharmacol Ther 2010;32(11–12):1351–6.
6. Perello A, Escorsell A, Bru C, et al. Wedged hepatic venous pressure adequately reflects portal pressure in hepatitis C virus-related cirrhosis. Hepatology 1999;30(6):1393–7.
7. La Mura V, Abraldes JG, Berzigotti A, et al. Right atrial pressure is not adequate to calculate portal pressure gradient in cirrhosis: a clinical-hemodynamic correlation study. Hepatology 2010;51(6):2108–16.
8. Groszmann RJ, Wongcharatrawee S. The hepatic venous pressure gradient: anything worth doing should be done right. Hepatology 2004;39(2):280–2.
9. Steinlauf AF, Garcia-Tsao G, Zakko MF, et al. Low-dose midazolam sedation: an option for patients undergoing serial hepatic venous pressure measurements. Hepatology 1999;29(4):1070–3.
10. Reverter E, Blasi A, Abraldes JG, et al. Impact of deep sedation on the accuracy of hepatic and portal venous pressure measurements in patients with cirrhosis. Liver Int 2014;34(1):16–25.
11. Tripodi A, Anstee QM, Sogaard KK, et al. Hypercoagulability in cirrhosis: causes and consequences. J Thromb Haemost 2011;9(9):1713–23.
12. Gluud C, Brok J, Gong Y, et al. Hepatology may have problems with putative surrogate outcome measures. J Hepatol 2007;46(4):734–42.
13. Garcia-Tsao G, Groszmann RJ, Fisher RL, et al. Portal pressure, presence of gastroesophageal varices and variceal bleeding. Hepatology 1985;5(3):419–24.
14. Groszmann RJ, Garcia-Tsao G, Bosch J, et al. Beta-blockers to prevent gastroesophageal varices in patients with cirrhosis. N Engl J Med 2005;353(21):2254–61.
15. Ripoll C, Groszmann R, Garcia-Tsao G, et al. Hepatic venous pressure gradient predicts clinical decompensation in patients with compensated cirrhosis. Gastroenterology 2007;133(2):481–8.
16. Ripoll C, Groszmann RJ, Garcia-Tsao G, et al. Hepatic venous pressure gradient predicts development of hepatocellular carcinoma independently of severity of cirrhosis. J Hepatol 2009;50(5):923–8.

17. Merkel C, Bolognesi M, Bellon S, et al. Prognostic usefulness of hepatic vein catheterization in patients with cirrhosis and esophageal varices. Gastroenterology 1992;102(3):973–9.

18. Vorobioff J, Groszmann RJ, Picabea E, et al. Prognostic value of hepatic venous pressure gradient measurements in alcoholic cirrhosis: a 10-year prospective study. Gastroenterology 1996;111(3):701–9.

19. Ripoll C, Banares R, Rincon D, et al. Influence of hepatic venous pressure gradient on the prediction of survival of patients with cirrhosis in the MELD era. Hepatology 2005;42(4):793–801.

20. Patch D, Armonis A, Sabin C, et al. Single portal pressure measurement predicts survival in cirrhotic patients with recent bleeding. Gut 1999;44(2):264–9.

21. Berzigotti A, Rossi V, Tiani C, et al. Prognostic value of a single HVPG measurement and Doppler-ultrasound evaluation in patients with cirrhosis and portal hypertension. J Gastroenterol 2011;46(5):687–95.

22. Garcia-Pagan JC, Escorsell A, Feu F, et al. Propranolol plus molsidomine vs propranolol alone in the treatment of portal hypertension in patients with cirrhosis. J Hepatol 1996;24(4):430–5.

23. Monescillo A, Martinez-Lagares F, Ruiz-del-Arbol L, et al. Influence of portal hypertension and its early decompression by TIPS placement on the outcome of variceal bleeding. Hepatology 2004;40(4):793–801.

24. Abraldes JG, Villanueva C, Banares R, et al. Hepatic venous pressure gradient and prognosis in patients with acute variceal bleeding treated with pharmacologic and endoscopic therapy. J Hepatol 2008;48(2):229–36.

25. de Franchis R. Evolving consensus in portal hypertension report of the Baveno IV consensus workshop on methodology of diagnosis and therapy in portal hypertension. J Hepatol 2005;43(1):167–76.

26. Garcia-Tsao G, Bosch J, Groszmann RJ. Portal hypertension and variceal bleeding–unresolved issues. Summary of an American Association for the study of liver diseases and European Association for the study of the liver single-topic conference. Hepatology 2008;47(5):1764–72.

27. de Franchis R. Revising consensus in portal hypertension: report of the Baveno V consensus workshop on methodology of diagnosis and therapy in portal hypertension. J Hepatol 2010;53(4):762–8.

28. Burroughs AK, Groszmann R, Bosch J, et al. Assessment of therapeutic benefit of antiviral therapy in chronic hepatitis C: is hepatic venous pressure gradient a better end point? Gut 2002;50(3):425–7.

29. Kumar M, Kumar A, Hissar S, et al. Hepatic venous pressure gradient as a predictor of fibrosis in chronic liver disease because of hepatitis B virus. Liver Int 2008;28(5):690–8.

30. Rincon D, Ripoll C, Iacono OL, et al. Antiviral therapy decreases hepatic venous pressure gradient in patients with chronic hepatitis C and advanced fibrosis. Am J Gastroenterol 2006;101(10):2269–74.

31. Roberts S, Gordon A, McLean C, et al. Effect of sustained viral response on hepatic venous pressure gradient in hepatitis C-related cirrhosis. Clin Gastroenterol Hepatol 2007;5(8):932–7.

32. Reiberger T, Rutter K, Ferlitsch A, et al. Portal pressure predicts outcome and safety of antiviral therapy in cirrhotic patients with hepatitis C virus infection. Clin Gastroenterol Hepatol 2011;9(7):602–8.e1.

33. Grace ND. Patients with clinically significant portal hypertension caused by hepatitis C virus cirrhosis respond poorly to antiviral therapy. Clin Gastroenterol Hepatol 2011;9(7):536–8.

34. Poynard T, Degott C, Munoz C, et al. Relationship between degree of portal hypertension and liver histologic lesions in patients with alcoholic cirrhosis. Effect of acute alcoholic hepatitis on portal hypertension. Dig Dis Sci 1987; 32(4):337–43.
35. Sen S, Mookerjee RP, Cheshire LM, et al. Albumin dialysis reduces portal pressure acutely in patients with severe alcoholic hepatitis. J Hepatol 2005;43(1): 142–8.
36. Rincon D, Lo Iacono O, Ripoll C, et al. Prognostic value of hepatic venous pressure gradient for in-hospital mortality of patients with severe acute alcoholic hepatitis. Aliment Pharmacol Ther 2007;25(7):841–8.
37. Altamirano J, Miquel R, Katoonizadeh A, et al. A histologic scoring system for prognosis of patients with alcoholic hepatitis. Gastroenterology 2014;146: 1231–9.e1–6.
38. Blasco A, Forns X, Carrion JA, et al. Hepatic venous pressure gradient identifies patients at risk of severe hepatitis C recurrence after liver transplantation. Hepatology 2006;43(3):492–9.
39. Samonakis DN, Cholongitas E, Thalheimer U, et al. Hepatic venous pressure gradient to assess fibrosis and its progression after liver transplantation for HCV cirrhosis. Liver Transpl 2007;13(9):1305–11.
40. Carrion JA, Navasa M, Bosch J, et al. Transient elastography for diagnosis of advanced fibrosis and portal hypertension in patients with hepatitis C recurrence after liver transplantation. Liver Transpl 2006;12(12):1791–8.
41. Kalambokis G, Manousou P, Samonakis D, et al. Clinical outcome of HCV-related graft cirrhosis and prognostic value of hepatic venous pressure gradient. Transpl Int 2009;22(2):172–81.
42. Carrion JA, Navasa M, Garcia-Retortillo M, et al. Efficacy of antiviral therapy on hepatitis c recurrence after liver transplantation: a randomized controlled study. Gartroenterology 2007;132:1746–56.
43. Bruix J, Sherman M. Management of hepatocellular carcinoma. Hepatology 2005;42(5):1208–36.
44. Bruix J, Castells A, Bosch J, et al. Surgical resection of hepatocellular carcinoma in cirrhotic patients: prognostic value of preoperative portal pressure. Gastroenterology 1996;111(4):1018–22.
45. Llovet JM, Fuster J, Bruix J. Intention-to-treat analysis of surgical treatment for early hepatocellular carcinoma: resection versus transplantation. Hepatology 1999;30(6):1434–40.
46. Forner A, Bruix J. East meets the West—portal pressure predicts outcome of surgical resection for hepatocellular carcinoma. Nat Clin Pract Gastroenterol Hepatol 2009;6(1):14–5.
47. Reig M, Berzigotti A, Bruix J. If portal hypertension predicts outcome in cirrhosis, why should this not be the case after surgical resection? Liver Int 2013;33(10):1454–6.
48. Casado M, Bosch J, Garcia-Pagan JC, et al. Clinical events after transjugular intrahepatic portosystemic shunt: correlation with hemodynamic findings. Gastroenterology 1998;114(6):1296–303.
49. Groszmann RJ, Bosch J, Grace ND, et al. Hemodynamic events in a prospective randomized trial of propranolol versus placebo in the prevention of a first variceal hemorrhage. Gastroenterology 1990;99(5):1401–7 [see comments].
50. Feu F, Garcia-Pagan JC, Bosch J, et al. Relation between portal pressure response to pharmacotherapy and risk of recurrent variceal haemorrhage in patients with cirrhosis. Lancet 1995;346(8982):1056–9.

51. Abraldes JG, Tarantino I, Turnes J, et al. Hemodynamic response to pharmacological treatment of portal hypertension and long-term prognosis of cirrhosis. Hepatology 2003;37(4):902–8.

52. Albillos A, Banares R, Gonzalez M, et al. Value of the hepatic venous pressure gradient to monitor drug therapy for portal hypertension: a meta-analysis. Am J Gastroenterol 2007;102(5):1116–26.

53. D'Amico G, Garcia-Pagan JC, Luca A, et al. Hepatic vein pressure gradient reduction and prevention of variceal bleeding in cirrhosis: a systematic review. Gastroenterology 2006;131(5):1611–24.

54. Villanueva C, Lopez-Balaguer JM, Aracil C, et al. Maintenance of hemodynamic response to treatment for portal hypertension and influence on complications of cirrhosis. J Hepatol 2004;40(5):757–65.

55. Stanley AJ, Jalan R, Ireland HM, et al. A comparison between gastric and oesophageal variceal haemorrhage treated with transjugular intrahepatic portosystemic stent shunt (TIPSS). Aliment Pharmacol Ther 1997;11(1):171–6.

56. Garcia-Pagan JC, Villanueva C, Albillos A, et al. Nadolol plus isosorbide mononitrate alone or associated with band ligation in the prevention of recurrent bleeding: a multicenter randomized controlled trial. Gut 2009;58(8):1144–50.

57. La Mura V, Abraldes JG, Raffa S, et al. Prognostic value of acute hemodynamic response to i.v. propranolol in patients with cirrhosis and portal hypertension. J Hepatol 2009;51(2):279–87.

58. Villanueva C, Aracil C, Colomo A, et al. Acute hemodynamic response to beta-blockers and prediction of long-term outcome in primary prophylaxis of variceal bleeding. Gastroenterology 2009;137(1):119–28.

59. D'Amico G, Pagliaro L, Bosch J. Pharmacological treatment of portal hypertension: an evidence-based approach. Semin Liver Dis 1999;19(4):475–505.

60. Bureau C, Peron JM, Alric L, et al. "A la carte" treatment of portal hypertension: adapting medical therapy to hemodynamic response for the prevention of bleeding. Hepatology 2002;36:1361–6.

61. Villanueva C, Aracil C, Colomo A, et al. Clinical trial: a randomized controlled study on prevention of variceal rebleeding comparing nadolol + ligation vs. hepatic venous pressure gradient-guided pharmacological therapy. Aliment Pharmacol Ther 2009;29(4):397–408.

62. Augustin S, Gonzalez A, Badia L, et al. Long-term follow-up of hemodynamic responders to pharmacological therapy after variceal bleeding. Hepatology 2012;56(2):706–14.

Endoscopic Band Ligation and Esophageal Stents for Acute Variceal Bleeding

Andrés Cárdenas, MD, MMSc, AGAF[a],*,
Alejandro Fernández-Simon, MD[a], Angels Escorcell, MD, PhD[b]

KEYWORDS

- Cirrhosis • Gastrointestinal bleeding • Esophageal varices
- Endoscopic band ligation • Esophageal stents • TIPS • Portal hypertension
- Acute variceal bleeding

KEY POINTS

- Acute variceal bleeding (AVB) is one of the most serious and feared complications of patients with portal hypertension.
- The management of AVB includes a stepped care approach aimed at resuscitation, restrictive transfusion policy, antibiotic prophylaxis, pharmacologic therapy with vasoconstrictors, and endoscopic therapy.
- The most accepted endoscopic method for treating bleeding varices is endoscopic band ligation, which is effective in approximately 90% of patients. Endoscopic sclerotherapy may be used if band ligation is not possible.
- Esophageal stents that cause tamponade of the esophagus are safer and more effective as a rescue therapy for AVB than balloon tamponade with Sengstaken Blakemore tubes.

 Video of Endoscopic band ligation technique accompanies this article at http://www.liver.theclinics.com/

Acute variceal bleeding (AVB) is a dreaded complication in patients with portal hypertension, and the first episode in a patient with cirrhosis constitutes a significant milestone in the progression of the hepatic disease with important implications in prognosis. Mortality rates due to AVB have decreased in the past 30 years, from 60% to 15% to 20% at 6 weeks, thanks to improvements in general management, medical treatment, and endoscopic therapy.[1] However, there is still a significant

Disclosure: None.

[a] GI/Endoscopy Unit, Institut de Malalties Digestives i Metaboliques, Hospital Clinic, University of Barcelona, Villarroel 170, Esc 3-2, Barcelona 08036, Spain; [b] ICU/Liver Unit, Institut de Malalties Digestives i Metaboliques, Hospital Clinic, University of Barcelona, Villarroel 170, Esc 3-2, Barcelona 08036, Spain
* Corresponding author. Institut de Malalties Digestives i Metaboliques, Hospital Clinic, University of Barcelona, Villarroel 170, Esc 3-2, 08036 Barcelona, Spain.
E-mail addresses: acardena@clinic.ub.es; acv69@hotmail.com

recurrence rate and that is why after an episode of AVB patients need secondary pro-phylaxis. Endoscopy by means of using endoscopic band ligation (EBL) plays a key role in the management of AVB. Current available methods, combined with vasoactive drugs, allow for the control of bleeding in approximately 90% of cases within the first days of the index bleed.[2,3] In cases in which AVB cannot be controlled with endos-copy, balloon tamponade of the esophagus may be required; however, there are significant complications with this method. The recent introduction of fully covered self-expandable metallic stents for AVB is useful in those cases in which balloon tam-ponade is considered as it is more effective and safer for the temporary control of bleeding. This article reviews the current management of AVB with particular emphasis on EBL and esophageal stents.

NATURAL HISTORY/DIAGNOSIS

Esophageal varices are present in nearly 30% to 40% of patients with compensated cirrhosis and in 60% to 80% of those with decompensated cirrhosis.[4] They initially develop as small varices that gradually dilate at a rate of 5% per year. Variceal bleeding usually occurs late in the natural history of portal hypertension, and for vari-ces to bleed, portal pressure as measured by the hepatic venous pressure gradient (HVPG) must rise above 12 mm Hg.[3,5] Certain characteristics such as the severity of liver disease, the size of the varix, and the presence of red wale marks (especially on thin areas of the variceal wall), place the varices at risk of bleeding, which can occur with an incidence of 4% to 15% per year.[4,6,7] Because patients with cirrhosis with an episode of upper gastrointestinal bleeding will have varices as the cause in 80% of cases, bleeding in this setting should be presumed to be of variceal origin.[8] The gold standard for diagnosis of AVB is gastroscopy, which may show active bleeding or oozing from a varix (present in nearly 10%–20% of patients) (**Fig. 1**), signs of a recent hemostasis with a white nipple or adherent clot on a varix, or blood in the stom-ach and/or presence of varices with no other explainable sources of bleeding. Early rebleeding rates within the first 48 to 72 hours after the index bleed can be high (30%–40%) if patients are not properly treated.[9–11] After 6 weeks, the risk of further bleeding is similar to that before the index bleed.[11,12] Mortality rates from an episode

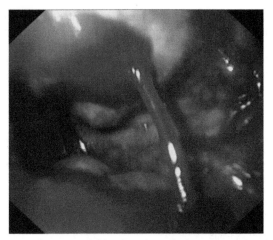

Fig. 1. Endoscopic view of an actively bleeding (spurting) esophageal varix in a patient with cirrhosis.

of variceal bleeding have significantly decreased in the past 3 decades, from 42% in the 1980s[11] to the current rates of 15% to 20%.[13–17] This is largely because of the implementation of standardized guidelines, advances in critical care, better pharmacologic and endoscopic therapies, use of transjugular intrahepatic portosystemic shunts (TIPS), restrictive transfusion policies, and use of prophylactic antibiotics for bacterial infections. Approximately one-third of the deaths are a direct consequence of bleeding, whereas the remaining are related to liver failure, infections, and renal failure.[8,18]

GENERAL MANAGEMENT

The current recommendations for the general management of patients with an episode of AVB have been reviewed elsewhere.[19] In short, the most important aspect is providing adequate resuscitation (ie, treatment of hypovolemia), avoiding aspiration by protecting the airway and intubation in selected cases, preventing bacterial infections, and stopping the hemorrhage with the use of vasoconstrictors and endoscopic therapy. Intubation always should be considered in patients with hepatic encephalopathy and actively vomiting blood.[20,21] Volume resuscitation with saline or other expanders should aim to keep systolic blood pressure between 90 and 100 mm Hg, which can help avoid shock and renal failure.[22] Overexpansion may induce rebound increases in portal pressure and facilitate rebleeding; therefore, a delicate fluid balance is needed in these cases and adequate monitoring in the intensive care unit is helpful. Red blood cell transfusion should aim for a hemoglobin level of 7 g/dL, except in patients with shock, ongoing bleeding, or ischemic heart disease.[23] A trial of a restrictive transfusion policy in which patients were transfused if hemoglobin levels dropped to lower than 7 g/dL (compared with transfusion if hemoglobin <9 g/dL) showed better survival in patients with cirrhosis (Child-Pugh A or B) transfused only if hemoglobin levels were lower than 7 g/dL.[23] There are no data to support the routine use of fresh frozen plasma to improve the elevated international normalized ratio in patients with cirrhosis unless they are anticoagulated with warfarin or heparin or other anticoagulants. Platelets should be transfused if they are below 50,000/μL.[24] Bacterial infections can occur in the setting of AVB, and thus all patients should receive antibiotics. This measure decreases the risk of infection and rebleeding and improves survival.[25–28] In most cases, either norfloxacin 400 mg orally, twice a day for 7 days or intravenous ceftriaxone 1–2 g per day should be given. Intravenous antibiotics are preferred in those patients with hypovolemic shock and advanced cirrhosis.[29] The rapid implementation of vasoconstrictors and performance of endoscopy should be instituted within the first 12 hours of admission.[30] This interval can be shortened to 6 hours in those actively vomiting blood once they are stabilized in a monitored unit. Finally, it is important to consider if the patient is a candidate for TIPS, as the early placement of TIPS (within 72 hours) for patients with AVB with Child-Pugh B actively bleeding or C cirrhosis (<13 points) is associated with a significant reduction in rebleeding and mortality and thus should be considered in such cases.[31]

HEMOSTATIC THERAPIES
Splanchnic Vasoconstrictors

There are 2 types of vasoconstrictors used in patients with AVB; the most commonly used are terlipressin (vasopressin analogue) and somatostatin and its analogue (octreotide). These drugs with specific splanchnic vasoconstrictor activity play a fundamental role in the management of AVB and need to be administered as soon as possible and before endoscopy. The early use of vasoconstrictors in most cases can initially arrest bleeding, which translates into better visualization at endoscopy. These drugs also reduce rebleeding and improve survival among patients with cirrhosis and AVB.[32–36] The available vasoconstrictors and their doses are shown in **Table 1**. A detailed analysis of the role of vasoconstrictors in AVB is out of the scope of this review and is detailed elsewhere.[36]

Endoscopic Therapy

Endoscopy is one of the cornerstones of the management of AVB because it confirms the diagnosis and allows specific therapy during the same session. An important consideration before considering endoscopy is choosing the type of sedation for the procedure as patients need to be fully sedated for the procedure to be successful. We recommend intravenous sedation with propofol, if possible, as it is safe and better tolerated than benzodiazepines (midazolam) plus an opiates (meperidine or fentanyl), which can trigger episodes of minimal hepatic encephalopathy.[37–39] Endoscopic therapies for varices are effective because they cause obliteration of the varix. The 2 endoscopic methods available for AVB are endoscopic sclerotherapy (ES) and EBL. ES consists of the injection of a sclerosing agent (sodium morrhuate 5%, ethanolamine oleate 5%, or polidocanol 1%–2%) into the variceal lumen or adjacent to it. This causes inflammation and thrombosis, creating a scar over the site of the varix. Although it is easy to perform (only need an injection catheter and the sclerosant) there are significant side effects related to the procedure. There are a number of local and systemic complications, which include esophageal ulcers, strictures, substernal chest pain, fever, dysphagia, and even the development of pleural effusions.[40,41] Another problem is the risk of bacteremia, which may arise in up to 30% to 55% of cases and can predispose to spontaneous bacterial peritonitis or distal abscesses.[42,43] Other rare complications include perforation, mediastinitis, pericarditis, chylothorax, and esophageal motility disorders.[40,41,44,45] Compared with EBL of varices, ES for AVB is associated with higher rebleeding rates and more side effects, such as ulcers and strictures.[46] Clinical trials have shown that EBL is better than ES for all major outcomes, including initial control of bleeding, recurrent bleeding, side effects, time to variceal eradication, and even survival.[47,48]

EBL

EBL was introduced an alternative with fewer complications to ES for the treatment of esophageal varices. The concept of using EBL for esophageal varices arose in the 1980s.[49] Given the anatomy and zones of venous return in the gastroesophageal junction Stiegmann and colleagues[50] sought out a means of blocking this drainage. The veins in the palisade zone, which extend proximal to the cardias into the lower esophagus, are the veins most likely to bleed because this is an area between the portal and systemic circulation with no perforating veins from the submucosa allowing for drainage or decompression to periesophageal veins. Thus, a way of "safely"

Table 1 Vasoconstrictors used in acute variceal bleeding	
Drug	**Dose**
Terlipressin	Intravenous bolus 2 mg/4 h for 24–48 h then 1 mg/4 h
Somatostatin	Intravenous bolus 250 μg followed by infusion of 250–500 μg/h
Octreotide	Intravenous bolus of 50–100 μg followed by infusion of 50 μg/h

All drugs are administered for a minimum of 2 days and may be prolonged for up to 5 days.

obliterating these vessels was that of placing rubber bands with endoscopy on the varices in the distal esophagus similar to what surgeons use for treating hemorrhoids. The rest is history, and currently EBL is considered the endoscopic treatment of choice for AVB. In brief, EBL consists of the placement of several elastic bands (range between 4–10) on the varices so as to occlude the varix and cause thrombosis. The technique is shown in Video 1. Ligation of the varix and surrounding mucosa eventually leads to necrosis of the mucosa. The bands fall off within 5 to 7 days, leaving a shallow ulcer that heals and subsequently scars. After the index treatment of an episode of AVB, scheduled repeat sessions need to be performed at 3-week to 4-week intervals to completely obliterate the varices and reduce the risk of rebleeding.[51]

There are several commercially available multiband devices. In Europe and the United States the most common are the Saeed Multiple Ligator (Wilson-Cook Medical, Inc, Winston-Salem, NC, USA) and the Speedband (Boston Scientific Corporation, Natick, MA, USA). They have between 4 and 10 preloaded bands. We prefer to always start the procedure with a 6-band or 7-band device. This allows for enough bands to be placed in a single session without having to repeatedly intubate the patient with the gastroscope. Band ligators have one principle: placement of elastic bands on a varix after it is sucked into a clear plastic cylinder attached to the tip of the endoscope (**Fig. 2**). After the index diagnostic endoscopy is performed in a patient with AVB and the suspected varix is identified, the endoscope is withdrawn and the ligation device is loaded. The device needs to be firmly attached to shaft of the scope near the knobs (**Fig. 3**). At this point, the patient needs to be reintubated and this sometimes can be difficult because the cap of the ligator makes the distal tip of the scope thicker and there is limited vision. It is better to perform a slight flexion of the patient's neck and then push very gently with slight torque to the left or right, always with direct visualization of the pharynx. Once the esophagus is intubated, the knob on the device needs to be on "forward-only" mode. After the varix is identified, the tip of the scope is pushed towards it and continuous suction applied so the mucosa of the varix fills the cap and causes a "red-out" sign; at this point, the band can be fired and a click must be felt (see **Fig. 3**, Video 1). Afterward, the scope should not be advanced distally so as to prevent dislodgement of band. This is the reason why ligation should always commence in the most distal portion of the esophagus near the gastroesophageal (GE) junction. Bands are applied in a spiral pattern, progressing up the esophagus until all major columns of varices of the lower third of the esophagus (no more than 8–10 cm above the GE junction) are banded. If there is a limited view because of ongoing bleeding, an option is to aggressively flush with water,

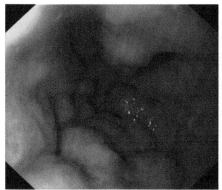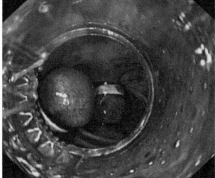

Fig. 2. Endoscopic view of large varices (*left*) and endoscopic view of successfully placed bands in the distal esophagus (*right*).

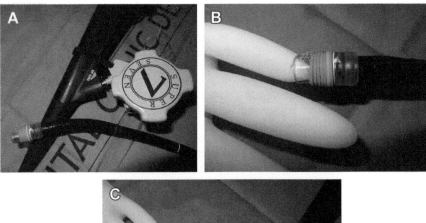

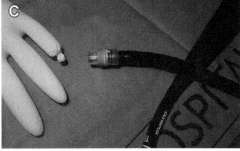

Fig. 3. (*A*) Band ligator placed on the shaft of the endoscope, the knob is attached to the working channel. (*B*) The proximal end of the endoscope has a cap with premounted bands that allows for suction of the varix (in this case a glove is used). (*C*) Once the varix is suctioned into the cap, the band is fired and the varix is ligated.

perform suction, and start placing bands at the GE junction. This reduces the heavy bleeding and further bands can be fired afterward.

The procedure is not exempt from complications either, and these include transient dysphagia and chest pain, which respond well to liquid analgesics (ie, acetaminophen), as well as an oral suspension of antacids or sucralfate. A liquid diet should be started the same day and soft foods the next day. Shallow ulcers at the site of bands are frequent and can bleed in up to 4% of cases.[52] The use of a proton pump inhibitor (ie, pantoprazole 40 mg per day for 10 days) decreases the size of ulcers but does not prevent them from bleeding.[53] Severe and rare complications, such as massive bleeding from ulcers or rarely from variceal rupture, esophageal perforation, esophageal strictures, or altered esophageal motility, may occur with EBL.[54] If a patient bleeds due to an ulcer after EBL, ES may be performed. Another option is applying Hemospray (a hemostatic powder) to the bleeding site. This powder, which is used for nonvariceal gastrointestinal bleeding, seems to be promising as a hemostatic technique for patients with portal gastropathy, variceal bleeding, and bleeding after EBL ulcers.[55–57]

EBL is highly effective in the control of AVB, with an immediate efficacy in 90% of cases.[2] Two randomized controlled trials that compared EBL and ES in AVB[47,48] have clearly shown that treatment with EBL along with vasoconstrictors is associated with higher efficacy, safety, and improved mortality than ES and vasoconstrictors. In addition, in 8 other trials, these 2 modalities also were compared in AVB and in the prevention of rebleeding. A meta-analysis of the 10 trials shows that EBL is better than ES in the initial control of bleeding, and is associated with fewer adverse events and improved mortality (**Fig. 4**).[58] Therefore, EBL is considered the endoscopic therapy

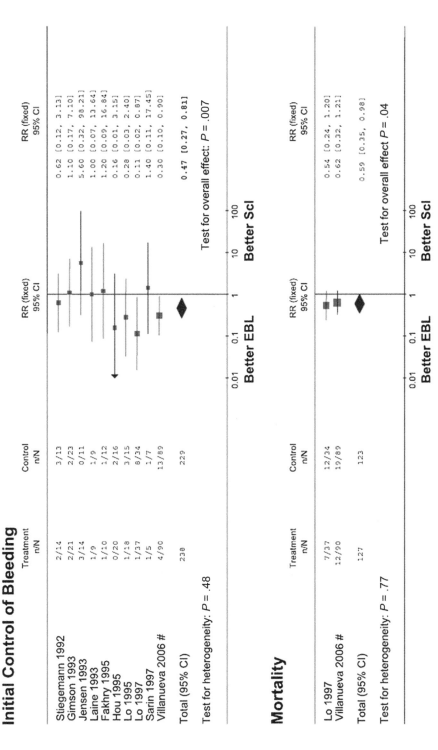

Fig. 4. Meta-analysis comparing the efficacy of urgent EBL versus ES for acute variceal bleeding. EBL is more effective in the initial control of bleeding and is associated with better mortality. # All patients received somatostatin.

of choice in AVB. Although EBL is preferred over ES for an episode of AVB, in the setting of active hemorrhage or torrential bleeding, EBL may be sometimes difficult to perform because of lack of visibility. Therefore, both techniques are reasonable options in the setting of AVB.

ESOPHAGEAL STENTS

Balloon tamponade of the esophagus is used in patients in whom endoscopic therapy cannot stop the bleeding or in those patients with a known history of esophageal varices in whom such profuse bleeding and hemodynamic status precludes an upper endoscopy. Current guidelines recommend using balloon tamponade only in massive bleeding, as a temporary "bridge" until definitive treatment can be instituted (for a maximum of 24 hours) in an intensive care unit.[22,59] Esophageal balloon tamponade, which is typically performed with a Sengstaken-Blakemore tube, causes hemostasis by direct compression of the bleeding varices. If placed properly, tamponade may provide initial control of bleeding in up to 85% of cases, but recurrence is observed in 50% of the patients after deflation of the balloon.[60] The most common complications include aspiration pneumonia and esophageal perforation, which may occur in 30% of patients, with a mortality rate of 5% mainly due to perforation.[60] The incidence of complications increases with the duration of tamponade and when tubes are inserted by inexperienced staff. Therefore, tamponade should be performed only by skilled and experienced personnel in intensive care facilities and with special caution in patients with respiratory failure or cardiac arrhythmias. Because of the high risk of aspiration pneumonia, tamponade should be preceded by prophylactic orotracheal intubation in most patients.

An alternative to balloon tamponade is placing fully covered self-expandable metal stents that act with a tamponade mechanism on the esophagus.[61] This certainly represents a promising therapeutic alternative to balloon tamponade. The main advantages include fewer side effects, ability to maintain enteral feeding, and the possibility to leave the stent in place for 1 week, which allows for stabilization of the patient so as to plan bridge therapies, such as TIPS. The SX-Ella Danis stent (135 × 25 mm; ELLA-CS, Hradec Kralove, Czech Republic) is a removable, fully covered, and self-expanding nitinol metal stent with atraumatic edges specifically designed for AVB (**Fig. 5**). It comes in a ready-to-use procedure pack that contains all items necessary for its placement. In

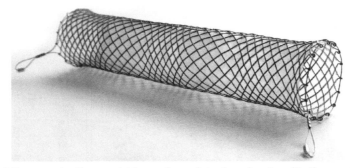

Fig. 5. A fully covered self-expandable esophageal stent can be placed in the esophagus as a rescue therapy in patients in whom variceal bleeding cannot be controlled by endoscopic therapy plus vasoactive drugs. The stent (SX-Ella Danis) is 135 mm long × 25 mm wide and has 2 threads in the distal and proximal end that allows the stent to be pulled endoscopically.

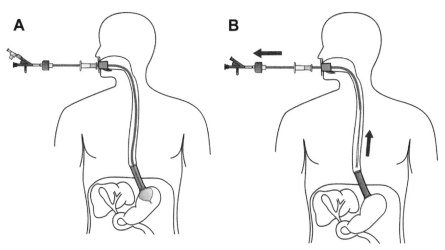

Fig. 6. (*A*) Once the stent is advanced into the stomach, a distal balloon at the proximal end is inflated with a syringe. (*B*) Then the stent is pulled back until it anchors in the cardias and lower esophagus and then deployed and the introducer is withdrawn.

Table 2
Case series reporting the efficacy of esophageal stents as a rescue therapy for the treatment of acute variceal bleeding

	No. Patients	SEMS Deployed, %	Initial Hemostasis, %	Rebleed, %	Migration, %	Mortality Follow-Up, d
Hubmann et al,[66] 2006	15	100	100	0	13	20% 60 d
Zehetner et al,[67] 2008	34	100	100	0	18	29% 60 d
Wright et al,[65] 2010	10	90	70	14	NR	50% 42 d
Dechêne et al,[63] 2012	8	100	100	38	0	75% 60 d
Holster et al,[68] 2013	5	100	100	20	20	40% 180 d
Zakaria et al,[69] 2013	16	94	88	0	38	25% NR
Fierz et al,[62] 2013	7	100	89	0	0	77% 42 d

Abbreviations: SEMS, self-expandable metal stents; NR, not reported.

addition, it has radiopaque markers at both ends and midportion for monitoring with plain chest radiographs. The stent can be deployed in the lower esophagus without radiological or endoscopic assistance; however, in some cases, a prior endoscopy is useful as a means to leave a rigid guidewire in the stomach, which later aids in placing the premounted stent. The procedure is relatively easy to perform but basic training is needed to understand how it is placed. Once the stent has been advanced to the stomach, a distal balloon at the proximal end is inflated with a syringe and then the stent is pulled back until it anchors in the cardias and lower esophagus. This then allows its deployment, thus no fluoroscopy is needed (**Fig. 6**). The stent can be removed 7 days later endoscopically using an overtube system (Extractor for SX-ELLA stent Danis) without causing trauma to the esophagus. Several case series have demonstrated its safety and efficacy in AVB (**Table 2**).[62–69] In most published cases, the stents have been successfully deployed in more than 90% of patients. The results on immediate hemostasis range between 70% and 100%. In most cases, patients can be offered a bridge therapy, such as TIPS or repeat endoscopic treatment with EBL or ES. A drawback of using the stent is migration, which can occur in 20% of cases.[61,65,66]

We recently performed a multicenter randomized controlled trial (published in abstract form) comparing esophageal stenting versus balloon tamponade in 28 patients with AVB refractory to medical and endoscopic treatment and/or with massive bleeding precluding endoscopy.[70] Fifteen patients were randomized to balloon tamponade and 13 to stent placement. Primary outcome measure was success of therapy, defined as survival at day 15 with control of bleeding and without serious adverse events. Our results showed that esophageal stents were more effective

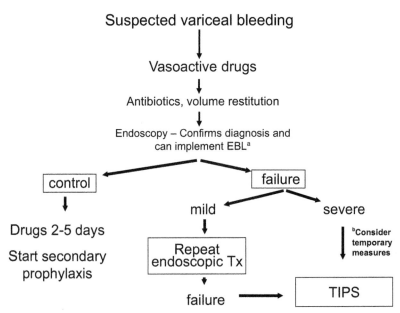

Fig. 7. Recommended algorithm for the treatment of an episode of acute variceal bleeding. [a] Placement of TIPS (within 72 hours) for patients AVB with Child B actively bleeding or C cirrhosis (<13 points) is associated with a significant reduction in rebleeding and mortality and can be considered in such cases. [b] Temporary measures include placement of an esophageal stent or balloon tamponade. Esophageal stents are preferred, as they are safer and more effective. The use of the balloon is associated with potentially lethal complications, such as aspiration and perforation of the esophagus. Tx, treatment.

than balloon tamponade for the temporary control of bleeding with absence of rebleeding at 15 days in 77% in the stent group versus 47% in the balloon tamponade group. Side effects occurred in 8% of patients in the stent group versus 52% in the balloon tamponade group. There were no differences in survival, but the primary end point of the study was on efficacy and safety and not survival. These better results were due to both a greater hemostatic effect and a lower rate of serious adverse events, especially aspiration pneumonia, with the use of esophageal stents.[70] These results favor the use of esophageal stents in patients with uncontrolled AVB, although further controlled studies are needed.

Failure to Control Bleeding

Approximately 10% to 15% of patients do not respond to the previously mentioned therapies. In such cases, if the patient is stable, a second therapeutic endoscopy may be performed. However, if this is unsuccessful or there is massive bleeding, the patient should be considered for other treatments, such as TIPS. This topic is discussed in detail in the article by Garcia-Pagan and colleagues, elsewhere in this issue.

SUMMARY

AVB is a dreaded complication of patients with cirrhosis and portal hypertension (**Fig. 7**). Initial management should focus on resuscitation with adequate volume replacement, careful blood transfusions to keep hemoglobin levels at 7 g/dL, antibiotic prophylaxis, and endotracheal intubation in selected cases. Standard of care mandates for early administration of vasoactive drugs and EBL within the first 12 hours of the index bleed. Patients who fail combined pharmacologic and endoscopic therapy may require temporary placement of balloon tamponade or esophageal stents until definitive treatment (preferably TIPS) can be instituted. Given the available data, esophageal stents in this setting are preferred. Patients who fail the previously mentioned therapies should undergo an evaluation for TIPS.

SUPPLEMENTARY DATA

Supplementary data related to this article can be found online at http://dx.doi.org/10.1016/j.cld.2014.07.003.

REFERENCES

1. Garcia-Tsao G, Bosch J. Management of varices and variceal hemorrhage in cirrhosis. N Engl J Med 2010;362:823–32. Available at: http://www.ncbi.nlm.nih.gov/pubmed/20200386. Accessed March 10, 2014.
2. Qureshi W, Adler DG, Davila R, et al. ASGE Guideline: the role of endoscopy in the management of variceal hemorrhage, updated July 2005. Gastrointest Endosc 2005;62:651–5. Available at: http://www.ncbi.nlm.nih.gov/pubmed/16246673. Accessed February 11, 2014.
3. O'Brien J, Triantos C, Burroughs AK. Management of varices in patients with cirrhosis. Nat Rev Gastroenterol Hepatol 2013;10:402–12. Available at: http://www.ncbi.nlm.nih.gov/pubmed/23545523. Accessed March 19, 2014.
4. De Franchis R, Primignani M. Natural history of portal hypertension in patients with cirrhosis. Clin Liver Dis 2001;5:645–63. Available at: http://www.ncbi.nlm.nih.gov/pubmed/11565135. Accessed February 27, 2014.

5. Merli M, Nicolini G, Angeloni S, et al. Incidence and natural history of small esophageal varices in cirrhotic patients. J Hepatol 2003;38:266–72. Available at: http://www.ncbi.nlm.nih.gov/pubmed/12586291. Accessed February 27, 2014.

6. Prediction of the first variceal hemorrhage in patients with cirrhosis of the liver and esophageal varices. A prospective multicenter study. N Engl J Med 1988;319:983–9. Available at: http://www.ncbi.nlm.nih.gov/pubmed/3262200. Accessed February 27, 2014.

7. Groszmann RJ, Bosch J, Grace ND, et al. Hemodynamic events in a prospective randomized trial of propranolol versus placebo in the prevention of a first variceal hemorrhage. Gastroenterology 1990;99:1401–7. Available at: http://www.ncbi.nlm.nih.gov/pubmed/2210246. Accessed February 27, 2014.

8. D'Amico G, De Franchis R. Upper digestive bleeding in cirrhosis. Post-therapeutic outcome and prognostic indicators. Hepatology 2003;38:599–612. Available at: http://www.ncbi.nlm.nih.gov/pubmed/12939586. Accessed February 7, 2014.

9. Bosch J, García-Pagán JC. Prevention of variceal rebleeding. Lancet 2003;361:952–4. Available at: http://www.ncbi.nlm.nih.gov/pubmed/12648985. Accessed February 27, 2014.

10. D'Amico G, Pagliaro L, Bosch J. Pharmacological treatment of portal hypertension: an evidence-based approach. Semin Liver Dis 1999;19:475–505. Available at: http://www.ncbi.nlm.nih.gov/pubmed/10643630. Accessed February 27, 2014.

11. Graham DY, Smith JL. The course of patients after variceal hemorrhage. Gastroenterology 1981;80:800–9. Available at: http://www.ncbi.nlm.nih.gov/pubmed/6970703. Accessed February 27, 2014.

12. Bosch J, Garcia-Pagán JC, Berzigotti A, et al. Measurement of portal pressure and its role in the management of chronic liver disease. Semin Liver Dis 2006;26:348–62. Available at: http://www.ncbi.nlm.nih.gov/pubmed/17051449. Accessed February 27, 2014.

13. Chalasani N, Kahi C, Francois F, et al. Improved patient survival after acute variceal bleeding: a multicenter, cohort study. Am J Gastroenterol 2003;98:653–9. Available at: http://www.ncbi.nlm.nih.gov/pubmed/12650802. Accessed February 27, 2014.

14. Carbonell N, Pauwels A, Serfaty L, et al. Improved survival after variceal bleeding in patients with cirrhosis over the past two decades. Hepatology 2004;40:652–9. Available at: http://www.ncbi.nlm.nih.gov/pubmed/15349904. Accessed February 27, 2014.

15. Stokkeland K, Brandt L, Ekbom A, et al. Improved prognosis for patients hospitalized with esophageal varices in Sweden 1969–2002. Hepatology 2006;43:500–5. Available at: http://www.ncbi.nlm.nih.gov/pubmed/16496319. Accessed March 6, 2014.

16. Bambha K, Kim WR, Pedersen R, et al. Predictors of early re-bleeding and mortality after acute variceal haemorrhage in patients with cirrhosis. Gut 2008;57:814–20. Available at: http://www.ncbi.nlm.nih.gov/pubmed/18250126. Accessed January 21, 2014.

17. Reverter E, Tandon P, Augustin S, et al. A MELD-based model to determine risk of mortality among patients with acute variceal bleeding. Gastroenterology 2014;146:412–9.e3. Available at: http://www.ncbi.nlm.nih.gov/pubmed/24148622. Accessed March 11, 2014.

18. Cárdenas A, Ginès P, Uriz J, et al. Renal failure after upper gastrointestinal bleeding in cirrhosis: incidence, clinical course, predictive factors, and short-term prognosis. Hepatology 2001;34:671–6. Available at: http://www.ncbi.nlm.nih.gov/pubmed/11584362. Accessed February 25, 2014.

19. Fortune B, Garcia-Tsao G. Current management strategies for acute esophageal variceal hemorrhage. Curr Hepatol Rep 2014;13:35–42. Available at: http://www.ncbi.nlm.nih.gov/pubmed/24955303. Accessed July 9, 2014.

20. Koch DG, Arguedas MR, Fallon MB. Risk of aspiration pneumonia in suspected variceal hemorrhage: the value of prophylactic endotracheal intubation prior to endoscopy. Dig Dis Sci 2007;52:2225–8. Available at: http://www.ncbi.nlm.nih.gov/pubmed/17385037. Accessed March 6, 2014.

21. Rudolph SJ, Landsverk BK, Freeman ML. Endotracheal intubation for airway protection during endoscopy for severe upper GI hemorrhage. Gastrointest Endosc 2003;57:58–61. Available at: http://www.ncbi.nlm.nih.gov/pubmed/12518132. Accessed March 6, 2014.

22. De Franchis R. Revising consensus in portal hypertension: report of the Baveno V consensus workshop on methodology of diagnosis and therapy in portal hypertension. J Hepatol 2010;53:762–8. Available at: http://www.ncbi.nlm.nih.gov/pubmed/20638742. Accessed February 24, 2014.

23. Villanueva C, Colomo A, Bosch A, et al. Transfusion strategies for acute upper gastrointestinal bleeding. N Engl J Med 2013;368:11–21. Available at: http://www.ncbi.nlm.nih.gov/pubmed/23281973. Accessed February 19, 2014.

24. Caldwell SH, Hoffman M, Lisman T, et al. Coagulation disorders and hemostasis in liver disease: pathophysiology and critical assessment of current management. Hepatology 2006;44:1039–46. Available at: http://www.ncbi.nlm.nih.gov/pubmed/17006940. Accessed June 3, 2014.

25. Hou MC, Lin HC, Liu TT, et al. Antibiotic prophylaxis after endoscopic therapy prevents rebleeding in acute variceal hemorrhage: a randomized trial. Hepatology 2004;39:746–53. Available at: http://www.ncbi.nlm.nih.gov/pubmed/14999693. Accessed March 6, 2014.

26. Soares-Weiser K, Brezis M, Tur-Kaspa R, et al. Antibiotic prophylaxis of bacterial infections in cirrhotic inpatients: a meta-analysis of randomized controlled trials. Scand J Gastroenterol 2003;38:193–200. Available at: http://www.ncbi.nlm.nih.gov/pubmed/12678337. Accessed March 6, 2014.

27. Fernández J, Ruiz del Arbol L, Gómez C, et al. Norfloxacin vs ceftriaxone in the prophylaxis of infections in patients with advanced cirrhosis and hemorrhage. Gastroenterology 2006;131:1049–56 [quiz: 1285]. Available at: http://www.ncbi.nlm.nih.gov/pubmed/17030175. Accessed February 4, 2014.

28. Chavez-Tapia NC, Barrientos-Gutierrez T, Tellez-Avila F, et al. Meta-analysis: antibiotic prophylaxis for cirrhotic patients with upper gastrointestinal bleeding—an updated Cochrane review. Aliment Pharmacol Ther 2011;34:509–18. Available at: http://www.ncbi.nlm.nih.gov/pubmed/21707680. Accessed July 9, 2014.

29. Rimola A, García-Tsao G, Navasa M, et al. Diagnosis, treatment and prophylaxis of spontaneous bacterial peritonitis: a consensus document. International Ascites Club. J Hepatol 2000;32:142–53. Available at: http://www.ncbi.nlm.nih.gov/pubmed/10673079. Accessed April 10, 2014.

30. Chen PH, Chen WC, Hou MC, et al. Delayed endoscopy increases re-bleeding and mortality in patients with hematemesis and active esophageal variceal bleeding: a cohort study. J Hepatol 2012;57:1207–13. Available at: http://www.ncbi.nlm.nih.gov/pubmed/22885718. Accessed July 9, 2014.

31. García-Pagán JC, Caca K, Bureau C, et al. Early use of TIPS in patients with cirrhosis and variceal bleeding. N Engl J Med 2010;362:2370–9. Available at: http://www.ncbi.nlm.nih.gov/pubmed/20573925. Accessed March 11, 2014.

32. Ioannou G, Doust J, Rockey DC. Terlipressin for acute esophageal variceal hemorrhage. Cochrane Database Syst Rev 2003;(1). CD002147. Available at: http://www.ncbi.nlm.nih.gov/pubmed/12535432. Accessed March 6, 2014.

33. Gøtzsche PC, Hróbjartsson A. Somatostatin analogues for acute bleeding oesophageal varices. Cochrane Database Syst Rev 2008;(3). CD000193. Available at: http://www.ncbi.nlm.nih.gov/pubmed/18677774. Accessed March 10, 2014.

34. Escorsell A, Ruiz del Arbol L, Planas R, et al. Multicenter randomized controlled trial of terlipressin versus sclerotherapy in the treatment of acute variceal bleeding: the TEST study. Hepatology 2000;32:471–6. Available at: http://www.ncbi.nlm.nih.gov/pubmed/10960437. Accessed March 10, 2014.

35. Corley DA, Cello JP, Adkisson W, et al. Octreotide for acute esophageal variceal bleeding: a meta-analysis. Gastroenterology 2001;120:946–54. Available at: http://www.ncbi.nlm.nih.gov/pubmed/11231948. Accessed March 10, 2014.

36. Wells M, Chande N, Adams P, et al. Meta-analysis: vasoactive medications for the management of acute variceal bleeds. Aliment Pharmacol Ther 2012;35: 1267–78. Available at: http://www.ncbi.nlm.nih.gov/pubmed/22486630. Accessed July 9, 2014.

37. Riphaus A, Lechowicz I, Frenz MB, et al. Propofol sedation for upper gastrointestinal endoscopy in patients with liver cirrhosis as an alternative to midazolam to avoid acute deterioration of minimal encephalopathy: a randomized, controlled study. Scand J Gastroenterol 2009;44:1244–51. Available at: http://www.ncbi.nlm.nih.gov/pubmed/19811337. Accessed July 9, 2014.

38. Khamaysi I, William N, Olga A, et al. Sub-clinical hepatic encephalopathy in cirrhotic patients is not aggravated by sedation with propofol compared to midazolam: a randomized controlled study. J Hepatol 2011;54:72–7. Available at: http://www.ncbi.nlm.nih.gov/pubmed/20934771. Accessed July 9, 2014.

39. Bamji N, Cohen LB. Endoscopic sedation of patients with chronic liver disease. Clin Liver Dis 2010;14:185–94. Available at: http://www.ncbi.nlm.nih.gov/pubmed/20682228. Accessed March 12, 2014.

40. Baillie J, Yudelman P. Complications of endoscopic sclerotherapy of esophageal varices. Endoscopy 1992;24:284–91. Available at: http://www.ncbi.nlm.nih.gov/pubmed/1612042. Accessed March 10, 2014.

41. Lee JG, Lieberman DA. Complications related to endoscopic hemostasis techniques. Gastrointest Endosc Clin N Am 1996;6:305–21. Available at: http://www.ncbi.nlm.nih.gov/pubmed/8673330. Accessed March 10, 2014.

42. Rolando N, Gimson A, Philpott-Howard J, et al. Infectious sequelae after endoscopic sclerotherapy of oesophageal varices: role of antibiotic prophylaxis. J Hepatol 1993;18:290–4. Available at: http://www.ncbi.nlm.nih.gov/pubmed/8228122. Accessed March 10, 2014.

43. Selby WS, Norton ID, Pokorny CS, et al. Bacteremia and bacterascites after endoscopic sclerotherapy for bleeding esophageal varices and prevention by intravenous cefotaxime: a randomized trial. Gastrointest Endosc 1994;40: 680–4. Available at: http://www.ncbi.nlm.nih.gov/pubmed/7859964. Accessed March 10, 2014.

44. Villanueva C, Colomo A, Aracil C, et al. Current endoscopic therapy of variceal bleeding. Best Pract Res Clin Gastroenterol 2008;22:261–78. Available at: http://www.ncbi.nlm.nih.gov/pubmed/18346683. Accessed March 10, 2014.

45. Park WG, Yeh RW, Triadafilopoulos G. Injection therapies for variceal bleeding disorders of the GI tract. Gastrointest Endosc 2008;67:313–23. Available at: http://www.ncbi.nlm.nih.gov/pubmed/18226695. Accessed March 10, 2014.

46. Laine L, el-Newihi HM, Migikovsky B, et al. Endoscopic ligation compared with sclerotherapy for the treatment of bleeding esophageal varices. Ann Intern Med 1993;119:1–7. Available at: http://www.ncbi.nlm.nih.gov/pubmed/8498757. Accessed March 10, 2014.
47. Villanueva C, Piqueras M, Aracil C, et al. A randomized controlled trial comparing ligation and sclerotherapy as emergency endoscopic treatment added to somatostatin in acute variceal bleeding. J Hepatol 2006;45:560–7. Available at: http://www.ncbi.nlm.nih.gov/pubmed/16904224. Accessed July 9, 2014.
48. Lo GH, Lai KH, Cheng JS, et al. Emergency banding ligation versus sclerotherapy for the control of active bleeding from esophageal varices. Hepatology 1997;25:1101–4. Available at: http://www.ncbi.nlm.nih.gov/pubmed/9141424. Accessed March 11, 2014.
49. Dzeletovic I, Baron TH. History of portal hypertension and endoscopic treatment of esophageal varices. Gastrointest Endosc 2012;75:1244–9. Available at: http://www.ncbi.nlm.nih.gov/pubmed/22624813. Accessed July 9, 2014.
50. Stiegmann GV, Goff JS, Michaletz-Onody PA, et al. Endoscopic sclerotherapy as compared with endoscopic ligation for bleeding esophageal varices. N Engl J Med 1992;326:1527–32. Available at: http://www.ncbi.nlm.nih.gov/pubmed/1579136. Accessed July 9, 2014.
51. Lo GH. The role of endoscopy in secondary prophylaxis of esophageal varices. Clin Liver Dis 2010;14:307–23. Available at: http://www.ncbi.nlm.nih.gov/pubmed/20682237. Accessed March 11, 2014.
52. Baron TH, Wong Kee Song LM. Endoscopic variceal band ligation. Am J Gastroenterol 2009;104:1083–5. Available at: http://www.ncbi.nlm.nih.gov/pubmed/19417747. Accessed March 10, 2014.
53. Shaheen NJ, Stuart E, Schmitz SM, et al. Pantoprazole reduces the size of postbanding ulcers after variceal band ligation: a randomized, controlled trial. Hepatology 2005;41:588–94. Available at: http://www.ncbi.nlm.nih.gov/pubmed/15726658. Accessed March 10, 2014.
54. Garcia-Pagán JC, Bosch J. Endoscopic band ligation in the treatment of portal hypertension. Nat Clin Pract Gastroenterol Hepatol 2005;2:526–35. Available at: http://www.ncbi.nlm.nih.gov/pubmed/16355158. Accessed March 10, 2014.
55. Ibrahim M, Lemmers A, Devière J. Novel application of Hemospray to achieve hemostasis in post-variceal banding esophageal ulcers that are actively bleeding. Endoscopy 2014;46(Suppl 1):E263. Available at: http://www.ncbi.nlm.nih.gov/pubmed/24906091. Accessed July 9, 2014.
56. Ibrahim M, El-Mikkawy A, Mostafa I, et al. Endoscopic treatment of acute variceal hemorrhage by using hemostatic powder TC-325: a prospective pilot study. Gastrointest Endosc 2013;78:769–73. Available at: http://www.ncbi.nlm.nih.gov/pubmed/24120338. Accessed March 19, 2014.
57. Holster IL, Poley JW, Kuipers EJ, et al. Controlling gastric variceal bleeding with endoscopically applied hemostatic powder (Hemospray). J Hepatol 2012;57:1397–8. Available at: http://www.ncbi.nlm.nih.gov/pubmed/22864337. Accessed July 9, 2014.
58. Abraldes JG, Bosch J. The treatment of acute variceal bleeding. J Clin Gastroenterol 2007;41(Suppl 3):S312–7. Available at: http://www.ncbi.nlm.nih.gov/pubmed/17975482. Accessed July 9, 2014.
59. Garcia-Tsao G, Sanyal AJ, Grace ND, et al. Prevention and management of gastroesophageal varices and variceal hemorrhage in cirrhosis. Hepatology 2007;46:922–38. Available at: http://www.ncbi.nlm.nih.gov/pubmed/17879356. Accessed January 21, 2014.

60. Avgerinos A, Armonis A. Balloon tamponade technique and efficacy in variceal haemorrhage. Scand J Gastroenterol Suppl 1994;207:11–6. Available at: http://www.ncbi.nlm.nih.gov/pubmed/7701261. Accessed March 11, 2014.

61. Escorsell A, Bosch J. Self-expandable metal stents in the treatment of acute esophageal variceal bleeding. Gastroenterol Res Pract 2011;2011: 910986. Available at: http://www.pubmedcentral.nih.gov/articlerender. fcgi?artid=3195306&tool=pmcentrez&rendertype=abstract. Accessed July 9, 2014.

62. Fierz FC, Kistler W, Stenz V, et al. Treatment of esophageal variceal hemorrhage with self-expanding metal stents as a rescue maneuver in a swiss multicentric cohort. Case Rep Gastroenterol 2013;7:97–105. Available at: http://www. pubmedcentral.nih.gov/articlerender.fcgi?artid=3617972&tool=pmcentrez& rendertype=abstract. Accessed July 9, 2014.

63. Dechêne A, El Fouly AH, Bechmann LP, et al. Acute management of refractory variceal bleeding in liver cirrhosis by self-expanding metal stents. Digestion 2012;85:185–91. Available at: http://www.ncbi.nlm.nih.gov/pubmed/22269340. Accessed July 9, 2014.

64. Mishin I, Ghidirim G, Dolghii A, et al. Implantation of self-expanding metal stent in the treatment of severe bleeding from esophageal ulcer after endoscopic band ligation. Dis Esophagus 2010;23:E35–8. Available at: http://www.ncbi. nlm.nih.gov/pubmed/20731698. Accessed July 9, 2014.

65. Wright G, Lewis H, Hogan B, et al. A self-expanding metal stent for complicated variceal hemorrhage: experience at a single center. Gastrointest Endosc 2010;71: 71–8. Available at: http://www.ncbi.nlm.nih.gov/pubmed/19879564. Accessed March 11, 2014.

66. Hubmann R, Bodlaj G, Czompo M, et al. The use of self-expanding metal stents to treat acute esophageal variceal bleeding. Endoscopy 2006;38:896–901. Available at: http://www.ncbi.nlm.nih.gov/pubmed/16981106. Accessed March 10, 2014.

67. Zehetner J, Shamiyeh A, Wayand W, et al. Results of a new method to stop acute bleeding from esophageal varices: implantation of a self-expanding stent. Surg Endosc 2008;22:2149–52. Available at: http://www.ncbi.nlm.nih.gov/pubmed/ 18622540. Accessed July 9, 2014.

68. Holster IL, Kuipers EJ, van Buuren HR, et al. Self-expandable metal stents as definitive treatment for esophageal variceal bleeding. Endoscopy 2013;45: 485–8. Available at: http://www.ncbi.nlm.nih.gov/pubmed/23468191. Accessed July 9, 2014.

69. Zakaria MS, Hamza IM, Mohey MA, et al. The first Egyptian experience using new self-expandable metal stents in acute esophageal variceal bleeding: pilot study. Saudi J Gastroenterol 2013;19:177–81. Available at: http://www. pubmedcentral.nih.gov/articlerender.fcgi?artid=3745660&tool=pmcentrez& rendertype=abstract. Accessed July 9, 2014.

70. Escorsell A, Cardenas A, Pavel O, et al. Self-expandable esophageal metal stent vs balloon tamponade in esophageal variceal bleeding refractory to medical and endoscopic treatment: a multicenter randomized controlled trial. Hepatology 2013;1386A–7A.

Endoscopic Treatment of Gastric Varices

Shiv K. Sarin, MD, DM, FNA, DSc*, Awinash Kumar, MD

KEYWORDS

- Portal hypertension • Gastric variceal sclerotherapy • Gastric variceal obturation
- Gastric variceal band ligation • Thrombin injection • Combined endoscopic therapy
- EUS-guided therapy

KEY POINTS

- Gastric variceal (GV) bleeding is the cause of upper gastrointestinal bleeding in 1 of 5 patients with portal hypertension and variceal bleeding.
- GV bleeding is associated with high morbidity and mortality and hence early detection and control of bleeding is important. An algorithmic approach to the management of GV bleeding is desirable.
- Endoscopic GV obturation by glue is the method of choice. Most often a single injection is effective but sometimes repeat sessions every 4 weeks may be needed for complete obturation of varices.

INTRODUCTION

Gastroesophageal varices are present in approximately 50% of patients with cirrhosis. Their presence correlates with severity of liver disease; although only 40% of patients who are Child A have varices, they are present in 85% of patients who are Child C.[1,2] Gastric varices are present in approximately 20% of patients with portal hypertension (PHT) either in isolation or in combination with esophageal varices (EVs).

Variceal hemorrhage occurs at yearly rate of 5% to 15%, and about 20% of cirrhotic patients with acute variceal bleeding die within 6 weeks.[3–5] Although variceal bleeding ceases spontaneously in 40% to 50% of patients, the incidence of early rebleeding ranges between 30% and 40% within the first 6 weeks, and about 40% of all rebleeding episodes occur in within the first 5 days.[4,6] Gastric varices bleed less frequently than EV and are the bleeding source in approximately 10% to 30% of patients with variceal hemorrhage.[7] However, gastric variceal (GV) bleeding tends to be more

Financial support: Nil.
The authors have nothing to disclose.
Department of Hepatology, Institute of Liver and Biliary Sciences, D1, Vasant Kunj, New Delhi 110010, India
* Corresponding author.
E-mail address: shivsarin@gmail.com

severe with higher mortality. In addition, a high proportion of patients, from 35% to 90%, rebleed after spontaneous hemostasis.

New endoscopic treatment options and interventional radiological procedures have broadened the therapeutic armamentarium for GV. This article provides background information on the classification and pathophysiology of formation of GV to help readers understand the management strategies primarily related to endoscopic approaches.

CLASSIFICATION OF GASTRIC VARICES

The most widely accepted and used classification system is the Sarin classification (**Fig. 1**).[7] This system has been recommended for use by the Asian Pacific Association for the Study of the Liver (APASL), American association for the study of liver diseases (AASLD), Baveno guidelines and by the expert panel because it is easy to use, has good correlation with pathophysiology, and guides therapy. It classifies GVs by their location in the stomach and their relationship with EVs. It also helps to propose treatment strategies.

Primary and Secondary GV

GVs may be considered primary or secondary. Primary GVs are present at initial examination or are seen in patients who have never had EV endoscopic variceal sclerotherapy (EVS) or endoscopic variceal band ligation (EVL). Secondary GVs are those that develop after endoscopic therapy (either EVS or EVL) for EV.

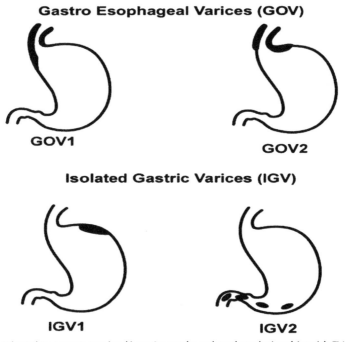

Fig. 1. Gastric varices are categorized into 4 types based on the relationship with EV, as well as by their location in the stomach: gastroesophageal varix (GOV) type 1, GOV type 2, isolated gastric varix (IGV) type 1, and IGV type 2. GOV type 1 is the most common type, accounting for 74% of all gastric varices. However, the incidence of bleeding is highest with IGV type 1 followed by GOV type 2.

HEMODYNAMIC FEATURES AND RELEVANT VASCULAR ANATOMY

Normal portal venous drainage of the stomach and lower esophagus and the pathologic drainage in PHT are shown in (**Figs. 2** and **3**). In PHT, there is a general enlargement of the veins draining the digestive tract.[8-11]

In the upper gastrointestinal (UGI) tract, the increased portal pressure is transmitted through 2 main venous pathways. First, through the right and left gastric veins, which drain varices around the distal esophagus and cardia (EV and gastroesophageal varix [GOV] 1)[12,13] into the portal vein, or when flow is reversed the blood flows cephalad into the azygous system. The second pathway is via the short and posterior gastric veins, which under normal circumstances drain blood from the fundus into the splenic vein, but in PHT the flow often is reversed and blood drains from the spleen toward the stomach into fundal varices (GOV2 and isolated gastric varix [IGV] 1).[12] IGV2 is caused by dilatation of branches of the gastroepiploic veins.

Spontaneous portosystemic splenorenal or gastrorenal shunts commonly develop between the splenic vein (splenorenal shunt) or gastric varices, respectively, and connect via the inferior phrenic or suprarenal vein to the left renal vein[12] Such shunts, collectively termed gastrorenal shunts (GRSs), are more common in GV (60%–85% of cases)[12,14] than in EV (17%–21% of cases).[12] Precisely what determines the predominant collateral pathways that develop in a given individual with PHT remains unknown; however, the size and length of the potential collateral vessel are likely to play a role.[12,15] Watanabe and colleagues[12] found that 78% of patients with PHT had predominant collateral flow though the left or right gastric vein, which correlated with the presence of EV or GOV1, whereas a minority of patients had predominant collateral flow through the short and posterior gastric veins, correlating with the presence of GV. These frequencies of flow patterns are in good agreement with the observed frequencies of EV and GV. Another study described blood flow patterns in patients with PHT based on the direction of flow in the left gastric vein and the presence or absence of a spontaneous GRS.[14]

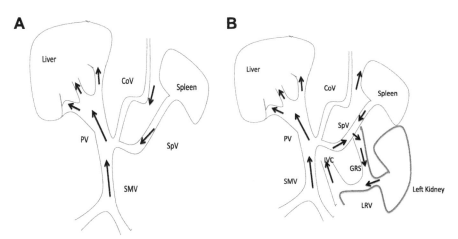

Fig. 2. (*A*) Normal portal venous blood flow. (*B*) Portal venous blood flow in the presence of portal hypertension and GRS. There is reversal of flow in the coronary vein (CoV) resulting in EV, and reversal of flow in the splenic vein resulting in gastric varices, which decompress via the GRS. GRS, gastrorenal shunt; IVC, inferior vena cava; LRV, left renal vein; PV, portal vein; SMV, superior mesenteric vein; SpV, splenic vein.

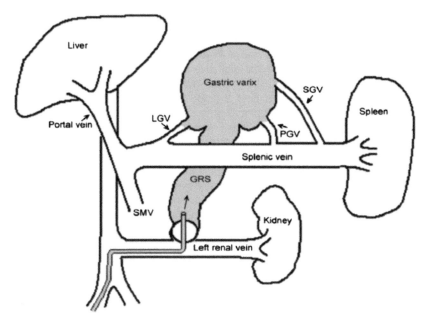

Fig. 3. Balloon-occluded retrograde transvenous obliteration (BRTO) of gastric varices. The balloon catheter was introduced by the femoral approach. Then the catheter was inserted into the GRS through the left renal vein. The balloon was inflated in place for 30 minutes to occlude the shunt. Then 5% ethanolamine oleate was injected into the gastric varices for obliteration. LGV, left gastric vein; PGV, posterior gastric vein; SGV, short gastric vein.

Segmental/Sinistral PHT

Segmental PHT resulting from splenic vein occlusion through thrombosis or, less commonly, stenosis,[16,17] often as a sequela of pancreatic disorder,[18] leads to the formation of IGV (IGV1 > IGV2). In segmental PHT, blood flows retrogradely through the short and posterior gastric veins and the gastroepiploic veins, resulting in the formation of GVs and ectopic varices. From the GV, blood flows hepatopetally through the left and right gastric veins to the portal vein.

MANAGEMENT
Primary Prophylaxis

Although primary prophylaxis has been studied and well established in managing EV, no guidelines are available for gastric varices. The hemodynamics of gastric varices differ from those of EV in that large gastric varices may develop at lower portal pressures because of the presence of gastrosystemic shunts. Because GV bleeding is more severe, being associated with high mortality, primary prophylaxis should be considered for high-risk varices and patients at high risk for bleeding (suggested to be those with an annual risk of $\geq$16%).[19] The therapeutic options include β-blockers and/or cyanoacrylate glue. Data on primary prophylaxis for GV are few and a recent randomized controlled trial (RCT) by Mishra and colleagues[20] showed that, in 30 patients receiving endoscopic tissue adhesive as primary prophylaxis, none had bled or died in 1 year of follow-up. The overall bleeding and mortality were 10% and 7%, respectively while on primary prophylaxis. Also, survival was significantly better in the cyanoacrylate group compared with the no-treatment group

(7% vs 26%; *P* =.048) and cyanoacrylate injection significantly reduced the GV bleeding rate compared with the β-blocker therapy without any significant survival benefit (mortality, 7% vs 17%; *P* = .393).

Risk Factors for GV Hemorrhage

1. Location of gastric varices (IGV1 > GOV2 > GOV1)[12,20]
2. Size of fundal varices (large > medium > small)
3. Severity of liver failure (Child class C > B > A) or MELD (Model for End-Stage Liver Disease) greater than or equal to 17
4. Presence of red color signs on GV
5. Concomitant hepatocellular carcinoma
6. Presence of portal hypertensive gastropathy

Patients with high-risk gastric varices should therefore be considered for primary prophylaxis. Cyanoacrylate injection should be the first line of treatment for primary prophylaxis of high-risk GV. Whether combined treatment with cyanoacrylate injection and β-blockers rather than either treatment given alone has any added advantages needs to be studied.

Management of Acute GV Bleeding

1. Medical management/general measures
2. Endoscopic therapies

Medical Management

According to the APASL guidelines on the management of acute variceal bleeding[21] and the Baveno consensus,[22] patients with suspected acute variceal hemorrhage and hemodynamic instability should be admitted to an intensive care unit setting. Blood volume resuscitation should be undertaken promptly but with caution, with a target hemoglobin of approximately 8 g/dL.[22] This recommendation is based on studies showing that restitution of all lost blood leads to increases in portal pressure to higher than baseline, with increased rebleeding and mortality.[22,23] Owing to the risk of aspiration of blood, tracheal intubation may be required before endoscopy. Coagulopathy and thrombocytopenia should be corrected. There is an increased risk of developing severe bacterial infections (both spontaneous bacterial peritonitis and other infections), which are associated with early rebleeding and a greater mortality.[24,25] The use of short-term prophylactic antibiotics (eg, norfloxacin 400 mg orally twice daily for 7 days) in patients with cirrhosis and gastrointestinal hemorrhage with or without ascites has been shown not only to decrease the rate of bacterial infections but also to increase survival.[26,27] Recent data suggest that the epidemiology of bacterial infections in cirrhotic patients with gastrointestinal bleeding is evolving.[28,29] Increasing quinolone resistance and more frequent gram-positive bacterial infections suggests that the third-generation cephalosporins (eg, intravenous ceftriaxone) may be most effective in this situation.

Vasoactive drugs

At present in the literature the evidence for the use of vasoactive drugs for acute GV bleed is limited. The efficacy of these drugs in controlling acute esophageal variceal bleed favors their use in the setting of acute GV bleed. RCTs comparing different pharmacologic agents (vasopressin, somatostatin, terlipressin, and octreotide) show no differences regarding control of hemorrhage and early rebleeding, and vasopressin is associated with a high incidence of adverse events.[30] The clinical efficacy of terlipressin versus placebo has been assessed in 7 RCTs, and a meta-analysis showed that terlipressin significantly reduced the incidence of failure to control bleed and mortality.[10] Terlipressin is the only pharmacologic agent that has been shown to reduce mortality (about 34% reduction). The vasoactive drugs are to be continued for 2 to 5 days.

Balloon Tamponade

Balloon tamponade has a role as a bridge to definitive therapy in certain situations. It is indicated in cases of massive bleed until the endoscopy is done or after endotherapy in cases of failure to control bleed until the salvage transjugular intrahepatic portosystemic shunt (TIPS)/balloon-occluded retrograde transvenous obliteration (BRTO) can be performed. Hemostasis can approach 80%, but with high rebleeding rates if used as the sole therapy. Owing to the larger gastric balloon in the Linton-Nachlas tube (600 mL), it is more desirable for GV bleeding than the Sengstaken-Blakemore tube (SBT).[31] Careful placement is essential, especially in sedated patients to reduce the risk of esophageal perforation from inflating the gastric balloon in the esophagus.

Although the use and practice of SBT has substantially decreased in the West, the utility of this simple device needs to be reemphasized. If placed properly, it provides an instant compression and control of esophageal variceal bleed, including bleeds from GOV1 and GOV2. Bleeds from GOV1 and GOV2 comprise nearly 90% of all GV bleeds and hence the relevance of SBT remains.

Endoscopic Therapies

Endoscopic therapy has now established itself as the initial and often the definitive treatment of GV bleeding.

Endoscopic treatment modalities for GV bleed are as follows:

1. GV sclerotherapy (GVS)
2. GV obturation (GVO) with glue
3. GV band ligation (GVL) with or without detachable snares
4. Thrombin injection (bovine or human)
5. Combined endoscopic therapy
6. Endoscopic ultrasonography (EUS)–guided therapy

GV Sclerotherapy

Endoscopic sclerotherapy has been effective in the treatment of EV bleeding and in eradication of EV,[32,33] but it has been less successful in the management of GV, probably because of the high volume of blood flow through GV compared with EV, resulting in rapid flushing away of the sclerosant in the bloodstream. GVS typically requires larger volumes of sclerosant than for EV[7,15] and fundal varices (GOV2 and IGV1) require significantly more sclerosant than GOV1.[10] This result may be associated with more side effects after GVS, such as fever, retrosternal and abdominal pain, and large ulcerations.[10] Perforations and mediastinitis are complications that are more serious, and the latter results in mortality in excess of 50%.

In acute GV bleeding, GVS has been reported to control bleeding in 60% to 100% of cases[10,34,35] but with unacceptably high rebleeding rates of up to 90%. Mucosal ulcers are also commonly seen, and cause rebleeding.[36] Approximately 50% of rebleeding is caused by sclerotherapy-induced ulcers and is difficult to control, with a success rate between 9% and 44%. GVS seems to be least successful in controlling acute fundal variceal bleeding.[34,37]

GVS is an effective and appropriate treatment of acute GOV1 hemorrhage and for attempting secondary prophylactic GOV1 obliteration. It is not appropriate for patients with fundal varices (GOV2 or IGV1) because of the low rate of primary hemostasis, the low success rate for secondary variceal eradication, and the high rate of rebleeding and complications.

GV Obturation

Obturation or obliteration is the term used for GVs treated by glue rather than eradication, because the varix can be visible even when it has been effectively treated. Endoscopic GV obliteration (GVO) is done by using tissue adhesives like N-butyl-2-cyanoacrylate and 2-octyl-cyanoacrylate, with the former being used more commonly. The door-to-needle time should preferably be less than 6 hours and no more than 12 hours.[21] N-butyl-2-cyanoacrylate is a monomer that rapidly undergoes exothermic polymerization on contact with the hydroxyl ions present in water. Before the glue injection it is worthwhile to pay attention to several key points (**Box 1**).

A disposable steel-hubbed sclerotherapy injection needle, 21-gauge and 6 to 8 mm long, is selected. After puncturing the varix lumen with the needle, cyanoacrylate is injected in 1-mL to 2-mL aliquots by using distilled water (about 1–2 mL, equal to the dead space) to flush the glue into the varix. As the needle is withdrawn from the varix, a steady stream of flush solution is aimed at the puncture site. Additional glue is injected until the varix is hard to palpation. When injected intravascularly, cyanoacrylate glue solidifies, producing a cast of the vessel. Subtotal occlusion is immediate, and total occlusion occurs later. After injection into a gastric varix, the overlying mucosa sloughs off and the cast of glue begins extruding into the gastric lumen after about a month, with complete extrusion by 3 months.[38] Initial hemostasis rates of more than 90% can be achieved.

Complications are well known but rare: thromboembolic phenomena (splenic, renal, pulmonary, cerebral, spinal, and coronary), the needle being stuck in the varix, gastric ulceration, retrogastric abscess, visceral fistula formation, bacteremia/sepsis, and (rarely) death. Embolic and thrombotic phenomena were associated with larger volumes of glue injection and it is recommended not to exceed 2 mL per session.[39] However, a larger volume could be injected (2 mL/column) if more than 1 column is to be injected. Repeat sessions are to be performed after about 4 weeks, until endoscopic obliteration is achieved. The GV obturation is assessed by blunt palpation using the hub of the same injector with the needle kept in. EUS is useful to identify the residual flow.[39] Rebleeding rates after cyanoacrylate injection vary from 7% to 65%, with most of the larger series reporting rates less than 15%, which are often seen in patients with associated portal vein thrombosis.

Box 1
GV glue: tricks and checks

- Glue (diluted with lipiodol or undiluted) 2-mL syringe
- DW, injectors 21 or 23 gauge (at least 2)
- Acetone, scissors, SBT, goggles for eye protection
- Continuous air insufflation during injection
- No suction during and for 20 seconds after injection
- Flush volume limited to the dead space volume of the injection catheter
- 2 mL per injection, and prompt removal of needle from the varix after injection

Abbreviation: DW, Dextrose water.

Oho and colleagues[40] performed a nonrandomized prospective study of 53 patients with acute GV bleeding. Glue achieved significantly better hemostasis (93% vs 67%). In a retrospective study, Ogawa and colleagues[41] found significantly better hemostasis with glue. In a randomized controlled trial by Sarin and colleagues[36] there was a trend toward better hemostasis (89% vs 62%) with glue compared with alcohol (n = 37).

Several recent long-term studies also reported hemostasis rates of 90% and low rebleeding rates of 15% to 30% with cyanoacrylate injection, with 1 to 3 injections needed to achieve obliteration, with higher eradication rates for GOV1 and GOV2 than for IGV1.[42–51] Even in young infants, the use of cyanoacrylate glue is safe and effective for the treatment of GV bleed.[52] At present, it is clear that GVO using tissue adhesives has high efficacy and safety for the control of acute GV bleed and for the prevention of GV rebleeding, and is the treatment of choice.[53] Complications with glue therapy are generally minor, but are occasionally serious and even life threatening (**Table 1**).

GV Band Ligation

Endoscopic variceal ligation is the gold standard endotherapy for EV but is less effective for gastric varices because of – (1) thick overlying mucosa, which makes suction difficult during band ligation; (2) larger sizes of varices, which are difficult to get into the suction hood of the EVL channel; (3) development of post-EVL ulcer bleed, which may be fatal, like the index bleed caused by underlying hemodynamic alteration; and (4) the overall higher rate of rebleed and reappearance of varices (lesser degree of deep fibrosis of the varices).[54]

EVL with nylon or stainless steel snares or standard rubber bands has been used. GV smaller than 2 cm in diameter can be ligated with standard rubber bands, whereas larger-diameter GV require the use of larger detachable snares.[55] Only 1 RCT, by Lo and colleagues,[56] compared the use of EVL using rubber bands with Endoscopic variceal obliteration (EVO) and showed that EVL was less effective than EVO in controlling acute GV bleeding (45% vs 87%) and had a higher rebleeding rate (54% vs 31%); the abilities to eradicate the varices were comparable (45% vs 51%). GV were eradicated successfully in almost all patients initially, but all patients subsequently developed recurrent GV within 2 years and needed EVO or EVS owing to difficulties in snaring the varices in a fibrosed mucosa.

Table 1
Complications reported with glue injection for gastric varices

Author, Study	No. of Cases	Pulmonary Embolism	SMV Thrombosis	Others
Belletrutti,[88] 2008	29	—	1	—
Hwang et al,[89] 2001	140	6	—	—
Gin-Ho-Lo et al,[90] 2001	31	—	—	CVA
Joo et al,[47] 2007	85	2	—	Splenic infarct, 1
Upadhyay et al,[91] 2005	1	—	—	Acute MI
Rickman,[92] 2004	1	1	—	—
Liu-fang Cheng et al,[93] 2010	753	1	—	Splenic vein thrombosis, 3; CVA, 1
Gin-Ho-Lo et al,[94] 2013	118	—	—	CVA, 1

Abbreviations: CVA, cerebrovascular accident; MI, myocardial infarction; SMV, superior mesenteric vein.

Thrombin

Thrombin is commercially available as a sterile, lyophilized powder. Thrombin principally affects hemostasis by converting fibrinogen to a fibrin clot. A 5-mL solution of thrombin containing 1000 units/mL of thrombin clots a liter of blood in less than 60 seconds. In a patient with bleeding GV, thrombin is reconstituted and a 1-mL aliquot is injected into the bleeding varix. The average dose of injected thrombin is between 1500 U and 2000 U. Ramesh and colleagues[57] showed that endoscopic treatment of bovine thrombin is effective in 92% of patients with bleeding GVs, without any rebleeding in a follow-up period of almost 2 years.

Daly[58] first reported the use of thrombin to treat gastric varices in 1947. A total of 8 uncontrolled studies to date have used thrombin or fibrin for the treatment of gastric varices, involving more than 200 patients in total.[59–62] Bovine thrombin was originally used, but because of concerns about prion transmission, it has been replaced by human thrombin. Initial hemostasis rates exceed 90% in most studies. Rebleeding rates vary from 0% to 50%. Studies showing use of thrombin in the treatment of gastric varices are shown in **Table 2**.

Complications have been reported infrequently, with anecdotal reports of nonfatal anaphylactic reactions related to bovine thrombin. With human thrombin, there remains a concern for unknown transmissible viruses, given that a vial of thrombin exposes a patient to roughly 4000 to 5000 plasma donations.[63] Another limitation of

Table 2 Use of thrombin in the treatment of gastric varices						
First Author, Year	No. of Patients	GV Type	Primary Hemostasis (%)	Rebleed (%)	Mortality (%)	Follow-up (mo)
Williams et al,[61] 1994	11 Cirrhosis, n = 10 PVT, n = 1	Cardia, n = 2 Fundus, n = 9	100	27	0	9
Przemioslo et al,[62] 1999	52 Cirrhosis, n = 49 Cirrhosis, with PVT, 3	GOV1, n = 31 GOV2, n = 21	94	16	8	15
Yang et al,[63] 2002	12 Cirrhosis, n = 9 PVT, n = 1 Hepatic metastasis, n = 1	GOV1, n = 1 GOV2, n = 10 Not reported, n = 1	100	25	17	17
Heneghan et al,[95] 2002	10 Cirrhosis, n = 10	GOV1, n = 4 GOV2, n = 6	70	50	50	8
Datta et al,[96] 2003	15 Cirrhosis, n = 12 PVT, n = 3	GOV1, n = 11 GOV2, n = 2 IGV1, n = 2	93	28	7	1
Ramesh,[57] 2008	13 Cirrhosis, n = 13	GOV, n = 12 IGV, n = 1	93	0	Not reported	22
Smith,[97] 2012	23 Cirrhosis, n = 17 Cirrhosis with PVT, n = 4	GOV2, n = 1 IGV1, n = 19 IGV2, n = 3	86	39	26	15

thrombin is its significantly higher cost compared with cyanoacrylate. One of the advantages of thrombin is the lack of mucosal damage and ulceration at the injection site, thus theoretically reducing the risk of rebleeding. Therefore, thrombin, although costly, is a promising therapy for the treatment of GV, given its ease of use, high efficacy, and excellent safety profile. Controlled studies comparing it with other modalities (especially cyanoacrylate) would be helpful before universally recommending it.

Combined Endoscopic Therapy

Combined endoscopic methods in the setting of acute GV bleed have been studied for the control of bleeding and to prevent rebleeding. Chun and Hyun[64] showed that endoscopic variceal ligation-injection sclerotherapy is safe and effective in achieving hemostasis and obliteration in all patients. Combination of variceal ligation and cyano-acrylate injection in GV effectively controlled acute bleed in 89% of patients; however, 33% rebled on follow-up.[65] Various studies have used different combination therapies for management of gastric varices (**Table 3**). Combination with sclerotherapy is unlikely to be accepted for the management of acute GV bleeding in view of the increased risk of iatrogenic complications and the need for greater technical skill and procedure time. Combination therapy is therefore not recommended for the control of acute GV bleed or prevention of rebleed.

EUS-guided Treatment

Along with color Doppler, EUS has been shown to be more sensitive than conventional endoscopy for detecting gastric varices. Iwase and colleagues[66,67] showed that linear Doppler EUS easily detect the persistence of blood flow in gastric varices after cyano-acrylate therapy and suggest the higher risk for recurrent bleeding. Lee and colleagues[39] compared patients with acute GV bleed receiving on-demand cyanoac-rylate injection for recurrent bleeding (n = 47) in one group with another group (n = 54) receiving scheduled biweekly EUS-guided glue injection until obliteration of all resid-ual varices. Repeated sessions on a scheduled basis significantly reduced the risk of late rebleeding compared with the on-demand approach (19% vs 45%). In a pro-spective case series[68] of 5 patients with bleeding gastric varices, EUS-guided injection of cyanoacrylate directed at the perforating veins achieved hemostasis in all patients, with no cases of recurrent bleeding over a 10-month follow-up. Variceal eradication was successful in 2 patients after 1 session and in 3 patients after 2 sessions (mean, 1.6).

Table 3
Randomized controlled studies of endoscopic treatment of gastric varices

First Author, Year	Classification (GOV1/GOV2/IGV1)	Treatment Modality	Hemostasis Rate (%)	Rebleeding Rate (%)	Follow-up
Sarin et al,[36] 2002	0/8/28	GVS (n = 17) GVO (n = 20))	62	33	15.4 mo
Tan et al,[98] 2006	53/25/19	GVL (n = 48) GVO (n = 49)	93 93	44 22	610 d 680 d
Lo et al,[99] 2007	36/33/0	TIPS (n = 35) GVO (n = 37)	93	11 38	32 mo
Mishra et al,[83] 2010	0/all GOV2 or IGV1	GVO (n = 33) β-Blocker (n = 34)	ND	15 55	26 mo

Abbreviation: ND, not disclosed.

In a novel approach, transesophageal EUS-guided coil embolization and cyanoacrylate injection[69] of GOV2 and IGV1 varices was shown to reduce the amount of glue needed and the number of sessions needed for complete GVO with control of acute bleeding in all cases. Among 24 patients with a mean follow-up of 193 days (range, 24–589 days), these difficult-to-treat GVs were obliterated after a single treatment session in 23 (96%) patients. There were no procedure-related complications and no symptoms or signs of cyanoacrylate glue embolization.

EUS can therefore be an important tool and its use is expanding in the management of GVs. It easily (1) localizes GV; (2) differentiates GV from other bleeding mucosal lesions; (3) detects perforating veins; (4) can guide the injection of sclerosants, glue, or thrombin both in amount as well as the site when adequate visualization is not possible with conventional endoscopy because of active ongoing bleed; and (5) can detect residual varices, perforators, and collaterals during follow-up to guide further sessions of endotherapy and may decrease the risk of rebleeding.

RADIOLOGIC INTERVENTIONS
Transjugular Intrahepatic Portosystemic Shunts

When patients with GV bleeding are unresponsive to initial endoscopic treatment, a second endoscopic therapy should be attempted if possible.[69] If a second attempt fails or the severity of bleeding precludes further endoscopic therapy, salvage therapy using surgical shunts or TIPSs should be considered for refractory GV bleeding. Most current studies of TIPS focus on treatment of refractory GV bleeding and prevention of GV rebleeding. A recent study showed that a primary hemostasis rate of 92.3% could be achieved with TIPS for acute GV bleeding.[70] Other studies have also shown initial hemostasis rates of 87% and 100% with the use of TIPS for acute refractory GV bleeding,[71–75] with an approximate rebleeding rate of 10% to 30%.[71–76]

Frequent complications of TIPS are encephalopathy and shunt stenosis/occlusion, with post-TIPS encephalopathy occurring in 4% to 16% of patients.[74–76] The shunt dysfunction can be reduced by using polytetrafluoroethylene (PTFE)-covered stent. Considering the currently available evidence, TIPS with PTFE-covered stent is the treatment of choice for patients who fail first-line medical and endoscopic therapy for management of GV bleeding.

BRTO

Kanagawa and colleagues[77] first introduced the BRTO procedure in 1996. GVs are associated with GRS in 60% to 85% of cases.[12,14] The GRS drains blood flow into systemic circulation and provides a pathway for radiologists to treat GV. The outflow of GRS was blocked by inflating the balloon, and 5% ethanolamine oleate iopamidol was injected in a retrograde manner.

The BRTO was used as either primary or secondary prophylaxis of GV in most series. Initial hemostasis of BRTO for acute GV bleeding ranges between 76.9% and 100%.[70,78,79] The rebleeding rate was from 0% to 15.4%.[70,78,79] BRTO had a similar initial hemostasis and lower rebleeding rate compared with GVO or band ligation for acute GV bleeding.[78,79] The BRTO had been shown to be as effective as TIPS for acute GV bleeding, without increasing hepatic encephalopathy.[70] Portal pressure has been shown to increase after BRTO, which can cause worsening of the size of EV.[14,80,81] Other common complications of BRTO are hemoglobinuria, abdominal pain, pyrexia, and pleural effusion, and occasionally hemodynamic shock and atrial fibrillation.

SECONDARY PROPHYLAXIS
Medical Therapies

There is little evidence for the use of drugs for secondary prevention of GV bleeding. Only a few studies have shown the efficacy of drug therapy for the prevention of GV rebleeding after successful endoscopic variceal obturation.[54,82] In a recent RCT by Mishra and colleagues,[83] the probability of GV rebleeding in the cyanoacrylate group was significantly lower than in the β-blocker group (15% vs 55%; $P = .004$) and the mortality was also lower (3% vs 25%; $P = .026$) during a median follow-up of 26 months. The median baseline and follow-up Hepatic Venous Pressure Gradient (HVPG) in the cyanoacrylate group were 15 (10–23) and 17 (11–24) mm Hg ($P = .001$) and in the β-blocker group were 14 (11–24) and 13 (8–25) mm Hg respectively ($P = .003$).

Thus, drug therapy with β-blockers should be continued (1) if it is well tolerated, (2) in the presence of concomitant EV, or (3) with a documented HVPG greater than 12 mm Hg as an adjunct to endoscopic therapy.

Endoscopic Therapies

After the index bleeding, the secondary prophylaxis of GV bleeding is better managed with endotherapy than drug therapy and the use of tissue adhesive is the modality of choice. New approaches to glue injection are continuously being tested.[84–86] Repeated tissue adhesive injection until obliteration of GV with or without β-blockers is the ideal approach for secondary prophylaxis of GV bleeding. In resource-constrained settings, because of nonavailability of facilities for glue injection or lack of expertise for endotherapy, GV sclerotherapy or band ligation may be considered because of the high risk of rebleeding.

Interventional Radiologic Approach

Interventional radiological techniques are routinely used for secondary prophylaxis of GV bleeding. The options include TIPS, BRTO, Balloon Occluded endoscopic injection sclerotherapy (BO-EIS). All these modalities achieve good control of acute bleeding as well as minimal rebleeding. The preferences include (1) to consider TIPS in cases with HVPG greater than 12; (2) BRTO for cases with low portal pressure (HVPG<12 mm Hg), presence of portal vein thrombosis, or large gastrorenal shunt; and (3) BO-EIS when it is difficult to perform the BRTO.[78,79,87]

Partial Splenic Embolization

Splenectomy or partial splenic embolization (PSE) has been considered as a modality for GV bleed per se or before BRTO to prevent rapid progression of EV. The procedure involves superselective catheterization and embolization of the intra-splenic arterial branches, usually with polyvinyl alcohol particles. PSE leads to reduction of portal venous pressures, reduction in splenic size with improvement of the hypersplenism-induced thrombocytopenia, enhanced hepatic function, and reduced encephalopathy.[87] From a standpoint of secondary prophylaxis against GV rebleeding, patients have been followed in 4 case series showing an 80% reduction in bleeding rates with follow-up times ranging from 3 to 50 months. Postembolization syndrome is almost universal with abdominal pain, fever, nausea, and anorexia.

Overall, the literature is limited in quality, but given the potential benefits of PSE further investigation is warranted to allow evidence-based evaluation of its use in the treatment of GV.

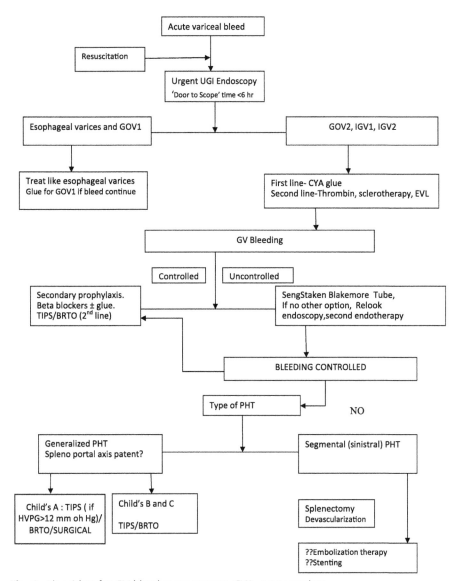

Fig. 4. Algorithm for GV bleed management. CYA, cyanoacrylate.

SUMMARY

GV bleeding is the cause of UGI bleed in 1 of 5 patients with portal hypertension and variceal bleeding. GV bleeding is associated with high morbidity and mortality and hence early detection and control of bleeding is important. An algorithmic approach to the management of GV bleeding is desirable (**Fig. 4**). The patient should be started with vasoactive drugs as soon as possible (door-to-needle time within 30 minutes) and early endoscopy after initial hemodynamic stabilization (door to scope time <6 hours) is recommended.[21] Endoscopic GV obturation by glue is the method of choice. Most often a single injection is effective but sometimes repeat sessions every 4 weeks may be needed for complete obturation of varices. Interventional radiological techniques such as TIPS or BRTO are effective rescue techniques. Secondary prophylaxis with β-blockers and endotherapy is ideal.

REFERENCES

1. Navasa M, Parés A, Bruguera M, et al. Portal hypertension in primary biliary cirrhosis. Relationship with histological features. J Hepatol 1987;5:292–8.
2. Sanyal AJ, Fontana RJ, Di Bisceglie AM, et al. The prevalence and risk factors associated with esophageal varices in subjects with hepatitis C and advanced fibrosis. Gastrointest Endosc 2006;64:855–64.
3. Carbonell N, Pauwels A, Serfaty L, et al. Improved survival after variceal bleeding in patients with cirrhosis over the past two decades. Hepatology 2004;40:652–9.
4. D'Amico G, De Franchis R, Cooperative Study Group. Upper digestive bleeding in cirrhosis. Post-therapeutic outcome and prognostic indicators. Hepatology 2003;38:599–612.
5. El-Serag HB, Everhart JE. Improved survival after variceal hemorrhage over an 11-year period in the Department of Veterans Affairs. Am J Gastroenterol 2000; 95:3566–73.
6. Graham DY, Smith JL. The course of patients after variceal hemorrhage. Gastro-enterology 1981;80:800–9.
7. Sarin SK, Lahoti D, Saxena SP, et al. Prevalence, classification and natural history of gastric varices: a long-term follow-up study in 568 portal hypertension patients. Hepatology 1992;16:1343–9.
8. Okuda K, Suzuki K, Musha H, et al. Percutaneous transhepatic catheterization of the portal vein for the study of portal hemodynamics and shunts: a preliminary report. Gastroenterology 1977;73:279–84.
9. Lunderquist A, Vang J. Transhepatic catheterization and obliteration of the coronary vein in patients with portal hypertension and esophageal varices. N Engl J Med 1974;291:646–9.
10. Vianna A, Hayes PC, Moscoso G, et al. Normal venous circulation of the gastro-esophageal junction: a route to understanding varices. Gastroenterology 1987; 93:876–89.
11. Anderson CA. GI magnetic resonance angiography. Gastrointest Endosc 2002; 55:S42–8.
12. Watanabe K, Kimura K, Matsutani S, et al. Portal hemodynamics in patients with gastric varices. A study in 230 patients with esophageal and/or gastric varices using portal vein catheterization. Gastroenterology 1988;95:434–40.
13. Hashizume M, Kitano S, Sugimachi K, et al. Three-dimensional view of the vascular structure of the lower oesophagus in clinical portal hypertension. Hepatology 1988;8:1482–7.
14. Matsumoto A, Hamamoto N, Nomura T, et al. Balloon-occluded retrograde transvenous obliteration of high-risk gastric fundal varices. Am J Gastroenterol 1999;94:643–9.
15. Sarin SK, Lahoti D. Management of gastric varices. Baillieres Clin Gastroenterol 1992;6:527–48.
16. Madsen MS, Petersen TH, Sommer H. Segmental portal hypertension. Ann Surg 1986;204:72–7.
17. Evan GR, Yellin AE, Weaver FA, et al. Sinistral (left-sided) portal hypertension. Am Surg 1990;56:758–63.

18. Little AG, Moosa AR. Gastrointestinal hemorrhage from left sided portal hypertension: an unappraised complication of pancreatitis. Am J Surg 1981;141:153–8.
19. Matsumoto A, Matsumoto H, Hamamoto N, et al. Management of gastric fundal varices associated with a gastrorenal shunt. Gut 2001;48:440–1.
20. Mishra SR, Sharma BC, Kumar A, et al. Primary prophylaxis of gastric variceal bleeding comparing cyanoacrylate injection and beta-blockers: a randomized controlled trial. J Hepatol 2011;54:1161–7.
21. Sarin SK, Kumar A, Angus PA, et al. For Asian Pacific Association for the Study of the Liver (APASL) Working Party on Portal Hypertension. Diagnosis and management of acute variceal bleeding: Asian Pacific Association for Study of the Liver recommendations. Hepatol Int 2011;5:607–24.
22. de Franchis R. Evolving consensus in portal hypertension report of the Baveno IV consensus workshop on methodology of diagnosis and therapy in portal hypertension. J Hepatol 2005;43:167–76.
23. Castaneda B, Morales J, Lionetti R, et al. Effects of blood volume restitution following a portal hypertensive-related bleeding in anesthetized cirrhotic rats. Hepatology 2001;33:821–5.
24. Bernard B, Cadranel JF, Valla D, et al. Prognostic significance of bacterial infection in bleeding cirrhotic patients: a prospective study. Gastroenterology 1995;108:1828–34.
25. Goulis J, Armonis A, Patch D, et al. Bacterial infection is independently associated with failure to control bleeding in cirrhotic patients with gastrointestinal hemorrhage. Hepatology 1998;27:1207–12.
26. Bernard B, Grange JD, Khac EN, et al. Antibiotic prophylaxis for the prevention of bacterial infections in cirrhotic patients with gastrointestinal bleeding: a meta-analysis. Hepatology 1999;29:1655–61.
27. Soares-Weiser K, Brezis M, Tur-Kaspa R, et al. Antibiotic prophylaxis for cirrhotic patients with gastrointestinal bleeding. Cochrane Database Syst Rev 2002;(2):CD002907.
28. Llovet JM, Rodriguez-Iglesias P, Moitinho E, et al. Spontaneous bacterial peritonitis in patients with cirrhosis undergoing selective intestinal decontamination. J Hepatol 1997;26:88–95.
29. Fernandez J, Navasa M, Gomez J, et al. Bacterial infections in cirrhosis: epidemiological changes with invasive procedures and norfloxacin prophylaxis. Hepatology 2002;35:140–8.
30. D'Amico G, Pagliaro L, Bosch J. Pharmacological treatment of portal hypertension: an evidence-based approach. Semin Liver Dis 1999;19:475–505.
31. Teres J, Cecilia A, Bordas JM, et al. Esophageal tamponade for bleeding varices. Controlled trial between the Sengstaken-Blakemore tube and the Linton-Nachlas tube. Gastroenterology 1978;75:566–9.
32. Paquet KJ, Feusener H. Endoscopic sclerosis and esophageal balloon tamponade in acute hemorrhage from esophagogastric varices. Hepatology 1985;5:580–3.
33. Jalan R, Hayes PC. UK guidelines on the management of variceal haemorrhage in cirrhotic patients. British Society of Gastroenterology. Gut 2000;46(Suppl 3–4):III1–15.
34. Korula J, Chin K, Ko Y, et al. Demonstration of two distinct subsets of gastric varices. Observations during a seven-year study of endoscopic sclerotherapy. Dig Dis Sci 1991;36:303–9.
35. Trudeau W, Prindiville T. Endoscopic injection sclerosis in bleeding gastric varices. Gastrointest Endosc 1986;32:264–8.

36. Sarin SK, Jain AK, Jain M, et al. A randomized controlled trial of cyanoacrylate versus alcohol injection in patients with isolated fundic varices. Am J Gastroenterol 2002;97:1010–5.
37. Millar AJ, Brown RA, Hill ID, et al. The fundal pile: bleeding gastric varices. J Pediatr Surg 1991;26:707–9.
38. Seewald S, Sriram PV, Nagra M, et al. The expert approach: cyanoacrylate glue in gastric variceal bleeding. Endoscopy 2002;34:926–32.
39. Lee YT, Chan FK, Ng EK, et al. EUS-guided injection of cyanoacrylate for bleeding gastric varices. Gastrointest Endosc 2000;52:168–74.
40. Oho K, Iwao T, Sumino M, et al. Ethanolamine oleate vs. butyl cyanoacrylate for bleeding gastric varices: a nonrandomized study. Endoscopy 1995;27: 349–54.
41. Ogawa K, Ishikawa S, Naritaka Y, et al. Clinical evaluation of endoscopic injection sclerotherapy using N-butyl-2-cyanoacrylate for gastric variceal bleeding. J Gastroenterol Hepatol 1999;14:245–50.
42. Belletrutti PJ, Romagnuolo J, Hilsden RJ, et al. Endoscopic management of gastric varices: efficacy and outcomes of gluing with N-butyl-2-cyanoacrylate in a North American patient population. Can J Gastroenterol 2008;22: 931–6.
43. Fry LC, Neumann H, Olano C, et al. Efficacy, complications and clinical outcomes of endoscopic sclerotherapy with N-butyl-2-cyanoacrylate for bleeding gastric varices. Dig Dis 2008;26:300–3.
44. Marques P, Maluf-Filho F, Kumar A, et al. Long-term outcomes of acute gastric variceal bleeding in 48 patients following treatment with cyanoacrylate. Dig Dis Sci 2008;53:544–50.
45. Cheng LF, Wang ZQ, Li CZ, et al. Treatment of gastric varices by endoscopic sclerotherapy using butyl cyanoacrylate: 10 years experience of 635 cases. Chin Med J (Engl) 2007;120:2081–5.
46. Mumtaz K, Majid S, Shah H, et al. Prevalence of gastric varices and results of sclerotherapy with N-butyl 2 cyanoacrylate for controlling acute gastric variceal bleeding. World J Gastroenterol 2007;13:1247–51.
47. Joo HS, Jang JY, Eun SH, et al. Long-term results of endoscopic (N-butyl 2 cyanoacrylate) injection for treatment of gastric varices—a 10 years experience. Korean J Gastroenterol 2007;49:320–6.
48. Kim JW, Baik SK, Kim KH, et al. Effect of endoscopic sclerotherapy using N-butyl-2-cyanoacrylate in patients with gastric variceal bleeding. Korean J Hepatol 2006;12(3):394–403.
49. Huang YH, Yeh HZ, Chen GH, et al. Endoscopic treatment of bleeding gastric varices by N-butyl-2-cyanoacrylate (Histoacryl) injection: long-term efficacy and safety. Gastrointest Endosc 2000;52:160–7.
50. Noophun P, Kongkam P, Gonlachanvit S, et al. Bleeding gastric varices: results of endoscopic injection with cyanoacrylate at King Chulalongkorn Memorial Hospital. World J Gastroenterol 2005;11:7531–5.
51. Akahoshi T, Hashizume M, Shimabukuro R, et al. Long-term results of endoscopic histoacryl injection sclerotherapy for gastric variceal bleeding: a 10-year experience. Surgery 2002;131:S176–81.
52. Rivet C, Robles-Medranda C, Dumortier J, et al. Endoscopic treatment of gastroesophageal varices in young infants with cyanoacrylate glue: a pilot study. Gastrointest Endosc 2009;69(6):1034–8.
53. Consolo P, Luigiano C, Giacobbe G, et al. Cyanoacrylate glue in the management of gastric varices. Minerva Med 2009;100(1):115–21.

54. Ryan BM, Stockbrugger R, Ryan MJ. A pathophysiologic, gastroenterologic, and radiologic approach to the management of gastric varices. Gastroenterology 2004;126:1175–89.
55. Sarin SK. Long-term follow-up of gastric variceal sclerotherapy: an eleven-year experience. Gastrointest Endosc 1997;46:8–14.
56. Lo GH, Lai KH, Cheng JS, et al. A prospective randomized trial of sclerotherapy versus ligation in the management of bleeding esophageal varices. Hepatology 1995;22:466–71.
57. Ramesh J, Limdi JK, Sharma V, et al. The use of thrombin injections in the management of bleeding gastric varices: a single-center experience. Gastrointest Endosc 2008;68:877–82.
58. Daly PM. Use of buffer thrombin in treatment of gastric varices: a preliminary report. Arch Surg 1947;55:208–12.
59. Kitano S, Hashizume M, Yamaga H, et al. Human thrombin plus 5 per cent ethanolamine oleate injected to sclerose oesophageal varices: a prospective randomized trial. Br J Surg 1989;76:715–8.
60. Snobl J, Van Buuren HR, Van Blankenstein M. Endoscopic injection using thrombin: an effective and safe method for controlling oesophagogastric variceal bleeding. Gastroenterology 1992;102:A891.
61. Williams SG, Peters RA, Westaby D. Thrombin—an effective treatment for gastric variceal haemorrhage. Gut 1994;35:1287–9.
62. Przemioslo RT, McNair A, Williams R. Thrombin is effective in arresting bleeding from gastric variceal hemorrhage. Dig Dis Sci 1999;44:778–81.
63. Yang WL, Tripathi D, Therapondos G, et al. Endoscopic use of human thrombin in bleeding gastric varices. Am J Gastroenterol 2002;97:1381–5.
64. Chun HJ, Hyun JH. A new method of endoscopic variceal ligation-injection sclerotherapy (EVLIS) for gastric varices. Korean J Intern Med 1995;10(2):108–19.
65. Sugimoto N, Watanabe K, Watanabe K, et al. Endoscopic hemostasis for bleeding gastric varices treated by combination of variceal ligation and sclerotherapy with N-butyl-2-cyanoacrylate. J Gastroenterol 2007;42:528–32.
66. Iwase H, Suga S, Morise K, et al. Color Doppler endoscopic ultrasonography for the evaluation of gastric varices and endoscopic obliteration with cyanoacrylate glue. Gastrointest Endosc 1995;41:150–4.
67. Romero-Castro R, Pellicer-Bautista FJ, Jimenez-Saenz M, et al. EUS-guided injection of cyanoacrylate in perforating feeding veins in gastric varices: results in 5 cases. Gastrointest Endosc 2007;66(2):402–7.
68. Binmoeller KF, Weilert F, Shah JN, et al. EUS-guided transesophageal treatment of gastric fundal varices with combined coiling and cyanoacrylate glue injection. Gastrointest Endosc 2011;74:1019–25.
69. de Franchis R, Faculty Baveno V. Revising consensus in portal hypertension: report of the Baveno V consensus workshop on methodology of diagnosis and therapy in portal hypertension. J Hepatol 2010;53:762–8.
70. Choi YH, Yoon CJ, Park JH, et al. Balloon occluded retrograde transvenous obliteration for gastric variceal bleeding its feasibility compared with transjugular intrahepatic portosystemic shunt. Korean J Radiol 2003;4:109–16.
71. Chau TN, Patch D, Chan YW, et al. "Salvage" transjugular intrahepatic portosystemic shunts: gastric fundal compared with esophageal variceal bleeding. Gastroenterology 1998;114:981–7.
72. Rees CJ, Nylander DL, Thompson NP, et al. Do gastric and oesophageal varices bleed at different portal pressures and is TIPS an effective treatment? Liver 2000;20:253–6.

73. Stanley AJ, Jalan R, Ireland HM, et al. A comparison between gastric and oesophageal variceal haemorrhage treated with transjugular intrahepatic porto-systemic stent shunt (TIPSS). Aliment Pharmacol Ther 1997;11:171–6.

74. Barange K, Péron JM, Imani K, et al. Transjugular intrahepatic portosystemic shunt in the treatment of refractory bleeding from ruptured gastric varices. Hepatology 1999;30:1139–43.

75. Gazzera C, Righi D, Doriguzzi Breatta A, et al. Emergency transjugular intrahepatic portosystemic shunt (TIPS): results, complications and predictors of mortality in the first month of followup. Radiol Med 2012;117:46–53 [in English, Italian].

76. Henderson JM, Boyer TD, Kutner MH, et al. Distal splenorenal shunt versus transjugular intrahepatic portal systematic shunt for variceal bleeding: a randomized trial. Gastroenterology 2006;130:1643–51.

77. Kanagawa H, Mima S, Kouyama H, et al. Treatment of gastric fundal varices by balloon occluded retrograde transvenous obliteration. J Gastroenterol Hepatol 1996;11:51–8.

78. Min SK, Kim SG, Kim YS, et al. Comparison among endoscopic variceal obliteration, endoscopic band ligation, and balloon-occluded retrograde transvenous obliteration for treatment of gastric variceal bleeding. Korean J Gastroenterol 2011;57:302–8.

79. Hong CH, Kim HJ, Park JH, et al. Treatment of patients with gastric variceal hemorrhage: endoscopic N-butyl-2-cyanoacrylate injection versus balloon-occluded retrograde transvenous obliteration. J Gastroenterol Hepatol 2009;24:372–8.

80. Akahane T, Iwasaki T, Kobayashi N, et al. Changes in liver function parameters after occlusion of gastrorenal shunts with balloon-occluded retrograde transvenous obliteration. Am J Gastroenterol 1997;92:1026–30.

81. Fukuda T, Hirota S, Sugimura K. Long-term results of balloon-occluded retrograde transvenous obliteration for the treatment of gastric varices and hepatic encephalopathy. J Vasc Interv Radiol 2001;12:327–36.

82. Tripathi D, Ferguson JW, Therapondos G, et al. Recent advances in the management of bleeding gastric varices. Aliment Pharmacol Ther 2006;24:1–17.

83. Mishra SR, Chander Sharma B, Kumar A, et al. Endoscopic cyanoacrylate injection versus beta-blocker for secondary prophylaxis of gastric variceal bleed: a randomised controlled trial. Gut 2010;59(6):729–35.

84. Nguyen AJ, Baron TH, Burgart LJ, et al. 2-Octyl-cyanoacrylate (Dermabond), a new glue for variceal injection therapy: results of a preliminary animal study. Gastrointest Endosc 2002;55:572–5.

85. Sharma M, Goyal A. Bleeding after glue injection in gastric varices. Gastroenterology 2012;142:e1–2.

86. Irani S, Kowdley K, Kozarek R. Gastric varices -an updated review of management. J Clin Gastroenterol 2011;45:133–48.

87. Saad WE, Sze YD. Variations of balloon-occluded retrograde transvenous obliteration (BRTO): balloon occluded antegrade transvenous obliteration (BATO) and alternative/adjunctive routes for BRTO. Semin Intervent Radiol 2011;28:314–24.

88. Belletrutti PJ, Romagnuolo J, Hilsden RJ, et al. Endoscopic management of gastric varices: efficacy and outcomes of gluing with N-butyl-2-cyanoacrylate in a North American patient population. Can J Gastroenterol 2008;22:931–6.

89. Hwang SS, Kim HH, Park SH, et al. N-butyl-2-cyanoacrylate pulmonary embolism after endoscopic injection sclerotherapy for gastric variceal bleeding. J Comput Assist Tomogr 2001;25:16–22.

90. Gin-Holo, Kwork H, Jin S, et al. Cyanoacrylate in management of bleeding gastric varices. Hepatology 2001;33:1060–4.
91. Upadhyay AP, Ananthasivan R, Radhakrishnan S, et al. Cortical Blindness and Acute Myocardial Infarction following injection of bleeding gastric varices with cyanacrylate glue. Endoscopy 2005;37:1034.
92. Rickman OB, Utz JP, Aughenbaugh GI, et al. Pulmonary Embolization of 2-Octyl Cyanoacrylate After Endoscopic Injection Therapy for Gastric Variceal Bleeding. Mayo Clin Proc. 2004;79(11):1455–8.
93. Cheng LF, Wang ZQ, Li CZ, et al. Clin Gastroenterol Hepatol 2010;8(9):760–6.
94. Lo GH, Lin CW, Perng DS, et al. Scand J Gastroenterol 2013;48(10):1198–204.
95. Heneghan MA, Byrne A, Harrison PM. An open pilot study of the effects of a human fibrin glue for endoscopic treatment of patients with acute bleeding from gastric varices. Gastrointest Endosc 2002;56:422–6.
96. Datta D, Vlavianos P, Alisa A, et al. Use of fibrin glue (beriplast) in the management of bleeding gastric varices. Endoscopy 2003;35:675–8.
97. Smith MR, Tidswell R, Tripathi D. Outcomes of endoscopic human thrombin injection in the management of gastric varices. Eur J Gastroenterol Hepatol 2014; 26(8):846–52.
98. Tan PC, Hou MC, Lin HC, et al. A randomized trial of endoscopic treatment of acute gastric variceal hemorrhage: n-butyl-2-cyanoacrylate injection versus band ligation. Hepatology 2006;43:690–7.
99. Lo GH, Liang HL, Chen WC, et al. A prospective, randomized controlled trial of transjugular intrahepatic portosystemic shunt versus cyanoacrylate injection in the prevention of gastric variceal rebleeding. Endoscopy 2007;39:679–85.

Endovascular Management of Gastric Varices

Wael E. Saad, MD, FSIR

KEYWORDS

- BRTO • TIPS • Gastric varices • Bleeding • Model for end-stage liver disease
- Hepatic encephalopathy

KEY POINTS

- The management of gastric varices is largely uncharted.
- Balloon-occluded retrograde transvenous obliteration (BRTO) for the management of gastric varices is safe and effective.
- Clinicians have not yet reached the stage where patients (stratified according to clinical presentation, endoscopic and/or vascular classifications, hepatic reserve, and comorbidities) undergo treatments that are tailored to their needs and based on evidence-based medicine.

INTRODUCTION

Bleeding from gastric varicesis a major complication of portal hypertension. Although less common than bleeding associated with esophageal varices, gastric variceal bleeding has a higher mortality.[1,2] Moreover, compared with endoscopic treatment of esophageal varices, endoscopic treatment of gastric varices is less effective.[3] Despite decades of varying endoscopic, percutaneous, and surgical treatment strategies, the literature is less established and overall is less effective.[3,4] From an endovascular perspective, transjugular intrahepatic portosystemic shunts (TIPSs) to decompress the portal circulation and/or transvenous obliteration are used to address bleeding gastric varices.[5-7] Until recently, there was a clear medical cultural divide between the strategy of decompressing the portal circulation (TIPS creation, for example) and transvenous obliteration for the management of gastric varices.[8,9] In Asia (predominantly Japan), the approach was obliteration and not decompression for cultural, historical, and financial reasons. In the West (United States and Europe), the approach was to decompress the portal circulation and not to obliterate the gastric varices due to the availability of the TIPS procedure and its clinical success (particularly with stent-grafts in the last decade) and the historical long-term clinical failures of

Department of Radiology, University of Michigan, 1500 East Medical Center Drive, Ann Arbor, MI 48109, USA
E-mail address: wsaad@med.umich.edu

Clin Liver Dis 18 (2014) 829–851
http://dx.doi.org/10.1016/j.cld.2014.07.005
1089-3261/14/$ – see front matter © 2014 Elsevier Inc. All rights reserved.
liver.theclinics.com

sclerosing (obliterating) varices in the 1970s in Europe and the United States.[8,9] In the past 5 to 7 years, and more so in the last 2 to 3 years, contemporary physicians (interventional radiologists, hepatologists, gastroenterologists, and surgeons) from both sides of this geocultural divide have entertained the other's strategy. Anecdotally, Japanese interventionalists are trying to reintroduce the concept of TIPSs to Japan, and American interventionalists and hepatologists are using transvenous obliteration to manage their patients either as an augment or alternative to decompression. There is resistance on both sides of the divide, which is understandable given the conservative nature of medicine and that this is the health and lives of humans. No one can argue, however, that there are advantages and disadvantages to both strategies.[9] What the author believes needs to be done is to define and stratify patients to understand which patients do better than others for each strategy in order to tailor treatments to patients' needs, morbidities, and risks.[8,9] Tailoring management strategy requires a more scientific multidisciplinary approach and considerably more and better clinical research to better understand and analyze this largely poorly understood and potentially mortal portal hypertension complication. To unintentionally compound the scientific debate and stratification further, combination therapy of transvenous obliteration and decompression can be performed and/or augmenting either strategy (or both strategies) with partial splenic arterial embolization can be performed.[9–12]

This article discusses the outcomes of transvenous obliteration and TIPSs for the management of gastric varices individually or in combination. Definitions, endovascular technical concepts, and contemporary vascular classifications of gastric variceal systems are described to help grasp the complexity of the hemodynamic pathology and hopefully help define the pathology better for future reporting and lay the ground for more defined stratification of patients not only based on comorbidity and hepatic reserve but also on anatomy and hemodynamic classifications.

ANATOMY, DEFINITIONS, AND CLASSIFICATIONS

Terminology and definitions of types of transvenous obliteration are discussed below in the BRTO-PROCEDURE section. The majority (>60%–80% of patients) of gastric varices are associated with a spontaneous portosystemic shunt that is to the left of the anatomic midline (left-sided portosystemic shunts).[9,13] These shunts include gastrorenal shunts, direct gastrocaval shunts, and gastrocaval shunts via the inferior phrenic vein.[9,13] More than 90% of these left-sided spontaneous portosystemic shunts are gastrorenal shunts. Morphologically, splenorenal shunts (or lienorenal shunts) are spontaneous left-sided portosystemic shunts that communicate the splenic vein with, most commonly, the left renal vein without passing through the gastrointestinal tract, thus without forming submucosal gastrointestinal varices (ectopic varices).[13] From a hemodynamic standpoint, gastrorenal shunts and splenorenal shunts are both splenorenal shunts: portal blood flow moves from portal to systemic circulations in gastrorenal shunts from the splenic vein siphoning up to form gastric varices and then descending to empty into the left renal vein (essentially it shunts from splenic to renal veins) (**Fig. 1**).[13] This is the source of interchangeable terminology and anatomic definition confusion.[13]

The gastric varices and the gastrorenal shunt are collectively termed, *the gastric variceal system or complex*.[13] The gastric variceal system can be simple with minimal portal venous feeders (afferent veins) and a singular draining portosystemic shunt (efferent vein) or complex, and commonly tortuous, with multiple afferent and efferent (collaterals included) veins. The detailed vascular components of the gastric variceal system can be seen in **Fig. 2**.[13] Morphologically and anatomically, gastric variceal

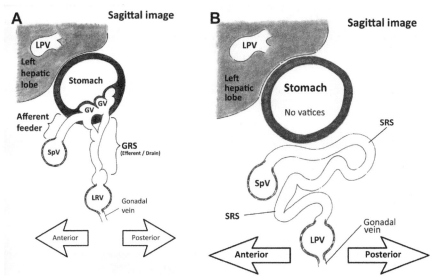

Fig. 1. Sagittal Illustrations depicting gastro-renal shunt and spleno-renal shunt anatomical features and hemodynamics. (*A*) Key labeled sagittal drawing of the basic anatomy of GV and their draining GRS. The afferent portal venous feeders comes off the SpV or porto-splenic venous axis. This supplies the GV which are in turn drained by the efferent systemic venous system. The most common efferent drainage is the GRS which commonly empties into the LRV. (*B*) Sagittal drawing of the basic anatomy of morphologic/anatomic SRS. The afferent portal venous feeders comes off the SpV or porto-splenic venous axis. The SRS does not supply any varices and does not run through the wall of the GIT. The most common efferent drainage is the LRV. The SRS, as depicted, commonly meanders (long and tortuous) and is not a straight, short porto-systemic shunt. GIT, gastro-intestinal tract; GRS, gastro-renal shunt; GV, gastric varices; LPV, intra-hepatic left portal vein; LRV, left renal vein; SRS, spleno-renal shunt; SpV, splenic vein. (*From* Saad WE. Vascular Anatomy and the morphologic and hemodynamic classifications of gastric varices and spontaneous portosystemic shunts relevant to the BRTO procedure. Tech Vasc Interventional Rad 2013;16:60–100; with permission.)

systems are widely heterogeneous and have varying degrees of complexity, tortuosity, size, and blood flow throughput (degree, velocity, and volume of portosystemic shunting). The degree of shunting/size of the gastric variceal system is invariably not reported by scientists and may be, in the author's opinion, the most important anatomic/hemodynamic variable potentially affecting outcome.[9] A hypothetical example is that small gastric variceal systems with small amount of portosystemic shunting may not have any hemodynamic and/or clinical consequences after a Balloon-occluded retrograde transvenous obliteration (BRTO) procedure; however, a large gastric variceal system with significant portosystemic shunting may require portal venous modulation (TIPS and/or splenic artery embolization) to compensate/temporize for the loss of the large gastrorenal shunt and temporize the increased portal flow diverted back to the portal circulation. If this hypothesis holds true, the next step is to define thresholds of significance of gastric variceal systems.[9]

In the same respect, the evolution of hemodynamics of spontaneous portosystemic shunts have been theorized based on the trophoblastic nature (or lack thereof) of the inline portal venous flow.[14,15] This has been collectively termed, *portosystemic shunt syndrome*.[16] To the best of the author's knowledge, the term was

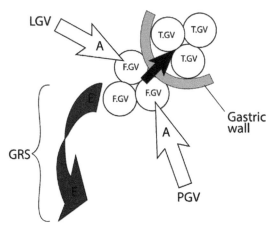

Fig. 2. Illustrations depicting the anatomical relationships of the different components of the gastric variceal system (GVS). GVS is composed of the afferent portal venous feeders (*hollow arrows with 'A'*), the central variceal part, and the gastro-renal shunt (systemic venous drainer/s). The central variceal part has the extra-gastric/F.GV, the intra-gastric submucosal/T.GV and a perforator vein/varix communicating between the false and true GVs (*black arrow*). The GRS is the efferent (*curved arrow with 'E'*) systemic venous drainage. Notice that the cluster of F.GV is the central part of the GVS where the T.GV, the afferent feeders (A) and GRS all communicate and exists outside the stomach. The complexity (tortuosity) of the F.GV varies considerably from one patient to the other varying from a simple varix (tubular venous structure) to a cluster of lakes of varices in a grape like morphology (hence the term: false gastric varices. E, efferent draining vein/shunt; F. GV, false gastric varices; GRS, gastro-renal shunt; LGV, left gastric vein; PGV, posterior gastric vein; T. GV, true gastric varices. (*From* Saad WE. Vascular Anatomy and the morphologic and hemodynamic classifications of gastric varices and spontaneous portosystemic shunts relevant to the BRTO procedure. Tech Vasc Interventional Rad 2013;16:60–100; with permission.)

originally coined by Kumamoto and coworkers[16] when describing the reduction of hepatic reserve over time (3–5 years) in patients with gastrorenal shunts. They had 3 groups that they followed longitudinally in a retrospective audit. One group was patients with no spontaneous portosystemic shunts; another had gastrorenal shunts that were occluded due to a BRTO procedure; and a third group had spontaneous gastrorenal shunts that were not treated and had patent shunts. Over time, the synthetic function of the third group (untreated shunt) deteriorated whereas the treated shunts (post-BRTO) group maintained their synthetic function similar to the control group (patients who never had a spontaneous shunt).[16] Saad and coworkers took this further and staged this syndrome based on their clinical experience.[14,15] In the early compensated stage, the spontaneous shunt is the result of portal hypertension and decompresses the portal circulation where there is mild hepatic dysfunction, no ascites, and potentially intermittent but medical manageable hepatic encephalopathy.[14,15] In the late stages, the shunt starts to grow and shunts more portal blood flow to the systemic circulation and starts contributing to the hepatic disease (vicious cycle is established) with a decline in hepatic reserve/synthetic function and worsening hepatic encephalopathy. As the shunt grows, there is reversal of flow in the portal vein (hepatofugal flow), diminution of the portal vein diameter, paucity of intrahepatic portal vein radicals, and the beginning of notable hepatic parenchymal atrophy (ascites still has not been established). In the terminal stages, there is overt hepatic atrophy accompanied by liver failure, portal vein thrombosis, and recalcitrant hepatic encephalopathy.[14,15] At the terminal stages, the spontaneous portosystemic shunts completely takes over the natural outflow of the portal venous circulation (the liver/hepatic sinusoids) and becomes the outflow of the splanchnic circulation (spleen and gastrointestinal tract).[14,15]

Several classifications associated with gastric varices have been described from endoscopic, clinical, vascular, and hemodynamic perspectives. Detailed classifications associated with gastric varices (with definitions, applications, and illustrations) are beyond the scope of this article but can be found in an article by Saad and co-workers.[13] The Sarin classification is the most common and most important endoscopic and possibly clinical classification.[1,13] Due to the limited scope of this article, the author highlights 3 vascular and/or hemodynamic classifications. The first classification is the modified Kiyosue classification, which is the most commonly described classification in the radiology literature (**Fig. 3**).[6,7,13] The application of this classification is technical for the BRTO procedure. It has no clinical or outcomes applications and thus would probably not have great applicability to readers of this article, but it is important to be aware of it due to its wide mention in the radiology literature.[6,7,13,17]

The second classification is the Saad-Caldwell classification for gastric varices (**Fig. 4**).[13] This is a vascular classification of gastric varices that is correlated with the Sarin endoscopioc classification of gastric varices. In essence, the classification system bridges between endoscopic findings (gastroenterology/hepatology discipline) and vascular findings (radiology discipline).[13] As a result, it helps hepatologists and gastroenterologist appreciate the variability in vasculature deeper than what they see in the mucosa and submucosa and helps in understanding the origins of the varices classified by Sarin and coworkers (see **Fig. 4**).[13] The third classification is a hemodynamic vascular classification of all ectopic varices (gastric varices included); however, it is important for all medical specialties to understand because it has management implications and applicability (**Fig. 5, Table 1**).[13,14,18]

THE BRTO PROCEDURE

Transvenous obliteration is a technique that not only is applied to the endovascular management of gastric varices but also is used for many other vascular beds/medical conditions, which include lower extremity varicose veins, vascular malformations, and pelvic or testicular varicoceles. Transvenous obliteration is the instilment of sclerosants and/or liquid embolic agents in vascular beds with the intent of thrombosis of the endoluminal blood, damage to the endothelial lining of the vascular bed, and scarring and reduction of the vascular bed, if not complete occlusion of the vascular bed. The most important principle in optimizing obliteration is to maximize the concentration and dwell time of the sclerosant in the target vascular bed. The principle is briefly summarized by the following quotation, "first you trap it, then you kill it."[17] Transvenous obliteration can be aided with balloon occlusion (common practice) but can also be aided with other means (eg, coils), which are less common means.[17] Additionally, how the catheter (or balloon approach) is advanced is a consideration for the technical nomenclature. Catheter and/or balloon approach in line with the direction of blood flow is referred to as antegrade approach and catheter and/or balloon approach in the opposite direction of blood flow is referred to as retrograde approach.[19,20] Due to the limited scope of the article, detailed techniques for transvenous sclerosis or obliteration are not discussed in the article.

The primary indications for BRTO are gastric variceal bleeding and hepatic encephalopathy refractory to medical management in the presence of a gastrorenal shunt.[1,5,16,21–50] Bleeding gastric varices can be defined as active bleeding, having a prior index bleed, or having impending bleeds due to high-risk gastric varices.[3] The latter is subject to interpretation because the endoscopic findings defining high-risk gastric varices are descriptive and subjective.[3]

With a focus on gastric varices, BRTO is commonly used. Due to the more readily accessible and less risky access of the systemic venous circulation (jugular and femoral veins) compared with the portal circulation, the common approach toward gastric varices with gastrorenal shunts is via the systemic veins going against

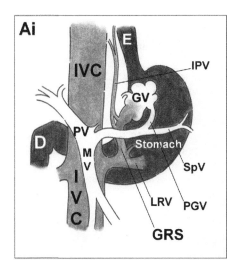
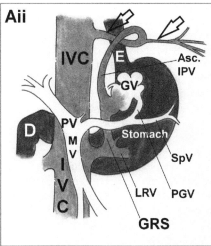
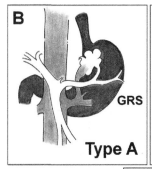
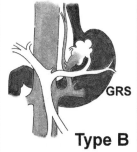
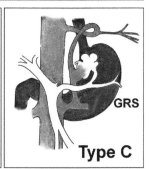
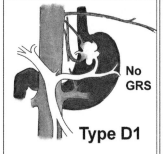
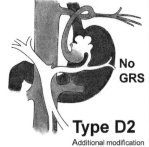

(retrograde) flow in the gastrorenal shunt.[19] Coupled with balloon occlusion, the procedure is referred to as BRTO.[17,19,20] Several techniques (alternatives or as an augment to BRTO) have been described, however, and are clinically successful in managing gastric varices by approaching the varices from the portal venous side in an antegrade approach using balloon occlusion. This technique is referred to as balloon-occluded antegrade transvenous obliteration (BATO).[19] The classic BRTO procedure is performed from a femoral (more common) or jugular venous percutaneous access with catheterization of the gastrorenal shunt via the left renal vein. Occlusion of the shunt (and thus stasis of blood flow) is commonly achieved using balloon occlusion catheters and is followed by coaxial (through the balloon occlusion catheter) placement of a microcatheter for administration of a sclerosing agent. At the completion of the BRTO procedure, the balloon is deflated and removed after confirmation of shunt thrombosis after a sclerosant dwell period (the dwell period is conventionally several hours with the balloon inflated). A detailed description of the BRTO procedure is described in the article by Saad and coworkers.[17] The byproduct of the BRTO procedure is thrombosis of the gastrorenal shunt, which is the source of controversies regarding which is the ideal

---

Fig. 3. Saad modification of the Kiyosue classification of the systemic venous drainage of gastric varices. (A) Key labeled drawings of the anatomy of GV and the draining systemic veins which includes the draining GRS, if present. The image is to help identify structures in the classification in **Fig. 3**B. The primary difference between (Ai) and (Aii) is the size and morphology of the IPV. In (Aii) the IPV has a vertical part and a horizontally oriented sub-diaphragmatic transverse part (Hollow black arrows). The vertical part is composed of an Asc. IPV and a descending portion. It is the descending portion, that when it anastomoses with the adrenal vein, forms the GRS. (3B) Schematic classification based on the anatomical classification of Kiyosue et al.[6,7] (Type-A) The simplest gastric variceal system drained by the GRS and without other systemic venous draining veins (significant or insignificant). (Type-B) Is a simple gastric variceal system drained by GRS and with insignificant (non-decompressive) systemic venous draining veins which are typically IPVs, but can also be other retroperitoneal veins (innominate veins, hemiazygous tributaries, intercostal veins, and adrenal veins) (see **Fig-3**Ai for detailed labeling). (Type-C) Is a more complex gastric variceal system drained by the GRS and with an additional significant (decompressive) systemic venous draining vein (IPV, usually >3mm in diameter, Saad interpretation of diameter estimate) (see **Fig-3**Aii for detailed labeling). (Type-D) Is a gastric variceal system that is not drained by the GRS. In other words, no GRS exists. However, there are significant systemic venous drainage by other retroperitoneal and/or phrenic vein(s). (Type-D1) The decompressive systemic venous draining veins have no particular predominance and include IPVs, but can also be other retroperitoneal veins such as innominate reroperitoneal veins, hemiazygous tributaries, intercostal veins, and adrenal veins. Type-D gastric varices represent more than 40% of technical failures (Saad Type-III failure). (Type-D2) Is the same as Type-D1, but there is a predominant systemic venous draining vein (usually >3mm in diameter) that can be accessible and is amenable to BRTO via unconventional systemic veins. These predominant draining routes include: Hemiazygous-azygous axis, inferior phrenic vein (usually the ascending portion leading to the transverse portion as drawn), and Pericardial vein (or pericardio-phrenic vein).Asc. IPV, ascending portion of the vertical part of the inferior phrenic vein; D, Duodenum; E, Esophagus; GRS, gastro-renal shunt; GV, gastric varices; IVC, Inferior vena cava; IPV, inferior phrenic vein; LRV, left renal vein; MV, mesenteric vein; PGV, posterior gastric vein; PV, main portal vein; SpV, splenic vein. (From Saad WE. Vascular Anatomy and the morphologic and hemodynamic classifications of gastric varices and spontaneous portosystemic shunts relevant to the BRTO procedure. Tech Vasc Interventional Rad 2013;16:60–100; with permission.)

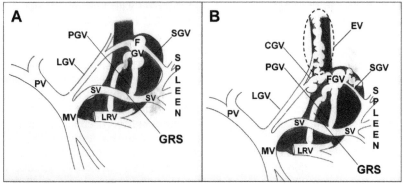

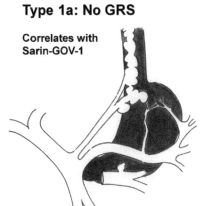

Ci

Type 1a: No GRS

Correlates with
Sarin-GOV-1

Cii

Type 1b: + GRS

Correlates with
Sarin-GOV-1

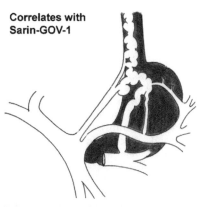

Di

Type 2a: No GRS

Correlates with
Sarin-IGV-1

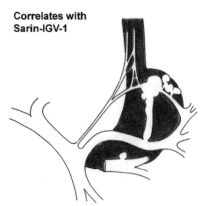

Dii

Type 2b: + GRS

Correlates with
• Sarin-IGV-1
• Fukuda-Hirota-1*

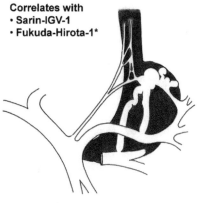

treatment of choice: BRTO versus TIPS (to compress or to decompress the portal circulation, respectively)[9,50] (see portosystemic shunt syndrome, discussed previously, and outcomes, discussed later).

OUTCOMES OF BRTO-ONLY FOR THE MANAGEMENT OF GASTRIC VARICES IN ASIAN INSTITUTIONS

The technical success rate of the BRTO procedure and complete obliteration rate (by cross-sectional imaging and/or endoscopic ultrasound) are greater than 80% and greater than 80%, respectively.[1,5,16,21–25,31–35,41–43,46,47,51–56] In a meta-analysis by Saad and Sabri,[55] the technical success rate and obliteration rate of BRTO from the Asian literature were 92% and 85%, respectively. BATO (approaching the gastric varices from the portal venous side via a trans-TIPS or transhepatic approach) significantly improves the technical success rate and obliteration rate to exceed 90% to 100%.[55] This is referred to as a BRTO intent with a BATO bailout.[55] Balloon rupture during the procedure or during the dwell time of the balloon has no statistically significant technical and/or clinical consequences.[57–59]

In the immediate post-BRTO period, transient fever, hemoglobinuria due to hemolysis (commonly mistakenly referred to as hematuria), and abdominal pain have

◀───

Fig. 4. Anatomical & hemodynamic classification of isolated gastric varices and gastro-esophageal varices as proposed by Saad and Caldwell. (*A-B*): This is the key labeled drawing of the basic anatomy of esophageal and gastric varices (GV) and their draining gastro-renal shunt (GRS). The drawings are key for the structure identification and labeling of the classification system illustrated and described in Fig. 4C-4F. The afferent portal venous feeders of the GV comes off the splenic vein (SV) or porto-splenic venous axis. These include the left (LGV), posterior (PGV), and short (SGV) gastric veins. The GV are in turn drained by the efferent systemic venous system which as drawn here is the GRS which empties into the left renal vein (LRV) The gastro-esophageal varices can be classified into esophageal varices (EV), and GV. The GV can be sub-classified into fundic (FGV) and cardia (CGV). (*4C*) Saad-Caldwell Type-1 GV are isolated CGV without fundic varices which probably correlate with Endoscopic Sarin Classification (GOV-1) (See **Fig-1**). The dominant portal venous feeder in these cases is the LGV which comes off the distal splenic vein, proximal main portal vein or the spleno-portal junction. The posterior and short gastric portal venous feeders are diminutive. Variations to Saad-Caldwell Type-1 is the presence or absence of associated esophageal varices and/or the presence (*Type-1b*) or absence (*Type-1a*) of a draining GRS. Due to that the main portal venous feeder is central or close to the main portal vein, the hemodynamics of this Type-1 varices are very similar to those of esophageal varices especially in the absence of a gastro-renal shunt (*Type-1a*). As a result, Type-1 gastric varices would probably respond favorably to a transjugular intrahepatic portosystemic shunt (TIPS) especially in the absence of a GRS (*Type-1a*). If a GRS is present (*Type-1b*), the GV may respond to TIPS with LGV embolization. Obviously a BRTO can be performed, however, if EV exist without endoscopic control, a TIPS is preferred. (*4D*) Saad-Caldwell Type-2 gastric varices are isolated FGV without CGV which probably correlate with Endoscopic Sarin Classification (IGV-1) and the Fukuda-Hirota Type-1. The dominant portal venous feeder in these cases is the PGV and SGV which come off the proximal splenic vein near the splenic hilum and distant from the liver and main portal vein. The left gastric portal venous feeder is diminutive. Variations to Saad-Caldwell Type-2 is the presence (*Type-2b*) or absence (*Type-2a*) of a draining GRS. Due to that the main PGV and/or SGV is at a distance from the main portal vein/liver, a TIPS may be less effective especially in the presence of a large (high flow) GRS. In the presence of a GRS (*Type-2b*), especially a large one, a BRTO is preferred. If there is no GRS (*Type-2a*), a TIPS with portal venous feeder embolization would be effective.

Ei
Type 3a: No GRS

Correlates with
Sarin-GOV-2

Eii
Type 3b: + GRS

Correlates with
• Sarin-GOV-2
• Fukuda-Hirota-3*

Fi
Type 4a: No GRS

Correlates with
Sarin-GOV-2

Fii
Type 4b: + GRS

Correlates with
• Sarin-GOV-2

Gi
Type 4a: No GRS

Correlates with
Sarin-GOV-2

Gii
Type 4b: + GRS

Correlates with
• Sarin-GOV-2

been observed in a large percentage of patients.[55] More serious procedure-related complications are rarely reported (<2%–5%) (**Box 1**) and include asymptomatic (image-proved) and symptomatic pulmonary embolus, anaphylactic reactions to ethanolamine oleate (not used in the United States), cardiac arrhythmia, and pulmonary edema.[55] Portal vein thrombosis and left renal vein thrombosis are also potential but rare complications of BRTO. There are no reports of left renal vein thrombosis of any clinical consequence (only an imaging finding).[55] Moreover, when intraprocedural and/or postprocedural imaging CT is routinely used, it demonstrates small overspill of sclerosant into the intrahepatic portal veins that is rarely of any clinical consequence.[25,55] Despite the lack of reports in the literature, anecdotally, certain severe complications should be discussed with the patient prior to undergoing the BRTO procedure.[55] These include stroke, particularly in patients with right to left shunts (a common finding in BRTO patients due to cirrhosis-related intrapulmonary shunting), aggravated and potentially life-threatening bleeding (there is a moment in the procedure where the balloon is inflated and the sclerosant has not been instilled where the gastric variceal system is pressurized), and paradoxic hepatic failure leading to death or liver transplantation within 30 to 60 days after the BRTO procedure (discussed later).[55,60]

Follow-up endoscopic examinations reveal localized mucosal changes in the region of treated gastric varices in a majority of patients (typically dusky discoloration of the mucosa overlying the obliterated gastric varices). A typical but not common ischemic gastric ulceration pattern with or without associated bleeding has also been reported.[3,42] The bleeding from these ischemic ulcers is usually occult and is an endoscopic finding only. These endoscopically visible changes usually respond to short-term conservative therapy.[3,50]

The bleeding control rate of actively bleeding gastricvarices after BRTO is reported as high as 91% to 100%.[3,21] Barring fatality, however, gastric variceal bleeding stops and it is unclear whether the cessation of active bleeding is actually due to intervention or spontaneous cessation. In the author's opinion, this applies to all other intervention

---

Fig. 4. (*continued*) (*4E*): Saad-Caldwell Type-3 gastric varices are complex cardio-fundic gastric varices with a high association with EV. All three portal venous feeders are involved and have variable dominance. These are usually complex and large variceal systems. Variations to Saad-Caldwell Type-3 is the presence (*Type-3b*) or absence (*Type-3a*) of a draining GRS. When the GRS is present (*Type-3b*), the GRS is usually large and has significant flow acting as an outflow to the 3 enlarged portal venous feeders (PGV, SGV, LGV). In the absence of a GRS (*Type-3a*) a TIPS is recommended with multiple portal venous feeder embolizations/trans-TIPS BATO-approach sclerosis. In the presence of a large GRS (*Type-3b*), a BRTO with or without a TIPS is recommended. (*4F*) Saad-Caldwell Type-4 gastric varices are like type-2 or type-3 (and are more likely to be similar to type-3), but is the presence of splenic +/− portal venous thrombosis. In these cases, the decisive factor is whether the portal vein is patent. If there is a patent portal vein and a GRS, a BRTO procedure would be reasonable. If the portal vein is occluded in the presence of a GRS, then the GRS most likely will be the outflow of the mesenteric and splenic veins and a BRTO is ill-advised unless the portal vein is recannulated (with or without a TIPS) or there is significant cavernous transformation of the portal vein that can replace the portal vein as a hepatic inflow and a mesenteric outflow. In the absence of a GRS and in the presence of splenic vein thrombosis +/− portal vein thrombosis, splenic artery embolization would be recommended. MV, mesenteric vein(s); PV,portal vein (main portal vein). (*From* Saad WE. Vascular Anatomy and the morphologic and hemodynamic classifications of gastric varices and spontaneous portosystemic shunts relevant to the BRTO procedure. Tech Vasc Interventional Rad 2013;16:60-100; with permission.)

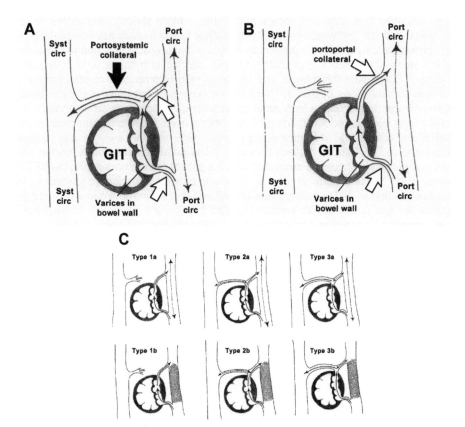

Fig. 5. Saad classification of ectopic varices (gastric, duodenal, mesenteric & stomal varices). (*A-B*) These are baseline labeled anatomy images to help interpret the images of the classification system. The image demonstrates a representative portal or mesenteric vein branch (Port Circ) on the right and a representative systemic vein branch (Syst Circ) on the left of a cross-section through a bowel loop which is a representative of the gastro-intestinal tract (GIT). Typical portal venous (splanchnic veins) branches would include the portal vein proper, the mesenteric vein (and tributaries) and the splenic vein. Typical systemic veins (but not confined to the examples given) include the inferior vena cava, the gonadal veins, renal veins, and retro-peritoneal and para-vertebral veins. Varices (ectopic varices) are seen in the wall of the bowel. (*A*) "ectopic varices" in this depicted instance is supplied and drained by portal collaterals (*white arrows with black outline*) and is also drained (efferent collateral) by a porto-systemic collateral (*black arrow*). (*B*) "ectopic varices" in this depicted instance is supplied and drained by portal collaterals (*white arrows with black outline*) and is not drained by a porto-systemic collateral. The efferent collateral drainage is portal and not systemic. In both (*Fig. A & B*), there is no portal venous occlusion. (*C*) Overview of the classification system. In short, Type-a is non-occlusive and is pressure driven (oncotic). *Type-a* are usually with some element of porto-systemic collaterals (*Type-2a and -3a*) to decompress the higher portal pressure. *Type-b* is the occlusive type and can have no porto-systemic collaterals; the varices can simply be part of a portal to portal "bypass" of a focal occlusion (*Type-b1*); however, porto-systemic collaterals can exist (*Type-b2 and -b3*).

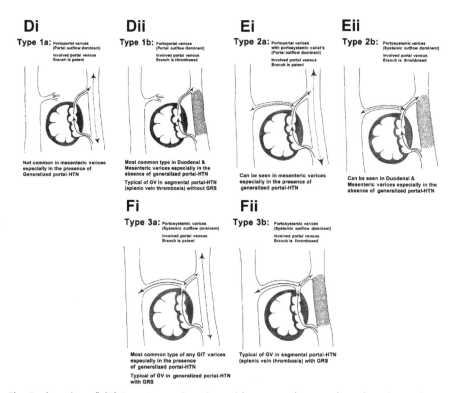

Di

Type 1a: Portoportal varices (Portal outflow dominant)

Involved portal venous Branch is patent

Not common in mesenteric varices especially in the presence of Generalized portal-HTN

Dii

Type 1b: Portoportal varices (Portal outflow dominant)

Involved portal venous Branch is thrombosed

Most common type in Duodenal & Mesenteric varices especially in the absence of generalized portal-HTN

Typical of GV in segmental portal-HTN (splenic vein thrombosis) without GRS

Ei

Type 2a: Portoportal varices with portosystemic collat's (Portal outflow dominant)

Involved portal venous Branch is patent

Can be seen in mesenteric varices especially in the presence of generalized portal-HTN

Eii

Type 2b: Portosystemic varices (Systemic outflow dominant)

Involved portal venous Branch is thrombosed

Can be seen in Duodenal & Mesenteric varices especially in the absence of generalized portal-HTN

Fi

Type 3a: Portosystemic varices (Systemic outflow dominant)

Involved portal venous Branch is patent

Most common type of any GIT varices especially in the presence of generalized portal-HTN

Typical of GV in generalized portal-HTN with GRS

Fii

Type 3b: Portosystemic varices (Systemic outflow dominant)

Involved portal venous Branch is thrombosed

Typical of GV in segmental portal-HTN (splenic vein thrombosis) with GRS

Fig. 5. (*continued*) (*D*) Type-1 ectopic varices without portal venous branch occlusion (*Type-1a*) and with portal venous branch occlusion (*Type-1b*). The portal venous branch can be any vein (location or size) in the portal circulation. This includes mesenteric vein and tributaries and portal vein tributaries as well as the main portal, mesenteric and splenic veins. Obviously, balloon-occluded retrograde transvenous obliteration (BRTO) of these ectopic varices (*Type-1*) is not feasible because, by definition, BRTO is via the porto-systemic collaterals from the systemic venous side and in *Type-1*, there are no porto-systemic collaterals. Any balloon obliteartion would be from the portal venous side (BATO: Balloon-occluded antegrade transvenous obliteration). In essence, Type-1b can be applied to gastric varices in the presence of splenic vein thrombosis (segmental or sentinel portal hypertension) and absence of a gastro-renal shunt (GRS). (*E*): Illustration demonstrating Type-2 ectopic varices without portal venous branch occlusion (*Type-2a*) and with portal venous branch occlusion (*Type-2b*). The portal venous branch can be any vein (location or size) in the portal circulation. BRTO of these ectopic varices (*Type-2*) is feasible because, by definition, BRTO is via the porto-systemic collaterals from the systemic venous side and in Type-2, there are rudimentary porto-systemic collaterals. Rudimentary means that it is not the main efferent outflow of the ectopic varices. The main efferent outflow of the ectopic varices in Type-2 is portal and not porto-systemic. Flow in the existing porto-systemic collaterals may be minimal and may even fluctuate. (*F*) Type-3 ectopic varices without portal venous branch occlusion (*Type-3a*) and with portal venous branch occlusion (*Type-3b*). The portal venous branch can be any vein (location or size) in the portal circulation. BRTO of these ectopic varices (Type-2) is feasible because, by definition, BRTO is via the porto-systemic collaterals from the systemic venous side and in Type-3, there are predominant porto-systemic collaterals. Predominant means that it is the main efferent outflow of the ectopic varices. The main efferent outflow of the ectopic varices in Type-3 is porto-systemic and not porto-portal. (*From* Saad WE. Vascular Anatomy and the morphologic and hemodynamic classifications of gastric varices and spontaneous portosystemic shunts relevant to the BRTO procedure. Tech Vasc Interventional Rad 2013;16:60–100; with permission.)

Table 1
Hemodynamic classification system

	Purely Portoportal Collaterals (Type 1)	Both Portoportal and Portosystemic Collaterals	
		Predominantly Portoportal Collaterals with Lesser Portosystemic Branches (Type 2)	Predominantly Portosystemic Collaterals with Lesser Portoportal Branches (Type 3)
Nonocclusive (oncotic) type (type a)	Type 1a	Type 2a	Type 3a
Occlusive type (type b)	Type 1b	Type 2b	Type 3b

The table contents (classification) is illustrated in **Fig. 5**.
From Saad WE, Lippert A, Saad NE, et al. Ectopic varices: anatomical classification, hemodynamic classification, and hemodynamic-based management. Tech Vasc Interv Radiol 2013;16:158–75; with permission.

(endoscopic or TIPS). The true gauge of success is longevity of outcome (rebleed rates). Longitudinally, gastric BRTOs in the Asian literature have recurrence rebleed rates of 0% to 10% and are commonly reported to be below 5%.[5,21,35,51–54] These outcomes are rarely, if at all, described, however, in an intent-to-treat basis specific to gastric variceal bleeding site.[55] Moreover, they commonly are not described along a particular timeline or, better yet, in a Kaplan-Meier method. When considering as an intent-to-treat basis, including technical failures, the upper gastrointestinal rebleed rate (all bleeding sources) ranges from 0% to 31.6%.[1,5,16,21–25,31–34,41–43,46,48,52,56] These studies do not clearly note whether rebleeding occurs from gastric varices versus from esophageal and duodenal varices or from portal hypertensive

Box 1
Procedure-related complications of BRTO for gastric varices

Study	Percentage (%)
Cho,[25] N = 49	
Death, 2/49	4.3%
Pulmonary embolus, 2/49	4.3%
Left renal vein thrombus, 1/49	2.2%
Hemoglobinuria, 26/49	53.1%
Spontanoeous bacterial peritonitis, 4/49	8.2%
Saad,[50] N = 39	
Partial portal vein thrombosis, 1/39	2.5%
Partial left renal vein thrombosis, 1/39	2.5%
Cardiac arrthymia, 1/39	2.5%
Pulmonary embolus, 1/39	2.5%
Jang,[63] N = 183	
Pumonary embolus, 5/183	2.7%
Left renal infarct, 1/183	0.5%
Gastrorenal shunt rupture, 1/183	0.5%
Watanabe,[71] N = 77	
Portal vein thrombosis, 3/77	3.9%
Renal vein thrombosis, 2/77	2.6%
Splenic vein thrombosis, 2/77	2.6%

Data from Refs.[25,50,63,71]

gastropathy. Three studies, evaluating a combined 141 patients, looked specifically at rates of gastric variceal recurrent bleed (3.2%–8.7%) versus global (all types/sources) variceal recurrent bleed (19%–31%) after BRTO.[21,23,24]

Due to the occlusion of the gastrorenal shunt after the BRTO procedure, blood flow is diverted back into the portal circulation and potentially into the liver; there is a favorable significant reduction in hepatic encephalopathy in most, if not all, patients treated with BRTO. Most of the studies evaluating hepatic encephalopathy after BRTO from Asia are retrospective, however, and thus do not have pre- and postprocedural objective criteria for assessing improvement of hepatic encephalopathy. In recent years, BRTO has become a reliable method for treating encephalopathy refractory to medical management. Complete obliteration of spontaneous gastrorenal shunt in these patients with portosystemic encephalopathy results in enhanced ammonia detoxification from the liver. Several studies have shown immediate reduction or complete resolution of encephalopathy in patients with portosystemic shunt encephalopathy.[5,16,36,46,61,62] Even with partial BRTO obliteration, the plasma ammonia levels significantly decrease after 24 to 48 hours. Six of seven patients with West Haven Criteria hepatic encephalopathy grades II and III were shown in 1 study to be completely resolved of symptoms at 1 and 4 months post-BRTO.[62]

Aside from gastric variceal bleeding, there are other outcomes (favorable or detrimental) that are encountered after the BRTO procedure that are based on hemodynamic pathogenesis.[55,60] Due to the loss of the spontaneous portosystemic shunt (occlusion/obliteration of the gastrorenal shunt) as a consequence of the BRTO procedure, the portal blood flow that had previously (pre-BRTO) been shunted into the systemic circulation is redirected back into the portal circulation and potentially toward the liver.[9,50] The loss of shunting and increased portal flow can reduce the risk of hepatic encephalopathy and may improve it and additionally may augment the trophoblastic nature of the portal venous flow improving, if not preserving, the hepatic synthetic function.[60] Unfortunately, diverting this portal blood flow into the portal circulation also increases the portal pressure and this can manifest in new-onset or worsening esophageal variceal bleeding (discussed previously) and/or hepatic hydrothorax and/or ascites.[50,55] In the author's opinion unfavorable outcomes after shunt loss are associated with portal pressure, and favorable outcomes after shunt loss are associated with portal blood flow.[9,50,55] It can be argued that ascites and hepatic hydrothorax are a consequence of worsening hepatic function and not related to oncotic causes; however, they usually occur in the presence of improved hepatic synthetic function.[9,50,55] Moreover, the importance of how much blood flow is directed back into the circulation (based on the original size of the gastric variceal system and how much it originally shunted portosystemically before BRTO) is emphasized (discussed previously).[9,50] Unfortunately, the cause and effect may not correlate that simply. There are other variables that temper the portal pressure and possibly the portal flow. These include the compliance of the splenic and portal vein, the compliance of the hepatic parenchyma, and the presence (or speed of development) and size of other portosystemic escape routes (shunting), such as esophageal varices. Maybe the most important factor that is difficult to predict and gauge is how this cirrhotic liver will respond to this excess antegrade portal flow. Will it rise to the occasion and drop its resistance (Does it have reserve?) and take the additional portal flow, or will it not?

Four studies evaluating 160 patients with repeated endoscopy over a 3-year period after BRTO reported 1-, 2-, and 3-year aggravation of esophageal varices rates of 27% to 35%, 45% to 66%, and 45% to 91%, respectively.[16,22,35,45] A large retrospective study of 177 patients undergoing BRTO found that new esophageal varices appeared in greater than 50% of patients who had no esophageal varices prior to BRTO. In addition, aggravation of esophageal varices was noted in approximately one-third of patients with preexisting esophageal varices.[63] Routine upper endoscopy is encouraged in regular intervals post-BRTO at which time band ligation may be required and even preemptive management prior to BRTO is advised (discussed later).[3] Two studies evaluating 117 patients found that bleeding from esophageal varices occurred in 36% to 57% of those patients who developed aggravation of esophageal varices after BRTO.[23,56]

Kaplan-Meier survival rates after BRTO range from 83% to 98% at 1 year, 76% to 79% at 2 years, 66% to 85% at 3 years, and 36% to 69% at 5 years.[5,31,35,39,44–46] Hepatic synthetic reserve is thought to be the most important prognostic factor for survival after BRTO. The presence of hepatocelluar carcinoma is considered the second most important prognostic factor.[55,64]

Ascites and hepatic hydrothorax have been reported after BRTO despite transient improvement or preservation of hepatic function. Several studies report these complications occurring within 30 to 60 days after BRTO in up to 8% of patients.[42,47,54] Massive or medically refractory ascites develops in up to 2.6% of patients and up to 5.8% of patients develop refractory hydrothorax. Investigators refer to a majority of these complications as transient but this is not supported by clear data in their studies. None of these findings is presented with clear definitions gauging significance or along particular timelines within the Asian literature[42,47,54] (discussed later).

There is controversy in the Asian literature whether BRTO improves, transiently improves, or just preserves the hepatic synthetic function/hepatic reserve.[16,39,54] The assessment of hepatic reserve in the Asian literature is based on the Child-Pugh score. All investigators agree that BRTO does not worsen the hepatic synesthetic function when looking at study cohorts as a whole.[16,39,54] Of those studies that show improvement in hepatic synthetic function, it is believed that the improvement in hepatic function is probably transient, reaching its maximal improvement effect at 3 to 6 months and returning to baseline pre-BRTO hepatic function within 9 months after BRTO.[16,39,54] The Child-Pugh score, however, includes ascites/hydrothorax, which occasionally increases after BRTO and potentially may mask the improvement in laboratory liver function tests. As a result, the Model for End-Stage Liver Disease (MELD) score may be a more sensitive indicator of hepatic reserve after BRTO[60] (discussed later).

OUTCOMES OF BRTO-ONLY FOR THE MANAGEMENT OF GASTRIC VARICES IN AMERICAN INSTITUTIONS

In 2012, the American College of Radiology Appropriateness Criteria Expert Panel on Interventional Radiology described BRTO for the management of gastric varices as a "viable alternative to TIPS in certain anatomic and medical conditions."[65] It did not, however, define these conditions.[65] BRTO in the United States is considerably different from BRTO in Japan. There are particular challenges that are unique to the United States, including differences in inventory and medical culture. Moreover, Japanese operators and the author anecdotally agree that the size of gastric varices and associated shunting in patients encountered in the United States is considerably larger in the United States, posing a particular challenge to balloon-size measurement and the ability to adequately occlude the shunts to achieve blood flow stasis. Moreover, there are no balloon occlusion catheters in the United States that are purposefully designed for BRTO of gastric varices, unlike in Asia. In addition, the United States does not have ethanolamine oleate in high concentrations nor its antidote, haptoglobin, which are readily available in Asia. In the United States, the most common sclerosing agent is 3% sodium tetradecyl sulfate (STS)[17,20,66] and American interventionalists have to make do with general-purpose balloon occlusion catheters. From a medical culture standpoint, performing the procedure (with a learning curve because the procedure is novel in this anatomic setting in the United States), then waiting for 4 to 12 hours for balloon and sclerosant dwell times, and then returning the patient to the angiography suite for balloon deflation is taxing to hospital resources and personnel, particularly when an alternative procedure (TIPS) or endoscopic therapy with cyanoacrylate is readily available, established over years, and does not require hours of intensive care. The patient would have an indwelling balloon occlusion catheter and sheath in the dwell period, thus a taxation for the hospital resources.[66] Despite these obstacles and challenges to medical culture, the practice of BRTO in the United States is growing significantly.[8]

The intent-to-treat (technical failures included) rebleeding rates after BRTO using 3% STS from gastric varices (in 30 consecutive patients) at 3, 6, 12, and 24 months were 5%, 5%, 5%, and 5%, respectively, due to one technical failure which led to continued bleeding from gastric varices.[50] Of the technically successful BRTOs (90%, n = 27/30), there was only 1 rebleed occurring 33 months after the procedure, which did not affect the 24-month Kaplan-Meier rebleed analysis.[50] No bleed from esophageal varices occurred after BRTO in the study period, giving an overall variceal rebleed rate (from any type of variceal source: gastric, esophageal, or ectopic) to be no different from the gastric variceal bleeding rate written immediately above. The overall upper gastrointestinal tract rebleed rates from all upper gastrointestinal tract sources and pathologies, however, at 3, 6, 12, and 24 months were 9%, 9%, 9%, and 21%, respectively. These sources and pathologies included portal hypertensive gastropathy and peptic ulcer disease that had no clinical consequences and were treated conservatively.[50] Patient survival rates, with a mean MELD score of all patients undergoing BRTO-only of 13 ± 4.2 (range 7–30), at 6, 9, and 12 months were 88%, 88%, and 88%, respectively.[50] An important distinction in this study was that BRTO was performed electively and without active gastric variceal bleeding. Anecdotally, this is an anomaly in the practice of BRTO in the United States. In other institutions in the United Sates, a majority of BRTOs are performed emergently for active bleeding. The explanation for the lack of esophageal variceal bleeding after BRTO was a hypervigilant and aggressive gastroenterology service that went to the length of preemptive banding of esophageal varices in preparation for the BRTO procedure.[50] Details of the pre-BRTO and post-BRTO imaging and clinical preparation and follow-up with management are beyond the scope of this article but are detailed in the article by Saad and coworkers.[3]

The rate of new-onset or worsening ascites and/or hydrothorax after BRTO is subject to definitions.[50] Any form of ascites, even detected by imaging, only occurs in 33% of patients post-BRTO and occurs at a mean interval of 4.6 months ± 6.0.[50] The ascites and/or hydrothorax (regardless of significance, discussed later) free rates at 3, 6, 12, and 24 months after the BRTO procedure were 87%, 58%, 43%, and 29%, respectively[50]: 44% of patients who developed worsening ascites were diagnosed within 30 days of the BRTO procedure and only 25% of them had transient self-limiting ascites; 25% had progressive ascites reaching clinical significance requiring parathentesis 8.0 months after the BRTO; the remaining 50% early (within 30 days from BRTO) were stable for 5 months; 44% of patients with new-onset or worsening ascites after BRTO had mild–moderate ascites that was subclinical (detected by imaging only); 22% had symptomatic ascites not requiring a procedure; and 33% of patients had clinically significant ascites requiring a procedure (paracentesis and/or TIPS).[50]

Saad and coworkers have described evaluating the effect of BRTO on the MELD score rather than relying on the Child-Pugh score, which considers ascites a means of differentiating complications that are oncotic driven from those related to hepatic synthetic dysfunction.[60] In their retrospective study of 26 patients undergoing technically successful BRTO procedures, they found a positive effect on hepatic reserve from 1.5 to 4 months after BRTO. Specifically, serum bilirubin and international normalized ratio were found to drop significantly below preprocedural baseline levels.[60] No significant changes in serum creatinine were observed in the 4-month study period (the baseline creatinine was normal).[60] These improved markers of hepatic synthetic function/components of the MELD score decreased MELD scores. Child-Pugh scores did not improve despite significant increases in serum albumin levels during the 1- to 4-month study period because of the onset of ascites in 31% of patients (n = 8/26 patients). The single predictor of improved MELD score after BRTO was a pre-BRTO MELD of less than 14.[60] In other words, people with relatively preserved hepatic function (Child-Pugh A or MELD <14) were more likely to further improve their hepatic synthetic function compared with patients with relatively worse hepatic function (MELD >14, probably Child-Pugh B and C).[60]

OUTCOMES OF TIPS-ONLY FOR THE MANAGEMENT OF GASTRIC VARICES

The literature addressing the management of gastric varices utilizing TIPS is scant, with limited sample sizes and emanates from Japan, Korea, and the United States. Unfortunately, variceal bleeding sources (esophageal and/or ectopic/gastric) are commonly amalgamated in the literature.[9] There are 7 studies addressing this subject. Six of these studies involve TIPSs created by bare stents and not covered stents. Only 1 study had a short-term (6–12 month) follow-up of patients undergoing TIPS for gastric varices with TIPSs created by covered stents.[67] In 2 studies using bare stents before the year 2000 (60 patients total), the 6-month and 12-month rebleed rates were 26% to 29% and 31%, respectively.[9,46,68] In the 4 studies published after the year 2000 (87 patients total), the 12- and 24-month gastric variceal rebleed rate at 12 to 24 months was 11% to 20%.[9,21,69,70] The only study (n = 27) of patients undergoing TIPS for gastric varices using covered stents had a gastric variceal rebleed rate of 10% to 11% at 6 to 12 months.[67] Three of these retrospective studies had an intrainstitutional comparison for bleeding outcomes with patients who underwent BRTO-only. One had a small sample size for any statistical comparative analysis (TIPSs: 13, BRTO: 8), and the other demonstrated a rebleed rate and hepatic encephalopathy rate in favor of BRTO (gastric variceal rebleed rate 15% vs 0% and hepatic encephalopathy rate of 31% vs 0%).[9,21] The study by Sabri and coworkers using covered stents for TIPSs did not show a statistical significance for rebleeding over a 6- to 12-month period (TIPSs: 10%–11% vs BRTO: 0%).[67]

OUTCOMES OF COMBINING TIPS WITH BRTO FOR THE MANAGEMENT OF GASTRIC VARICES

The combination therapy of TIPS and BRTO is an interesting approach and possibly a middle ground for the debate of TIPS versus BRTO. Unfortunately, the literature presents 1 study with a small sample size comparing outcomes of patients undergoing BRTO-only (BRTO + TIPS: 9 and BRTO-only: 27).[50] Patients with both TIPS and BRTO pose a unique hemodynamic entity. In theory, the increased portal pressure burden to the liver and portal circulation could be buffered by the TIPS, which might be an ideal situation, replacing the lost/occluded spontaneous portosystemic shunt (gastrorenal shunt) after BRTO with an artificial portosystemic shunt (TIPS).[50] In this retrospective study, patients were placed into 2 groups, BRTO alone and BRTO + TIPS. Two patients in the BRTO + TIPS group had combined procedures (performed concomitantly in the same procedural setting) whereas the other 7 had BRTO in the setting of preexisting TIPS (average 4.9 months, range 0–14 months). One-year survival in both groups was similar. No patients in the BRTO + TIPS group experienced recurrent variceal bleeding. Recurrent bleeding for the BRTO-only group at 3, 6, 12, and 24 months was 5% ($P<.03$).[50] Moreover, ascites and/or hydrothorax did not occur in the BRTO + TIPS group (100% ascites-free rate 3–24 months post-BRTO) whereas the ascites and/or hydrothorax free rates for BRTO alone at 3, 6, 12, and 24 months were 87%, 58%, 43%, and 29%, respectively ($P = .01$), which seems to demonstrate a protective role for TIPS against the development of ascites and/or hydrothorax after BRTO and suggests that if refractory ascites or hydrothorax develops after BRTO, TIPS may prove beneficial.[50]

SUMMARY

The management of gastric varices is largely uncharted. BRTO for the management of gastric varices is safe and effective and thus is a viable management option for this difficult clinical setting. When the BRTO procedure should be considered an alternative or an augment to TIPS or other treatment options requires further clinical research. The stage is not yet reached where patients (stratified according to clinical presentation, endoscopic and/or vascular classifications, hepatic reserve, and comorbidities) undergo treatments that are tailored to their needs and based on evidence-based medicine. A more contemporary management approach to addressing this clinical condition is required to achieve this. It is the hope that this stage can be achieved with more meaningful and collaborative research for the betterment of patients' health.

REFERENCES

1. Sarin SK, Lahoti D, Saxena SP, et al. Prevalence, classification and natural history of gastric varices: a long term follow-up study in 568 portal hypertension patients. Hepatology 1992;16(6):1343–9.
2. Ryan BM, Stockbrugger RW, Ryan JM. A pathophysiologic, gastroenterologic, and radiologic approach to the management of gastric varices. Gastroenterology 2004;126:1175–89.
3. Saad WE, Al-Osaimi AM, Caldwell SH. Pre- and post-balloon-occluded retrograde transvenous obliteration clinical evaluation, management, and imaging: indications, management protocols and follow-up. Tech Vasc Interv Radiol 2012;15:165–202.
4. Sarin SK, Agarwal SR. Gastric varices and portal hypertensive gastropathy. Clin Liver Dis 2001;5:727–67.
5. Hirota S, Matsumoto S, Tomita M, et al. Retrograde transvenous obliteration of gastric varices. Radiology 1999;211(2):349–56.
6. Kiyosue H, Mori H, Matumoto S, et al. Transcatheter obliteration of gastric varices. Part 1. Anatomic classification. Radiographics 2003;23(4):911–20.
7. Kiyosue H, Mori H, Matsumoto S, et al. Transcatheter obliteration of gastric varices. Part 2. Strategy and techniques based on hemodynamic features. Radiographics 2003;23(4):921–37.
8. Saad WE. The history and evolution of balloon-occluded retrograde tranvenous obliteration (BRTO): from the United States to Japan and back. Semin Intervent Radiol 2011;28:283–7.

9. Saad WE, Darcy MD. Transjugular intrahepatic portosystemic shunt (TIPS) versus balloon-occluded retrograde transvenous obliteration (BRTO) for the management of gastric varices. Semin Intervent Radiol 2011;28:339–49.

10. Saad WE, Anderson CL, Patel RS, et al. Management of gastric varices in the pediatric population with balloon-occluded retrograde tranvenousobliteration (BRTO) utilizing sodium tetradecyl sulfate foamsclerosis with or without partial splenic artery embolization. Cardiovasc Intervent Radiol 2014. [Epub ahead of print].

11. Yoshimatsu R, Yamagami T, Tanaka O, et al. Hemodynamic changes after balloon occlusion of the splenic artery during balloon-occluded retrograde transvenous obliteration for gastric varices. J Vasc Interv Radiol 2012;23:1207–12.

12. Kiyosue H, Tanoue S, Kondo Y, et al. Balloon-occluded retrograde transvenous obliteration of complex gastric varices assisted by temporary balloon occlusion of the splenic artery. J Vasc Interv Radiol 2011;22:1045–8.

13. Saad WE. Vascular anatomy and the morphological and hemodynamic classifications of gastric varices and spontaneous portosystemic shunts relevant to the BRTO procedure. Tech Vasc Interv Radiol 2013;16(2):60–100.

14. Saad WE, Lippert A, Saad NE, et al. Ectopic varices: anatomical classification, hemodynamic classification, and hemodynamic-based management. Tech Vasc Interv Radiol 2013;16:158–75.

15. Saad WE. Portosystemic shunt syndrome and the management of hepatic encephalopathy. Semin Intervent Radiol 2014;31(3):262–5.

16. Kumamoto M, Toyonaga A, Inoue H, et al. Long-term results of balloon-occluded retrograde transvenous obliteration for gastric fundal varices: hepatic deterioration links to portosystemic shunt syndrome. J Gastroenterol Hepatol 2010;25(6):1129–35.

17. Saad WE, Hirota S, Kitanosono T. The Conventional Balloon-occluded Retrograde Transvenous Obliteration (BRTO) Procedure: Indications, Contraindications and Technical Applications. Tech Vasc Interv Radiol 2013;16(2):101–5.

18. Saad WE, Schwaner S, Lippert A, et al. Management of stomalvarices with transvenous obliteration utilizing sodium tetradecyl sulfate foam sclerosis. Cardiovasc Intervent Radiol 2014. [Epub ahead of print].

19. Saad WE, Sze DH. Variations of balloon-occluded transvenous obliteration (BRTO): balloon-occluded antegradetransvenous obliteration (BATO) and alternative/adjunctive routes for BRTO. Semin Intervent Radiol 2011;28:314–24.

20. Saad WE, Nicholson D, Koizumi J. Inventory used for balloon-occluded retrograde (BRTO) and antegrade (BATO) tranvenous obliteration (BRTO) inventory: sclerosants and balloon-occlusion devices. Tech Vasc Interv Radiol 2012;15:226–40.

21. Kitamoto M, Imamura M, Kamada K, et al. Balloon-occluded retrograde transvenous obliteration of gastric fundal varices with hemorrhage. AJR Am J Roentgenol 2002;178(5):1167–74.

22. Ibukuro K, Sugihara T, Tanaka R, et al. Balloon-occluded retrograde transvenous obliteration (BRTO) for a direct shunt between the inferior mesenteric vein and the inferior vena cava in a patient with hepatic encephalopathy. J Vasc Interv Radiol 2007;18(1 Pt 1):121–5.

23. Ninoi T, Nishida N, Kaminou T, et al. Balloon-occluded retrograde transvenous obliteration of gastric varices with gastrorenal shunt: long-term follow-up in 78 patients. AJR Am J Roentgenol 2005;184(4):1340–6.

24. Akahoshi T, Hashizume M, Tomikawa M, et al. Long-term results of balloon-occluded retrograde transvenous obliteration for gastric variceal bleeding and risky gastric varices: a 10-year experience. J Gastroenterol Hepatol 2008;23(11):1702–9.

25. Cho SK, Shin SW, Lee IH, et al. Balloon-occluded retrograde transvenous obliteration of gastric varices: outcomes and complications in 49 patients. AJR Am J Roentgenol 2007;189(6):W365–72.

26. deFranchis R, Primignani M. Natural history of portal hypertension in patients with cirrhosis. Clin Liver Dis 2001;5(3):645–63.

27. Hayashi S, Saeki S, Hosoi H, et al. A clinical and portal hemodynamic analysis for obliteration of gastric-renal shunt communicated with gastric fundicvarices. Nippon Shokakibyo Gakkai Zasshi 1998;95(7):755–63.

28. Tanihata H, Minamiguchi H, Sato M, et al. Changes in portal systemic pressure gradient after balloon-occluded retrograde transvenous obliteration of gastric varices and aggravation of esophageal varices. Cardiovasc Intervent Radiol 2009;32(6):1209–16.

29. Choi YS, Lee JH, Sinn DH, et al. Effect of balloon-occluded retrograde transvenous obliteration on the natural history of coexisting esophageal varices. J Clin Gastroenterol 2008;42(9):974–9.

30. Nakamura S, Torii N, Yatsuji S, et al. Long-term follow up of esophageal varices after balloon-occluded retrograde transvenous obliteration for gastric varices. Hepatol Res 2008;38(4):340–7.

31. Yamagami T, Kato T, Hirota T, et al. Infusion of 50% glucose solution before injection of ethanolamine oleate during balloon-occluded retrograde transvenous obliteration. Australas Radiol 2007;51(4):334–8.

32. Ninoi T, Nakamura K, Kaminou T, et al. TIPS versus transcathetersclerotherapy for gastric varices. AJR Am J Roentgenol 2004;183(2):369–76.

33. Sonomura T, Sato M, Kishi K, et al. Balloon-occluded retrograde transvenous obliteration for gastric varices: a feasibility study. Cardiovasc Intervent Radiol 1998;21(1):27–30.

34. Kiyosue H, Matsumoto S, Onishi R, et al. Balloon-occluded retrograde transvenous obliteration (B-RTO) for gastric varices: therapeutic results and problems. Nippon Igaku Hoshasen Gakkai Zasshi 1999;59(1):12–9.

35. Koito K, Namieno T, Nagakawa T, et al. Balloon-occluded retrograde transvenous obliteration for gastric varices with gastrorenal or gastrocaval collaterals. AJR Am J Roentgenol 1996;167(5):1317–20.

36. Chikamori F, Kuniyoshi N, Kawashima T, et al. Gastric varices with gastrorenal shunt: combined therapy using transjugular retrograde obliteration and partial splenic embolization. AJR Am J Roentgenol 2008;191(2):555–9.

37. Chikamori F, Kuniyoshi N, Shibuya S, et al. Transjugular retrograde obliteration for chronic portosystemic encephalopathy. Abdom Imaging 2000;25(6):567–71.

38. Chikamori F, Kuniyoshi N, Shibuya S, et al. Combination treatment of transjugular retrograde obliteration and endoscopic embolization for portosystemic encephalopathy with esophageal varices. Hepatogastroenterology 2004;51(59):1379–81.

39. Miyamoto Y, Oho K, Kumamoto M, et al. Balloon-occluded retrograde transvenous obliteration improves liver function in patients with cirrhosis and portal hypertension. J Gastroenterol Hepatol 2003;18(8):934–42.

40. Sugimori K, Morimoto M, Shirato K, et al. Retrograde transvenous obliteration of gastric varices associated with large collateral veins or a large gastrorenal shunt. J Vasc Interv Radiol 2005;16(1):113–8.

41. Fukuda T, Hirota S, Matsumoto S, et al. Application of balloon-occluded retrograde transvenous obliteration to gastric varices complicating refractory ascites. Cardiovasc Intervent Radiol 2004;27(1):64–7.

42. Shimoda R, Horiuchi K, Hagiwara S, et al. Short-term complications of retrograde transvenous obliteration of gastric varices in patients with portal hypertension: effects of obliteration of major portosystemic shunts. Abdom Imaging 2005;30(3):306–13.

43. Takuma Y, Nouso K, Makino Y, et al. Prophylactic balloon-occluded retrograde transvenous obliteration for gastric varices in compensated cirrhosis. Clin Gastroenterol Hepatol 2005;3(12):1245–52.

44. Arai H, Abe T, Takagi H, et al. Efficacy of balloon-occluded retrograde transvenous obliteration, percutaneous transhepatic obliteration and combined techniques for the management of gastric fundal varices. World J Gastroenterol 2006;12(24):3866–73.

45. Arai H, Abe T, Shimoda R, et al. Emergency balloon-occluded retrograde transvenous obliteration for gastric varices. J Gastroenterol 2005;40(10):964–71.

46. Choi YH, Yoon CJ, Park JH, et al. Balloon-occluded retrograde transvenous obliteration for gastric variceal bleeding: its feasibility compared with transjugular intrahepatic portosystemic shunt. Korean J Radiol 2003;4(2):109–16.

47. Park KS, Kim YH, Choi JS, et al. Therapeutic efficacy of balloon-occluded retrograde transvenous obliteration in patients with gastric variceal bleeding. Korean J Gastroenterol 2006;47(5):370–8.

48. Kim ES, Park SY, Kwon KT, et al. The clinical usefulness of balloon occluded retrograde transvenous obliteration in gastric variceal bleeding. Taehan Kan Hakhoe Chi 2003;9(4):315–23.

49. Matsumoto A, Hamamoto N, Nomura T, et al. Balloon-occluded retrograde transvenous obliteration of high risk gastric fundal varices. Am J Gastroenterol 1999;94(3):643–9.

50. Saad WE, Wagner C, Lippert A, et al. Protective value of TIPS against the development of acites and/or bleeding after balloon-oclluded reytrograde transvenous obliteration of gastric varices. Am J Gastroenterol 2013;108:1612–9.

51. Kanagawa H, Mima S, Kouyama H, et al. Treatment of gastric fundal varices by balloon-occluded retrograde transvenous obliteration. J Gastroenterol Hepatol 1996;11(1):51–8.

52. Fukuda T, Hirota S, Sugimura K. Long-term results of balloonoccluded retrograde transvenous obliteration for the treatment of gastric varices and hepatic encephalopathy. J Vasc Interv Radiol 2001;12(3):327–36.

53. Akahane T, Iwasaki T, Kobayashi N, et al. Changes in liver function parameters after occlusion of gastrorenal shunts with balloon-occluded retrograde transvenous obliteration. Am J Gastroenterol 1997;92(6):1026–30.

54. Chikamori F, Kuniyoshi N, Shibuya S, et al. Eight years of experience with transjugular retrograde obliteration for gastric varices with gastrorenal shunts. Surgery 2001;129(4):414–20.

55. Saad WE, Sabri SS. Balloon-occluded retrograde transvenous obliteration (BRTO): technical results and outcomes. Semin Intervent Radiol 2011;28:333–8.

56. Hong CH, Kim HJ, Park JH, et al. Treatment of patients with gastric variceal hemorrhage: endoscopic N-butyl-2-cyanoacrylate injection versus balloon-occluded retrograde transvenous obliteration. J Gastroenterol Hepatol 2009; 24(3):372–8.

57. Park SJ, Chung JW, Kim HC, et al. The prevalence, risk factors, and clinical outcome of balloon rupture in balloon–occluded retrograde transvenous obliteration of gastric varices. J Vasc Interv Radiol 2010;21(4):503–7.

58. Saad WE, Nicholson D, Lippert A, et al. Balloon–occlusion catheter rupture during balloon-occluded retrograde transvenous obliteration of gastric varices

utilizing sodium tetradecyl sulfate: incidence and consequences. Vasc Endo-vascular Surg 2012;46(8):664–70.

59. Patel A, Fischamn A, Saad WE. Balloon-occluded obliteration of gastric varices. Am J Roentgenol 2012;199:721–9. http://dx.doi.org/10.2214/AJR.12.9052.

60. Saad WE, Wagner C, Al-Osaimi A, et al. The effect of balloon-ocludedtransvenous obliteration of gastric varices and gastrorenal shunts on the hepatic synthetic fun-citon: a comparison between child-pugh and model for end-stage liver disease scores. Vasc Endovascular Surg 2013;47(4):281–7.

61. Araki T, Hori M, Motosugi U, et al. Can Balloon –occluded retrograde transve-nous obliteration be performed for gastric varices without gastrorenal shunts? J Vasc Interv Radiol 2010;21(5):663–70.

62. Kato T, Uematsu T, Nishigaki Y, et al. Therapeutic effects of BRTO on portal –sys-temic encephalopathy in patietns with liver cirrhosis. Intern Med 2001;40:688–91.

63. Jang SY, Kim GH, Park SY, et al. Clinical outcomes of balloon-occluded retro-grade transvenous obliteration for the treatment of gastric variceal hemorrhage in Korean patients with Liver Cirrhosis: a retrospective multicenter study. Clin Mol Hepatol 2012;18:368–74.

64. Saad WE, Bleibel W, Adenaw N, et al. Thrombocytopenia in patients with gastric varices and the effect of balloon-occluded retrograde transvenous obliteration on the platelet count. J Clin Imaging Sci 2014;30:24.

65. Saad WE, Al-Osaimi AM, Caldwell S, et al, for the Expert Panel on Interventional Radiology for the American College of Radiology. ACR appropriateness criteria(r): radiologic management of gastric varices. Available at: http://www.acr. org/~/media/ACR/Documents/AppCriteria/Interventional/RadiologicManagement GastricVarices.pdf. Accessed July 23, 2012.

66. Saad WE, Nicholson DB. Optimizing logistics for balloon-occluded retrograde transvenous obliteration (BRTO) of gastric varices by doing away with the indwelling balloon: concept and techniques. Tech Vasc Interv Radiol 2013;16: 152–7.

67. Sabri SS, Abi-Jaoudeh N, Swee W, et al. Short-term rebleeding rate for isolated gastric varices managed by transjugular intrahepatic shunt versus balloon-occluded retrograde transvenous obliteration. J Vasc Interv Radiol 2014;25:355–61.

68. Chau TN, Patch D, Chan YW, et al. "Salvage" transjugular intrahepatic portosys-temic shunts: gastric fundal compared with esophageal variceal bleeding. Gastroenterology 1998;114:981–7.

69. Barange K, Peron JM, Imani K, et al. Transjugular intrahepatic portosystemic shunt in the treatment of refractory bleeding from ruptured gastric varices. Hep-atology 1999;30:1139–43.

70. Lo GH, Liang HL, Chen WC, et al. A prospective randomized controlled trial of transjugular intrahepatic portosystemic shunt versus cyanoacrylate injection in the prevention of gastric varicealrebleeding. Endoscopy 2007;39:679–85.

71. Watanabe M, Shiozawa K, Ikehara T, et al. Short-term effects and early com-plications of balloon-occluded retrograde transvenous obliteration for gastric varices. ISNR Gastroenterol 2012. [Epub ahead of print].

Transjugular Intrahepatic Portosystemic Shunt

Kavish R. Patidar, DO[a], Malcolm Sydnor, MD[b,c,d], Arun J. Sanyal, MD[e,*]

KEYWORDS

- Transjugular intrahepatic portosystemic shunt • Esophageal varices • Ascites
- Hepatic hydrothorax • Hepatorenal syndrome • Hepatopulmonary syndrome
- Venoocclusive disease • Budd-Chiari syndrome

KEY POINTS

- The largest body of evidence supports the use of transjugular intrahepatic portosystemic shunt (TIPS) in recurrent or refractory esophageal variceal bleeding followed by refractory ascites. Its use may also be beneficial for other conditions, including hepatic hydrothorax, Budd-Chiari syndrome, Hepatorenal syndrome, and Hepatopulmonary syndrome.
- Contraindications for TIPS placement include systolic and diastolic cardiac disease, severe pulmonary hypertension, and primary prevention of variceal bleed.
- Numerous innovative supporting techniques have evolved over recent years to address problematic anatomy, improve the safety profile of the procedure, and to improve outcomes.

INTRODUCTION

Portal hypertension is one of the major complications of cirrhosis. It results from increased intrahepatic resistance and increased splanchnic blood flow leading to a hyperdynamic circulatory state. The transjugular intrahepatic portosystemic shunt (TIPS) has been an established procedure in the treatment of the complications of portal hypertension, including bleeding esophageal varices; refractory cirrhotic ascites; hepatic hydrothorax; hepatorenal syndrome (HRS) and hepatopulmonary syndrome

Funding Sources: T32 training grant (Dr A.J. Sanyal); none (Dr M. Sydnor, Dr K.R. Patidar). Conflicts of Interest: See last page of the article (Dr A.J. Sanyal); none (Dr A.J. Sydnor, Dr K.R. Patidar).

[a] Department of Internal Medicine, Virginia Commonwealth University Hospital, 1200 East Broad Street, MCV Box 980342, Richmond, VA 23298-0342, USA; [b] Radiology, Virginia Commonwealth University Hospital, 1200 East Broad Street, MCV Box 980615, Richmond, VA 23298-0615, USA; [c] Surgery, Virginia Commonwealth University Hospital, 1200 East Broad Street, Richmond, VA 23298, USA; [d] Vascular Interventional Radiology, Virginia Commonwealth University Hospital, 1200 East Broad Street, Richmond, VA 23298, USA; [e] Division of Gastroenterology, Department of Internal Medicine, Virginia Commonwealth University School of Medicine, 1200 East Broad Street, MCV Box 980342, Richmond, VA 23298-0342, USA
* Corresponding author.
E-mail address: asanyal@mcvh-vcu.edu

Clin Liver Dis 18 (2014) 853–876
http://dx.doi.org/10.1016/j.cld.2014.07.006
1089-3261/14/$ – see front matter © 2014 Elsevier Inc. All rights reserved.

(HPS); and, more recently, Budd-Chiari syndrome (BCS) and venoocclusive disease. However, despite these broad applications, refractory acute variceal hemorrhage and control of refractory cirrhotic ascites are the only 2 indications subjected to numerous controlled trials.

The TIPS procedure, first described by Rosch and colleagues[1] in 1979, is a percutaneous image-guided procedure in which a tract or conduit is constructed within the liver between the systemic venous system and portal system with an intent for portal decompression (**Fig. 1**).[2] The most common conduit is between the right hepatic vein (HV) and the right portal vein (PV). Patency was originally achieved by bare metal stents. The advent of polytetrafluoroethylene (PTFE)–covered stents in recent years has dramatically improved patency rates[3] and are preferred over bare metal stents.[4]

In this section, the authors review the indications, recommended patient selection, postoperative care, common complications, and clinical outcomes related to the TIPS procedure. They also provide a detailed stepwise technique to the TIPS procedure as well as a description on advanced TIPS techniques.

INDICATIONS FOR TRANSJUGULAR INTRAHEPATIC PORTOSYSTEMIC SHUNT CREATION

TIPS reduces the portosystemic pressure gradient by shunting of blood from the PV to the HV. Its creation successfully reduces the portosystemic pressure gradient in more than 90% of cases.[5–11] Indications for TIPS are summarized in **Table 1**.

Primary Prevention of Variceal Hemorrhage

The development of esophageal varices is a common complication of portal hypertension, with subsequent hemorrhage representing a major cause of morbidity and mortality in patients with cirrhosis.[56,57] The highest rate of development occurs in Child–Turcotte–Pugh (CTP) class B and C disease,[58] with an increasing risk for hemorrhage occurring in larger varices (5% for small varices and 15% for large varices[59]), appearance of red-whale marks,[11] and severity of disease (CTP class B and C). Currently, beta-blockers and endoscopic variceal ligation (EVL) are considered the best

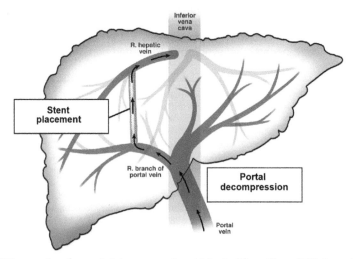

Fig. 1. TIPS procedure for portal decompression. (*Adapted from* Bhogal HK, Sanyal AJ. Using transjugular intrahepatic portosystemic shunts for complications of cirrhosis. Clin Gastroenterol Hepatol 2011;9(11):937; with permission.)

Table 1
Indications for TIPS

Indication	References
Refractory or recurrent esophageal variceal hemorrhage[a]	4,7–9,12–19
Refractory ascites[a]	20–25
Acute esophageal variceal bleeding	26,27
HRS (types 1 and 2)	28–31
Refractory bleeding gastric varices	32–36
Portal hypertensive gastropathy	37,38
Hepatic hydrothorax	39–45
HPS	46,47
BCS	48–51
Hepatic venoocclusive disease	52–55

[a] Strongest evidence for TIPS based on controlled trials.

approach for the primary prevention for variceal hemorrhage. There are no trials to date comparing TIPS with other forms of therapy for the prevention of variceal hemorrhage. Thus, in the absence of evidence in light of its risks (hepatic encephalopathy, procedural complications), TIPS is not indicated for the primary prevention for variceal hemorrhage.

Acute Variceal Bleeding

The use of TIPS in the setting of acute variceal hemorrhage is limited. In a study by Monescillo and colleagues,[60] 116 cirrhotic patients were randomized within 24 hours of acute variceal hemorrhage to either receive endoscopic sclerotherapy or the TIPS procedure based on a hepatic venous pressure gradient (HVPG) of less than 20 or more, respectively. Patients who received early TIPS were found to have reduced treatment failure rates as well as better in-hospital and 1-year survival. In a similar multicenter center study, comparing TIPS with PTFE-covered stents versus medical therapy with propranolol/nadolol and EVL, early use of TIPS (within 72 hours of randomization) was found to have lower rates of rebleeding, with 3% in the early TIPS group and 45% in the pharmacotherapy plus EVL group.[61] Furthermore, survival at 1 year was significantly better in the TIPS group at 86% versus 61% in the pharmacotherapy plus EVL group. The aforementioned studies suggest that if early risk stratification can be performed (via measurement of HVPG), early TIPS insertion could improve the overall outcomes for patients who present with an acute variceal bleed.

Refractory Acute Variceal Bleeding

Combined treatment with EVL, prophylactic antibiotics, and vasoactive drugs is the suggested standard of care for the treatment of acute esophageal bleeding.[56] Patients who survive an initial episode of variceal hemorrhage are at a high risk for rebleeding (more than 60% at 1 year[62]). Factors that contribute to recurrent hemorrhage include severity of liver disease, severity of initial hemorrhage, presence of encephalopathy, impaired renal function, and increasing age.[63–67] In addition, patients with a HVPG greater than 20 mm Hg are likely to have severe or recurrent bleeding and are more likely to fail initial medical or endoscopic therapy.[12]

Numerous randomized controlled trials have compared the use of TIPS with endoscopic therapy for refractory or recurrent variceal bleeding.[4,7–9,13–19,68] The results of multiple meta-analyses (**Table 2**[7]) of TIPS compared with various forms of endoscopic

Table 2
TIPS versus endoscopic treatment in secondary prophylaxis for variceal bleeding: results from multiple meta-analysis

	References			
Study Findings	Luca et al,[69] 1999	Papatheodoridis et al,[70] 1999	Burroughs & Vangeli,[71] 2002	Zheng et al,[72] 2008
No. of pts	750	811	948	883
No. of randomized trials	11	11	13	12
No. of TIPS	372	403	472	440
No. endoscopic therapies	378	408	476	443
Recurrent bleeding				
TIPS, No. (%)	81 (21)	76 (18.9)	88 (18.6)	86 (19)
Endoscopic therapy, No. (%)	196 (52)	190 (46.6)	210 (44.1)	194 (43.8)
NNT with TIPS	3.3	4	4	Not reported
Posttreatment encephalopathy				
TIPS, No. (%)	119 (35)	126 (34.0)	134 (28.4)	148 (33.6)
Endoscopic therapy, No. (%)	65 (19)	70 (18.7)	83 (17.3)	86 (19.4)
Mortality				
TIPS, No. (%)	109 (28)	110 (27.3)	130 (27.5)	111 (25.2)
Endoscopic therapy, No. (%)	98 (26)	108 (26.5)	118 (24.8)	98 (22.1)

Abbreviations: NNT, number needed to treat; pts, patients.

therapies have shown a significant decrease in the risk of recurrent bleeding after the insertion of TIPS. Mortality rates were found to be similar between the endoscopy and TIPS groups, though the development of posttreatment hepatic encephalopathy (HE) was almost twofold in the TIPS group.

TIPS has also been compared with pharmacotherapy[73] for the prevention of recurrent variceal hemorrhage. In a prospective, randomized controlled trial, a total of 91 cirrhotic patients (CTP B and C) who survived their first variceal hemorrhage were randomized to receive TIPS (n of 47) or pharmacotherapy (n of 44, to receive propranolol plus isosorbide-5-mononitrate). With a mean follow-up of 15 months, rebleeding rates were 39% and 17% in the pharmacotherapy and TIPS groups, respectively. Survival was the same in both groups (72%); however, the investigators noted improved CTP class in the pharmacotherapy group (72%) versus the TIPS group (45%).

Overall, many of the aforementioned trials included bare metal stents (vs PTFE-covered stents); endoscopic therapy mostly consisted of sclerotherapy (vs EVL); thus, the literature should be kept in perspective when analyzing primary and secondary outcomes. Amid the present use of PTFE-covered stents, data regarding survival, patency rates, and the development of posttreatment HE seem to be improved.[3,74–76] Furthermore, the results of a recent meta-analysis of 6 published controlled trials comparing clinical outcomes of TIPS with PTFE-covered stents versus bare metals stents showed significant improvement of primary patency rates, significant reduction in the risk of developing HE, and a significant decrease in mortality.[77]

Lastly, it is worth mentioning that TIPS has also been compared with surgical shunts in the management of recurrent variceal bleeding. In a meta-analysis including 3 prospective randomized trials and one retrospective case-controlled study, 30-day and 1-year survival were found to be the equivalent between the two groups,[26] though the 2-year survival rate was significantly better in the surgical patients with an odds ratio (OR) of 2.5. Less frequent shunt failure was also significantly reduced in the surgical patients with an OR of 0.3. However, with the use of PTFE-covered stents, the ease and efficacy of TIPS has made surgical shunts rare; there is limited expertise in the United States to perform such shunts, whereas TIPS is widely available.

Refractory Bleeding from Gastric Varices and Portal Hypertensive Gastropathy

Few studies have shown the efficacy of TIPS in refractory bleeding gastric varices.[27,32,33,78] In one series, 28 patients with gastric fundal varices unresponsive to vasoconstrictor therapy underwent emergent TIPS placement. Bleeding was controlled in most patients, comparable with the success rate for bleeding esophageal varices.[78] In another small series with 32 patients with refractory bleeding gastric varices, TIPS placement achieved homeostasis in 90% in those with active bleeding; the rebleeding rates were 14%, 26%, and 31%, respectively at 1 month, 6 months, and 1 year.[34] In addition, TIPS has also been compared with glue therapy for bleeding gastric varices.[34,35] In a prospective, randomized control trial comparing TIPS with cyanoacrylate therapy, TIPS was found to be more effective with less rebleeding rates (11%) versus the cyanoacrylate group (38%).[33] Both groups were also found to have similar survival rates and frequencies of complications. It is also important to note that another endovascular procedure, balloon-occluded retrograde transvenous obliteration for gastric varices, has recently shown promising results for refractory bleeding from gastric varices.[36]

Portal hypertensive gastropathy (PHG) is common in patients in portal hypertension, and its prevalence parallels with the severity of liver disease.[79] The diagnosis of PHG is made endoscopically with gastric mucosa having a snakeskin appearance of the fundus and body of the stomach. Although bleeding from PHG is uncommon, TIPS has been evaluated in several small studies.[37,38] In these studies, there was 75% to 90% endoscopic improvement in PHG following TIPS; one series demonstrated a decreased need for transfusions.[37]

Refractory Ascites

Management of refractory ascites includes large-volume paracentesis (LVP) and TIPS. The mechanism of action of how TIPS may improve ascites is through increased natriuresis via reductions in proximal tubular sodium reabsorption and in the renin-angiotensin-aldosterone system.[80] There have been a total of 6 randomized controlled trials comparing LVP with TIPS (**Table 3**[20–23,81,82]) involving 396 patients, of which 197 underwent TIPS. The findings from these studies have shown that TIPS improved control of ascites (range of 38%–84%, mean of 64%) versus LVP (range 0%–43%, mean of 24%). However, there were also increased rates of post-TIPS HE (range of 23%–77%, mean of 53%), with no effect on survival in 4 of the 6 studies. From the results of multiple meta-analyses,[24,25,83–85] the insertion of TIPS showed similar improvement of ascites; however, the survival benefit seemed to be inconclusive, as 3 of the 5 meta-analysis did not show improved survival.

Table 3
TIPS versus LVP in treatment of refractory ascites

Study Findings	References					
	Lebrec et al[81]	Rossle et al[82]	Gines et al[20]	Sanyal et al[21]	Salnero et al[22]	Narahara et al[23]
No. of pts	25	66	70	109	66	60
No. of TIPS pts	13	29	35	52	33	30
No. of LVP pts	12	31	35	57	33	30
Improvement of ascites						
TIPS No. (%)	5 (38)	16 (84)	18 (51)	30 (53)	26 (79)[a]	24 (80)
LVP No. (%)	0 (0)	9 (43)	6 (17)	9 (16)	14 (42)[a]	8 (27)
Survival						
TIPS (%)	29[b]	58[b]	26[b]	26	59[b]	64[b]
LVP (%)	56[b]	32[b]	30[b]	30	29[b]	35[b]
Posttreatment encephalopathy						
TIPS No. (%)	3 (23)	15 (51)	27 (77)	22 (39)	20 (61)	20 (66)
LVP No. (%)	0 (0)	11 (35)	23 (66)	13 (23)	13 (39)	5 (17)

Abbreviation: pts, patients.
[a] Defined as treatment failure, which was defined as when a patient received at least 4 LVP within 1 month for episodes of recurrent tense ascites.
[b] Transplant-free survival after 2 years.

Refractory Hepatic Hydrothorax

Hepatic hydrothorax occurs in about 6% to 10% of patients with advanced cirrhosis.[86] The treatment of hepatic hydrothorax includes medical therapy, repeated thoracentesis, chest tube placement, and diaphragmatic defect repair.[87] Refractory hepatic hydrothorax poses a significant therapeutic challenge and is limited to video-assisted thoracoscopic surgery and TIPS for those who are not transplant candidates.

TIPS has been evaluated for refractory hepatic hydrothorax in numerous small noncontrolled trials.[39–41,88–90] On the whole, 198 patients underwent TIPS, with a response rate (both complete and partial) ranging from 59% to 82%. Survival, however, could not be reliably determined given that there were no control groups and that most of the studies were retrospective studies. Nevertheless, the 30-day mortality ranged from 5% to 25%, with 2 studies[42,43] reporting a 1-year survival of 64% and 48%, respectively. In summary, given its response rate and limited therapeutic options, TIPS is an adequate management strategy for refractory hepatic hydrothorax.

Hepatopulmonary Syndrome

HPS is complication of advanced cirrhosis and is caused by the development of intrapulmonary vascular dilatation resulting in hypoxia.[42] There have been several case reports and small series of studies evaluating TIPS in HPS.[43,44] In one series, 7 patients with HPS underwent TIPS placement, of which only 1 patient had transient improvement in arterial oxygenation.[46] Thus, given the limited data available, TIPS insertion is currently not recommended for HPS.[3]

Hepatorenal Syndrome

There are 2 types of HRS, type 1 and type 2; its development confers a poor prognosis. Type 1 is a rapid, progressive decline in renal function (less than 2 weeks); type 2 is characterized as gradual decline in renal function.[45] There have been 4 small studies (n of 61) evaluating the role of TIPS in HRS.[28,46,47,91] In these studies, TIPS insertion was found to improve renal function through enhanced glomerular filtration rates and renal plasma flow as well as via reductions in serum creatinine and plasma aldosterone levels. Because none of these studies were controlled, a survival benefit cannot be fully elucidated. In the largest series,[29] the 1- and 2-year survival rates were 20% for type 1 and 70% and 45% for type 2, respectively. In addition, TIPS may have a role in maintenance therapy in patients who initially respond to vasoconstrictor therapy[31] and as a bridge to liver transplantation.[30]

Budd-Chiari Syndrome

BCS is caused by hepatic venous outflow obstruction or thrombosis HVs or hepatic portion of the inferior vena cava (IVC) leading to a clinical constellation of liver injury, abdominal pain, and ascites.[29] There have been only a small number of studies evaluating the utility of TIPS for the management of BCS.[30,31,48,92] In one of the larger series,[51] 124 patients (of which included patients with severe BCS who did not respond to medical treatment and recanalization) underwent TIPS placement. The overall 5-year survival was 84% and transplant-free survival at 1 and 5 years after TIPS was 88% and 78%, respectively.

From a technical aspect, the creation of TIPS may be difficult if the HVs are occluded. This difficulty can be overcome with a transcaval approach using ultrasound guidance through the caudate lobe with subsequent implantation of a covered stent.[51] Furthermore, a larger diameter of the shunt is recommended to allow for decompression of sinusoidal and splanchnic beds.[51] A transmesenteric approach may also be performed in this situation, but this approach is limited to few centers.[49]

Hepatic Venoocclusive Disease

Venoocclusive disease (also known as sinusoidal obstruction syndrome) is usually seen after bone marrow transplantation.[50] The disease is similar to BCS; however, hepatic venous outflow obstruction occurs at the level of the hepatic venules and sinusoids. In a limited number of patients,[51,52,93,94] TIPS insertion had shown improvement in liver disease, although it did not improve survival. Given the limited data, the value of TIPS in venoocclusive disease is unclear and should be approached on a case-by-case basis.

PATIENT SELECTION AND PRE–TRANSJUGULAR INTRAHEPATIC PORTOSYSTEMIC SHUNT EVALUATION

Patients who are being considered for a TIPS procedure should be under the care of a gastroenterologist or hepatologist with consultation from interventional radiology. Absolute and relative contraindications[3] are listed in **Box 1**. Absolute contraindications include heart failure, severe tricuspid regurgitation, and severe pulmonary hypertension (mean pulmonary wedge pressure >45 mm Hg). Relative contraindications include anatomic issues that can complicate the creation of the shunt or reduce technical success (ie, obstruction of HVs, PV thrombosis, hepatic masses, hepatic cysts),

Box 1	
Contraindications for TIPS	
Relative	**Absolute**
Hepatocellular carcinoma, especially centrally located	Primary prevention of variceal bleeding
Obstruction of all HVs	Congestive heart failure
PV thrombosis	Severe tricuspid regurgitation
Moderate pulmonary hypertension	Severe pulmonary hypertension
Severe coagulopathy (international normalized ration >5)	Multiple hepatic cysts
Thrombocytopenia of <20,000 cells/cm^3	Uncontrolled systemic infection or sepsis
Hepatic encephalopathy	Unrelieved biliary obstruction

severe coagulopathy, and HE. Even though TIPS can be created in the aforementioned situations, the risk, benefit, and difficulty with creating the shunt needs to be balanced with patient care and the clinical scenario. Examples of this include palliative treatment of patients with Hepatocellular carcinoma (HCC) with refractory variceal bleeding, recanalization of occluded PVs in patients with recurrent variceal bleeding, and treatment of patients with BCS and progressive liver failure. In addition, patients with a history of HE are at an increased risk for exacerbation of HE after shunt creation[53]; they should be aware of this risk-benefit scenario.

There have been numerous models created in predicting post-TIPS survival.[54,55,95–97] Among these, the modified Model for End-Stage Liver Disease score (MELD)[98] has proved to be superior to CTP score and Emory score.[99] A MELD score above 18 predicts a significantly higher mortality 3 months after TIPS as compared to a score of less than 18.[98,100] In addition, mortality also depends on the original TIPS indication.

Like with any procedure, the TIPS procedure carries its risks and benefits; a clear understanding of these risks and benefits must be understood and agreed on by patients. A detailed history and physical examination is required. In addition, pre-TIPS laboratory studies should be obtained 24 hours before the procedure. These studies include serum electrolytes, complete blood count, coagulation studies, and liver and kidney function panel.

Cross-sectional imaging (liver ultrasound with Doppler, computer tomography, or magnetic resonance imaging) should be reviewed; if not current (>1 month), a repeat study should be obtained to evaluate vascular patency and to look for hepatic masses that may complicate the procedure. In patients who have suspected or known cardiac or pulmonary disease, an echocardiogram should be obtained to exclude diastolic/systolic dysfunction and pulmonary arterial hypertension because TIPS is known to increase central venous pressure, pulmonary capillary wedge pressure, and exacerbate known cardiac dysfunction.[99] In addition, a paracentesis should be performed for refractory ascites before the procedure in order to reduce the risk of periprocedural bleeding. Furthermore, a thoracentesis may benefit patients with hepatic hydrothorax, as it may improve respiratory function and assist with sedation.

CONVENTIONAL TECHNIQUE

In the United States, the TIPS procedure is performed by interventional radiologists. The procedure is either performed under conscious sedation or under general anesthesia with endotracheal intubation.[5] The later is preferred by many for patient control and comfort because of the potentially prolonged nature of the procedure.

Hepatic Venous Access

A right internal jugular (IJ) approach is preferred, as it allows a direct path to the IVC. Secondary options include left IJ vein[101] and femoral vein[102] approaches, but these are reserved for unusual anatomy or in cases of central venous occlusive disease. After the neck is cleaned and draped in a sterile fashion, IJ venous access is obtained via sonographic guidance. A catheter is then advanced beyond the right atrium into the HV under fluoroscopic guidance. The right HV is chosen whenever possible, as it allows for an anterior inferior transhepatic puncture of the right PV, thus providing the safest approach for the TIPS. A wedged hepatic venogram is then obtained using carbon dioxide (CO_2) to demonstrate the portal venous anatomy (**Fig. 2**).

Portal Venous Access and Transjugular Intrahepatic Portosystemic Shunt Insertion

There are several commercial sets available for portal puncture: Haskal (Cook Medical, Bloomington, IN) and Ring (Cook Medical) transjugular intrahepatic access sets, which both include a 16-gauge modified Colapinto puncture needle; Rosch-Uchida transjugular liver access set (Cook Medical), which contains a 14-gauge needle; and Angiodynamic transjugular access set (Angiodynamics Medical, Latham, NY) containing 14- and 21-gauge needles. After the CO_2 portogram has been performed and a target identified, the needle (which is constrained in a hard inner sheath and softer 10-French outer sheath) is directed anteriorly and inferiorly from the right HV into the right PV (**Fig. 3**). Once access is achieved, the needle is removed and a wire and catheter are advanced into the splenic or mesenteric vein. Portal venography (**Fig. 4**) and pressure measurements are performed.

An angioplasty balloon is then used to dilate the tract (**Fig. 5**), allowing for passage of the 10-French sheath into the PV. The PTFE-covered stent (Viatorr, W.L. Gore, Newark, DE), which is the standard TIPS stent, is then deployed and postdilated to 8 mm. This stent is unique because the caudal 2 cm, which resides in the PV, is uncovered and the variable cranial length of the stent, which traverses the liver and HV, is covered by PTFE. After stent deployment and dilation, trans-TIPS portal

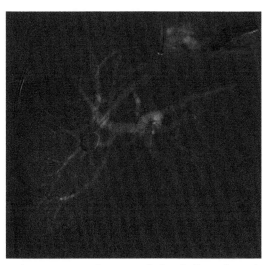

Fig. 2. Wedged hepatic venogram using an occlusion balloon from the right HV demonstrating normal portal venous anatomy.

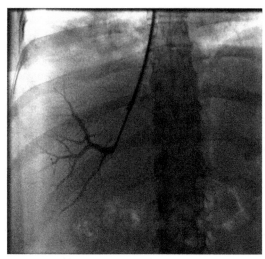

Fig. 3. Injection of contrast confirming placement of needle in a branch of the right PV.

venography (**Fig. 6**) and pressure measurements are repeated. If the pressure remains higher than desired, the stent can be further dilated to 10 or 12 mm. A portal pressure gradient (PPG) less than 12 mm Hg[3] should be achieved in patients with a history of bleeding esophageal varices and refractory ascites. However, the optimal PPG for re-fractory ascites is still under much debate, with some investigators suggesting a PPG of less than 8 mm Hg.[22] In patients with preexisting HE, a higher gradient may be appropriate to reduce post-TIPS HE[103]; more data are needed to elucidate this.

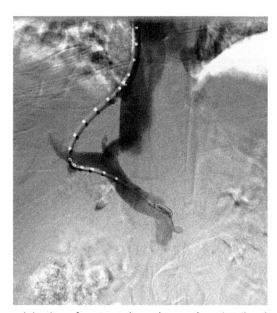

Fig. 4. Simultaneous injection of contrast through a marker pigtail catheter in the PV and sheath in the right HV demonstrating appropriate anatomy.

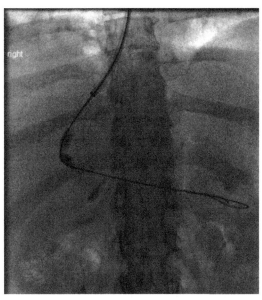

Fig. 5. Angioplasty balloon dilating the transhepatic tract to 8 mm before stent placement.

Selective Embolization of Portosystemic Collaterals

At the discretion of the interventionalist, selective embolization of varices or other portosystemic collaterals can be performed after TIPS placement. This procedure may benefit patients with a history of bleeding esophageal varices, as embolization at the time of TIPS placement has been found to decrease the rate of recurrent esophageal bleeding (84% and 81% at 2 and 4 years, respectively) versus TIPS alone (61% and 53% at 2 and 4 years, respectively).[104] Furthermore, selective embolization can also be performed in cases when the gradient is not reduced to less than 12 mm Hg. There

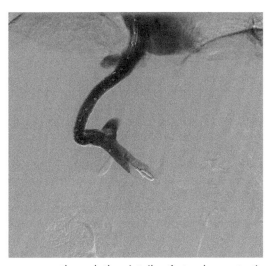

Fig. 6. Completion venogram through the pigtail catheter demonstrating appropriate flow from the PV through the TIPS shunt into the right HV and right atrium.

is a wide variety of embolic devices that can be used, including coils and Amplatzer Vascular Plugs (St Jude Medical, Saint Paul, MN).

Immediate Postprocedural Management

After TIPS placement, patients should be observed for a minimum of 12 hours in a hospital unit. Vital signs should be closely monitored for evidence of intraperitoneal hemorrhage. Post-TIPS laboratory values should be obtained, including a complete blood count (to monitor for hemorrhage and infection), coagulation panel, and kidney and hepatic function tests. A liver sonogram with Doppler can be obtained a day after the shunt placement to evaluate for shunt patency.

ADVANCED AND ALTERNATIVE TRANSJUGULAR INTRAHEPATIC PORTOSYSTEMIC SHUNT TECHNIQUES

Numerous options exist when difficult anatomy prohibits the right hepatic to right PV approach. These options include a left hepatic to left portal approach or an IVC to right portal approach through the caudate lobe with or without the aid of transabdominal or intravascular ultrasound. The gunsight technique[105] can be used when success has not been achieved with traditional transvascular methods. This technique involves placement of a loop snare in the IVC from the IJ access and placement of a loop snare in the PV from a percutaneous approach. A needle is then advanced from a second percutaneous approach using lateral fluoroscopy through both loop snares into the IVC. A wire is passed through the needle into the IVC and snared from above, thus establishing systemic to portal access for placement of the shunt.

Occasionally, patients with PV thrombosis will present and require recanalization of the portal system. This recanalization can be achieved through a variety of techniques using a percutaneous or transhepatic approach in order to relieve the portal obstruction and facilitate flow through the shunt (**Fig. 7**).

COMPLICATIONS

The most common complications following the TIPS procedure are listed in **Box 2**.[2] These complications can be divided into 3 major categories: technical related, portosystemic related, and other unique complications.

Technical-Access Related

Puncture of the liver capsule is common, occurring up to 30% of patients[106]; however, serious intraperitoneal bleeding is rare. Liver capsule puncture is likely in patients with a small liver and when multiple needle punctures are required. Biliary puncture and fistula formation is also a rare complication, occurring with an incidence of less than 5%.[107] Fistula formation between the biliary and vascular systems could result in hemobilia, cholangitis, sepsis, and stent infection.[1,108] If fistula formation occurs between a stent and the biliary system, early stent occlusion may ensue because of marked psuedointimal hyperplasia.[106] Fistulous communication may be decreased by using controlled needle passage and number of needle punctures. Biliary diversion via an internal or external drainage catheter may be used to address biliary-vascular fistulas; embolization can be performed in cases of hemobilia; and biliary-stent fistulas can be treated with the placement of a PTFE-covered stent to reline the hepatic parenchymal tract.[106]

Hepatic infarction is a rare complication that can result from a reduction in sinusoidal flow. It can also occur secondary to stent compression of the hepatic artery. A low PPG after TIPS placement can increase the incidence of hepatic infarction. This

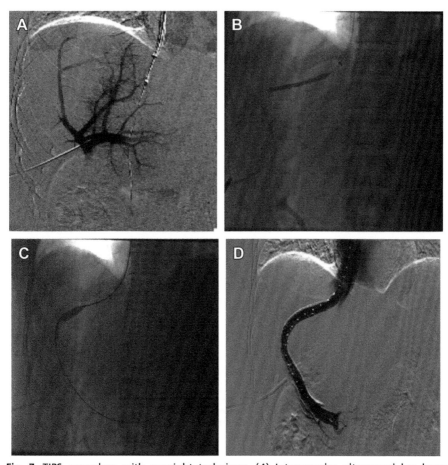

Fig. 7. TIPS procedure with gunsight technique. (*A*) Intravascular ultrasound has been placed in the IVC, and percutaneous access into the portal system has been obtained and confirmed with an injection of contrast through the needle. (*B*) After puncturing through loop snares in the right PV and IVC from a second percutaneous access, the wire was pulled through the IVC sheath and the tract between the two sheaths is being angioplastied with a small-diameter balloon. (*C*) The wire was pulled into the PV and advanced into the splenic vein from above and the tract is now being dilated to 8 mm. (*D*) Completion venogram through the pigtail catheter demonstrating appropriate flow from the PV through the TIPS shunt into the right HV and right atrium.

problem can be treated with the placement of stents within the primary stent to reduce the shunt caliber.

Technical-Stent Related

With the use of PTFE-covered stents, thrombosis, occlusion, and stent migration are infrequently seen.[2,3] Before the use of PTFE-covered stents, the most common site for shunt stenosis was at the hepatic venous end. Midstent stenosis is thought to be secondary to pseudointimal hyperplasia within bare metal stents,[109] with rates of stenosis ranging from 18% to 78%.[3] In a randomized controlled trial[110] comparing covered and bare metal stents, the rates of primary patency in the covered and bare metal stent groups were 86% and 47%, respectively, at 1 year. At 2 years, the patency rates

---

Box 2
Complications from TIPS

Technical complications

  Related to access

    Capsule puncture

    Intraperitoneal bleed

    Hepatic infarction

    Fistula

    Hemobilia

  Related to the stent

    Thrombosis

    Occlusion

    Stent migration

    Sepsis

Related to portosystemic shunting

  HE

  Hemodynamic consequences

  Sepsis

Unique complications

  Intravascular hemolysis

  Endotipsitis

From Bhogal HK, Sanyal AJ. Using transjugular intrahepatic portosystemic shunts for complications of cirrhosis. Clin Gastroenterol Hepatol 2011;9(11):943; with permission.

---

were 80% and 19% for covered and bare metal stents, respectively. In another large nonrandomized series,[111] the primary patency rates were similar, with 87% and 81% at 6 and 12 months, respectively.

Portosystemic-Shunting Related

HE is the most frequent medical complication that usually occurs 2 to 3 weeks after TIPS insertion.[112] The pathophysiology of post-TIPS HE is complex, though mainly caused by diverted portal flow away from the liver caused by TIPS and into the arterial system[55,113] and decreased liver metabolic capacity. The frequency of new or worsening HE ranges from 10% to 44%,[3] and factors associated with post-TIPS HE development include prior history of HE, increasing age, shunt caliber, high creatinine levels, low serum sodium concentration, and liver dysfunction.[55,114] Previously, studies with bare metal stents found an increased risk for the development of HE after TIPS insertion for ascites.[20–25] Consequently, studies with covered stents were found to have lower rates of HE after TIPS placement.[112,115] A meta-analysis further confirms this statement.[69] However, it should be mentioned that most of these studies were not designed to test post-TIPS HE. In addition, the methodology used to access for HE was highly variable and subjective based.

The prevention of post-TIPS HE includes possibly having a higher PPG[105] (especially in patients with a high risk of HE) and treating precipitating factors before

TIPS placement. Post-TIPS HE can be treated with standard therapy; in refractory cases, the shunt can be reduced or occluded.[55,105,115,116]

Unique Complications

Intravascular hemolysis and endotipsitis (infection of TIPS stent) are rare complications of TIPS[106,117,118] and infrequently occur with covered stents. If present, intravascular hemolysis is usually self-limiting, resolving in 3 to 4 weeks. Endotipsitis presents with fever and abdominal pain; laboratory evaluation reveals positive blood cultures and an elevated white blood cell count. Treatment is with prolonged antibiotics.

POST–TRANSJUGULAR INTRAHEPATIC PORTOSYSTEMIC SHUNT FOLLOW-UP AND MAINTENANCE

The recurrence of portal hypertension symptoms could indicate shunt dysfunction. Prompt sonogram with Doppler of the liver should be obtained to evaluate shunt velocity. Velocities of 50 cm/s or less or 250 cm/s are associated with shunt dysfunction, with greater than 90% sensitivity and specificity.[119] If a patient is asymptomatic, sonogram with Doppler of the liver is usually performed within 4 weeks of placement and every 6 months to a year. The gold standard to evaluate shunt patency is portal venography. However, this is reserved to evaluate shunt occlusion seen on the sonogram, as it is invasive and carries its own complications. If a bare metal stent was used, revision with a covered stent can be performed.[119]

FUTURE CONSIDERATIONS

The use of TIPS in the management of end-stage liver disease has been refined, and it is now an integral part of the treatment armamentarium for this condition. A key challenge that remains to be resolved is how to prevent further hepatic decompensation in those who already have some hyperbilirubinemia before TIPS. The impact of TIPS on the systemic microcirculatory dysfunction associated with cirrhosis also needs to be better understood. Although it is much less common than before, acute on chronic liver failure (ACLF) still occurs with TIPS; better methods to prevent this are needed. As expected, portosystemic shunting increases the risk of infection; the role of selective gut decontamination or ways to improve intestinal barrier functions in preventing ACLF after TIPS is now needed. There have also been reports of an increased risk of HCC after TIPS. These reports need to be definitively confirmed or refuted.

SUMMARY

TIPS has become a valuable option in the management of the complications of portal hypertension. The best available evidence for the use of TIPS includes refractory or recurrent esophageal variceal bleeding and refractory ascites. In addition, TIPS insertion could improve outcomes for patients who present with an acute variceal bleed, hepatic hydrothorax, and HRS. With the use of covered stents, long-term patency has dramatically improved, further advocating early use. The insertion of TIPS unfortunately comes with complications, with HE being one of the most common. A possible solution to this includes thorough selection of patients and careful attention to the final portosystemic gradient. Lastly, with advanced and alternative techniques, TIPS could play a larger role in the future treatment of patients with complications of portal hypertension.

CONFLICT OF INTEREST DISCLOSURE TABLE, JANUARY 2014 (BASED ON INCOMES OVER LAST 24 MONTHS)

Company	Stock	Employment	Speaker	Consulting Advisor	Research Grants	Travel Grants	Intellectual Property	Royalties
Abbott	A	A	A	B	A	A	A	A
Exhalenz	A	A	A	A	A	A	A	A
Conatus	A	A	A	A	C[a]	A	A	A
Genentech	A	A	A	B[b]	A	A	A	A
Genfit	A	A	A	A[c]	A	A	A	A
Gilead	A	A	A	B	F	A	A	A
Echosens-Sandhill	A	A	A	A[c]	A[d]	A	A	A
Ikaria	A	A	A	B	E	A	A	A
Immuron	A	A	A	A[e]	A	A	A	A
Intercept	A	A	A	A[c]	A	A	A	A
Merck	A	A	A	B	A	A	A	A
Norgine	A	A	A	B	A	A	A	A
Roche	A	A	A	B	A	A	A	A
Salix	A	A	A	C	E	A	A	A
Uptodate	A	A	A	A	A	A	A	C
Takeda	A	A	A	B	D	A	A	A
Astellas	A	A	A	A	D	A	A	A
Novartis	A	A	A	A[f]	E	A	A	A
Nimbus	A	A	A	B	A	A	A	A
Galectin	A	A	A	A[f]	E	A	A	A
Nitto Denko	A	A	A	B	A	A	A	A
Sequana	A	A	A	A[c]	A	A	A	A
Bristol Myers	A	A	A	B	A	A	A	A

The research grants listed above for Salix, Gilead, and Exhalenz represent the site budgets for Virginia Commonwealth University clinical trials involving these companies and do not support the author directly.

Research collaborations without any funding from the commercial entity: Regulus, CSL Behring, Ferring, Zora Lipidomics, and Metabolon.

A, no interest; B, less than $5000; C, $5001 to 10,000; D, $10,001 to $50,000; E, $50,001 to 100,000; F, more than $100,000.

[a] They will provide drug and laboratory costs for a National Institute on Alcohol Abuse and Alcoholism–sponsored study of a caspase inhibitor for alcoholic hepatitis. The author has no personal financial conflict of interest.

[b] The author is consulting with Genentech regarding nonalcoholic steatohepatitis and fibrosis.

[c] The author is a consultant but has divested himself. The author has no financial conflict of interest.

[d] Echosens has provided a fibroscan machine for dedicated research use for nonalcoholic steatohepatitis (NASH)–related studies via the National Institute of Diabetes and Digestive and Kidney Diseases, NASH Clinical Research Network.

[e] The author will be the principal investigator of the Immuron upcoming trial for alcoholic hepatitis as part of the National Institute on Alcohol Abuse and Alcoholism–funded TREAT consortium. Immuron will provide the drug and no additional funding.

[f] The author has provided advice but not taken any personal remuneration.

REFERENCES

1. Rosch J, Hanafee W, Snow H, et al. Transjugular intrahepatic portacaval shunt. An experimental work. Am J Surg 1971;121(5):588–92.
2. Bhogal HK, Sanyal AJ. Using transjugular intrahepatic portosystemic shunts for complications of cirrhosis. Clin Gastroenterol Hepatol 2011;9(11):936–46. http://dx.doi.org/10.1016/j.cgh.2011.06.013 [quiz: e123].
3. Tripathi D, Redhead D. Transjugular intrahepatic portosystemic stent-shunt: technical factors and new developments. Eur J Gastroenterol Hepatol 2006; 18(11):1127–33. http://dx.doi.org/10.1097/01.meg.0000236871.78280.a7.
4. Boyer TD, Haskal ZJ, American Association for the Study of Liver Diseases. The role of transjugular intrahepatic portosystemic shunt (TIPS) in the management of portal hypertension: update 2009. Hepatology 2010;51(1):306. http://dx.doi.org/10.1002/hep.23383.
5. Rossle M, Haag K, Ochs A, et al. The transjugular intrahepatic portosystemic stent-shunt procedure for variceal bleeding. N Engl J Med 1994;330(3): 165–71. http://dx.doi.org/10.1056/NEJM199401203300303.
6. Boyer TD. Transjugular intrahepatic portosystemic shunt: current status. Gastroenterology 2003;124(6):1700–10.
7. Luketic VA, Sanyal AJ. Esophageal varices. II. TIPS (transjugular intrahepatic portosystemic shunt) and surgical therapy. Gastroenterol Clin North Am 2000;29(2): 387–421, vi.
8. Cello JP, Ring EJ, Olcott EW, et al. Endoscopic sclerotherapy compared with percutaneous transjugular intrahepatic portosystemic shunt after initial sclerotherapy in patients with acute variceal hemorrhage. A randomized, controlled trial. Ann Intern Med 1997;126(11):858–65.
9. Sanyal AJ, Freedman AM, Luketic VA, et al. Transjugular intrahepatic portosystemic shunts compared with endoscopic sclerotherapy for the prevention of recurrent variceal hemorrhage. A randomized, controlled trial. Ann Intern Med 1997;126(11): 849–57.
10. Cabrera J, Maynar M, Granados R, et al. Transjugular intrahepatic portosystemic shunt versus sclerotherapy in the elective treatment of variceal hemorrhage. Gastroenterology 1996;110(3):832–9.
11. Barton RE, Rosch J, Saxon RR, et al. TIPS: short- and long-term results: a survey of 1750 patients. Semin Intervent Radiol 1995;12:364–7.
12. Moitinho E, Escorsell A, Bandi JC, et al. Prognostic value of early measurements of portal pressure in acute variceal bleeding. Gastroenterology 1999;117(3):626–31.
13. Sauer P, Theilmann L, Stremmel W, et al. Transjugular intrahepatic portosystemic stent shunt versus sclerotherapy plus propranolol for variceal rebleeding. Gastroenterology 1997;113(5):1623–31.
14. Jalan R, Forrest EH, Stanley AJ, et al. A randomized trial comparing transjugular intrahepatic portosystemic stent-shunt with variceal band ligation in the prevention of rebleeding from esophageal varices. Hepatology 1997;26(5):1115–22. http://dx.doi.org/10.1002/hep.510260505.
15. Merli M, Salerno F, Riggio O, et al. Transjugular intrahepatic portosystemic shunt versus endoscopic sclerotherapy for the prevention of variceal bleeding in cirrhosis: a randomized multicenter trial. Gruppo Italiano Studio TIPS (G.I.S.T.). Hepatology 1998;27(1):48–53. http://dx.doi.org/10.1002/hep.510270109.
16. Sauer P, Hansmann J, Richter GM, et al. Endoscopic variceal ligation plus propranolol vs. transjugular intrahepatic portosystemic stent shunt: a long-term randomized trial. Endoscopy 2002;34(9):690–7. http://dx.doi.org/10.1055/s-2002-33565.

17. Garcia-Villarreal L, Martinez-Lagares F, Sierra A, et al. Transjugular intrahepatic portosystemic shunt versus endoscopic sclerotherapy for the prevention of variceal rebleeding after recent variceal hemorrhage. Hepatology 1999;29(1): 27–32. http://dx.doi.org/10.1002/hep.510290125.

18. Pomier-Layrargues G, Villeneuve JP, Deschenes M, et al. Transjugular intrahepatic portosystemic shunt (TIPS) versus endoscopic variceal ligation in the prevention of variceal rebleeding in patients with cirrhosis: a randomised trial. Gut 2001;48(3):390–6.

19. Narahara Y, Kanazawa H, Kawamata H, et al. A randomized clinical trial comparing transjugular intrahepatic portosystemic shunt with endoscopic sclerotherapy in the long-term management of patients with cirrhosis after recent variceal hemorrhage. Hepatol Res 2001;21(3):189–98.

20. Gines P, Uriz J, Calahorra B, et al. Transjugular intrahepatic portosystemic shunting versus paracentesis plus albumin for refractory ascites in cirrhosis. Gastroenterology 2002;123(6):1839–47. http://dx.doi.org/10.1053/gast.2002.37073.

21. Sanyal AJ, Genning C, Reddy KR, et al. The North American Study for the Treatment of Refractory Ascites. Gastroenterology 2003;124(3):634–41. http://dx.doi.org/10.1053/gast.2003.50088.

22. Salerno F, Merli M, Riggio O, et al. Randomized controlled study of TIPS versus paracentesis plus albumin in cirrhosis with severe ascites. Hepatology 2004; 40(3):629–35. http://dx.doi.org/10.1002/hep.20364.

23. Narahara Y, Kanazawa H, Fukuda T, et al. Transjugular intrahepatic portosystemic shunt versus paracentesis plus albumin in patients with refractory ascites who have good hepatic and renal function: a prospective randomized trial. J Gastroenterol 2011;46(1):78–85. http://dx.doi.org/10.1007/s00535-010-0282-9.

24. D'Amico G, Luca A, Morabito A, et al. Uncovered transjugular intrahepatic portosystemic shunt for refractory ascites: a meta-analysis. Gastroenterology 2005; 129(4):1282–93. http://dx.doi.org/10.1053/j.gastro.2005.07.031.

25. Albillos A, Banares R, Gonzalez M, et al. A meta-analysis of transjugular intrahepatic portosystemic shunt versus paracentesis for refractory ascites. J Hepatol 2005;43(6):990–6. http://dx.doi.org/10.1016/j.jhep.2005.06.005.

26. Clark W, Hernandez J, McKeon B, et al. Surgical shunting versus transjugular intrahepatic portasystemic shunting for bleeding varices resulting from portal hypertension and cirrhosis: a meta-analysis. Am Surg 2010;76(8):857–64.

27. Chau TN, Patch D, Chan YW, et al. "Salvage" transjugular intrahepatic portosystemic shunts: gastric fundal compared with esophageal variceal bleeding. Gastroenterology 1998;114(5):981–7.

28. Wong F, Pantea L, Sniderman K. Midodrine, octreotide, albumin, and TIPS in selected patients with cirrhosis and type 1 hepatorenal syndrome. Hepatology 2004;40(1):55–64. http://dx.doi.org/10.1002/hep.20262.

29. Valla DC. The diagnosis and management of the Budd-Chiari syndrome: consensus and controversies. Hepatology 2003;38(4):793–803. http://dx.doi.org/10.1053/jhep.2003.50415.

30. Perello A, Garcia-Pagan JC, Gilabert R, et al. TIPS is a useful long-term derivative therapy for patients with Budd-Chiari syndrome uncontrolled by medical therapy. Hepatology 2002;35(1):132–9. http://dx.doi.org/10.1053/jhep.2002.30274.

31. Mancuso A, Fung K, Mela M, et al. TIPS for acute and chronic Budd-Chiari syndrome: a single-centre experience. J Hepatol 2003;38(6):751–4.

32. Tripathi D, Therapondos G, Jackson E, et al. The role of the transjugular intrahepatic portosystemic stent shunt (TIPSS) in the management of bleeding gastric varices: clinical and haemodynamic correlations. Gut 2002;51(2):270–4.

33. Barange K, Peron JM, Imani K, et al. Transjugular intrahepatic portosystemic shunt in the treatment of refractory bleeding from ruptured gastric varices. Hepatology 1999;30(5):1139–43. http://dx.doi.org/10.1002/hep.510300523.

34. Lo GH, Liang HL, Chen WC, et al. A prospective, randomized controlled trial of transjugular intrahepatic portosystemic shunt versus cyanoacrylate injection in the prevention of gastric variceal rebleeding. Endoscopy 2007;39(8):679–85. http://dx.doi.org/10.1055/s-2007-966591.

35. Procaccini NJ, Al-Osaimi AM, Northup P, et al. Endoscopic cyanoacrylate versus transjugular intrahepatic portosystemic shunt for gastric variceal bleeding: a single-center U.S. analysis. Gastrointest Endosc 2009;70(5):881–7. http://dx.doi.org/10.1016/j.gie.2009.03.1169.

36. Sabri SS, Swee W, Turba UC, et al. Bleeding gastric varices obliteration with balloon-occluded retrograde transvenous obliteration using sodium tetradecyl sulfate foam. J Vasc Interv Radiol 2011;22(3):309–16. http://dx.doi.org/10.1016/j.jvir.2010.11.022 [quiz: 316].

37. Kamath PS, Lacerda M, Ahlquist DA, et al. Gastric mucosal responses to intrahepatic portosystemic shunting in patients with cirrhosis. Gastroenterology 2000;118(5):905–11.

38. Urata J, Yamashita Y, Tsuchigame T, et al. The effects of transjugular intrahepatic portosystemic shunt on portal hypertensive gastropathy. J Gastroenterol Hepatol 1998;13(10):1061–7.

39. Siegerstetter V, Deibert P, Ochs A, et al. Treatment of refractory hepatic hydrothorax with transjugular intrahepatic portosystemic shunt: long-term results in 40 patients. Eur J Gastroenterol Hepatol 2001;13(5):529–34.

40. Wilputte JY, Goffette P, Zech F, et al. The outcome after transjugular intrahepatic portosystemic shunt (TIPS) for hepatic hydrothorax is closely related to liver dysfunction: a long-term study in 28 patients. Acta Gastroenterol Belg 2007;70(1):6–10.

41. Dhanasekaran R, West JK, Gonzales PC, et al. Transjugular intrahepatic portosystemic shunt for symptomatic refractory hepatic hydrothorax in patients with cirrhosis. Am J Gastroenterol 2010;105(3):635–41. http://dx.doi.org/10.1038/ajg.2009.634.

42. Machicao VI, Balakrishnan M, Fallon MB. Pulmonary complications in chronic liver disease. Hepatology 2013. http://dx.doi.org/10.1002/hep.26745.

43. Martinez-Palli G, Drake BB, Garcia-Pagan JC, et al. Effect of transjugular intrahepatic portosystemic shunt on pulmonary gas exchange in patients with portal hypertension and hepatopulmonary syndrome. World J Gastroenterol 2005;11(43):6858–62.

44. Paramesh AS, Husain SZ, Shneider B, et al. Improvement of hepatopulmonary syndrome after transjugular intrahepatic portasystemic shunting: case report and review of literature. Pediatr Transplant 2003;7(2):157–62.

45. Salerno F, Gerbes A, Gines P, et al. Diagnosis, prevention and treatment of hepatorenal syndrome in cirrhosis. Gut 2007;56(9):1310–8. http://dx.doi.org/10.1136/gut.2006.107789.

46. Guevara M, Gines P, Bandi JC, et al. Transjugular intrahepatic portosystemic shunt in hepatorenal syndrome: effects on renal function and vasoactive systems. Hepatology 1998;28(2):416–22. http://dx.doi.org/10.1002/hep.510280219.

47. Brensing KA, Textor J, Perz J, et al. Long term outcome after transjugular intrahepatic portosystemic stent-shunt in non-transplant cirrhotics with hepatorenal syndrome: a phase II study. Gut 2000;47(2):288–95.

48. Garcia-Pagan JC, Heydtmann M, Raffa S, et al. TIPS for Budd-Chiari syndrome: long-term results and prognostics factors in 124 patients. Gastroenterology 2008;135(3):808–15. http://dx.doi.org/10.1053/j.gastro.2008.05.051.

49. Rozenblit G, DelGuercio LR, Savino JA, et al. Transmesenteric-transfemoral method of intrahepatic portosystemic shunt placement with minilaparotomy. J Vasc Interv Radiol 1996;7(4):499–506.

50. DeLeve LD, Shulman HM, McDonald GB. Toxic injury to hepatic sinusoids: sinusoidal obstruction syndrome (veno-occlusive disease). Semin Liver Dis 2002; 22(1):27–42. http://dx.doi.org/10.1055/s-2002-23204.

51. Smith FO, Johnson MS, Scherer LR, et al. Transjugular intrahepatic portosystemic shunting (TIPS) for treatment of severe hepatic veno-occlusive disease. Bone Marrow Transplant 1996;18(3):643–6.

52. Zenz T, Rossle M, Bertz H, et al. Severe veno-occlusive disease after allogeneic bone marrow or peripheral stem cell transplantation–role of transjugular intrahepatic portosystemic shunt (TIPS). Liver 2001;21(1):31–6.

53. Riggio O, Nardelli S, Moscucci F, et al. Hepatic encephalopathy after transjugular intrahepatic portosystemic shunt. Clin Liver Dis 2012;16(1):133–46. http://dx. doi.org/10.1016/j.cld.2011.12.008.

54. Jalan R, Elton RA, Redhead DN, et al. Analysis of prognostic variables in the prediction of mortality, shunt failure, variceal rebleeding and encephalopathy following the transjugular intrahepatic portosystemic stent-shunt for variceal haemorrhage. J Hepatol 1995;23(2):123–8.

55. Chalasani N, Clark WS, Martin LG, et al. Determinants of mortality in patients with advanced cirrhosis after transjugular intrahepatic portosystemic shunting. Gastroenterology 2000;118(1):138–44.

56. North Italian Endoscopic Club for the Study and Treatment of Esophageal Varices. Prediction of the first variceal hemorrhage in patients with cirrhosis of the liver and esophageal varices. A prospective multicenter study. N Engl J Med 1988;319(15):983–9. http://dx.doi.org/10.1056/NEJM198810133191505.

57. Garcia-Tsao G, Sanyal AJ, Grace ND, et al, Practice Guidelines Committee of the American Association for the Study of Liver Diseases, Practice Parameters Committee of the American College of Gastroenterology. Prevention and management of gastroesophageal varices and variceal hemorrhage in cirrhosis. Hepatology 2007;46(3):922–38. http://dx.doi.org/10.1002/hep.21907.

58. Kovalak M, Lake J, Mattek N, et al. Endoscopic screening for varices in cirrhotic patients: data from a national endoscopic database. Gastrointest Endosc 2007; 65(1):82–8. http://dx.doi.org/10.1016/j.gie.2006.08.023.

59. D'Amico G, Pagliaro L, Bosch J. Pharmacological treatment of portal hypertension: an evidence-based approach. Semin Liver Dis 1999;19(4):475–505. http:// dx.doi.org/10.1055/s-2007-1007133.

60. Monescillo A, Martinez-Lagares F, Ruiz-del-Arbol L, et al. Influence of portal hypertension and its early decompression by TIPS placement on the outcome of variceal bleeding. Hepatology 2004;40(4):793–801. http://dx.doi.org/10.1002/ hep.20386.

61. Garcia-Pagan JC, Caca K, Bureau C, et al. Early use of TIPS in patients with cirrhosis and variceal bleeding. N Engl J Med 2010;362(25):2370–9. http://dx. doi.org/10.1056/NEJMoa0910102.

62. Bosch J, Garcia-Pagan JC. Prevention of variceal rebleeding. Lancet 2003; 361(9361):952–4. http://dx.doi.org/10.1016/S0140-6736(03)12778-X.

63. D'Amico G, De Franchis R, Cooperative Study Group. Upper digestive bleeding in cirrhosis. post-therapeutic outcome and prognostic indicators. Hepatology 2003;38(3):599–612. http://dx.doi.org/10.1053/jhep.2003.50385.

64. de Franchis R, Primignani M. Why do varices bleed? Gastroenterol Clin North Am 1992;21(1):85–101.

65. Burroughs AK, Mezzanotte G, Phillips A, et al. Cirrhotics with variceal hemorrhage: the importance of the time interval between admission and the start of
analysis for survival and rebleeding rates. Hepatology 1989;9(6):801–7.
66. Graham DY, Smith JL. The course of patients after variceal hemorrhage. Gastroenterology 1981;80(4):800–9.
67. Lebrec D, De Fleury P, Rueff B, et al. Portal hypertension, size of esophageal varices, and risk of gastrointestinal bleeding in alcoholic cirrhosis. Gastroenterology
1980;79(6):1139–44.
68. Gulberg V, Schepke M, Geigenberger G, et al. Transjugular intrahepatic portosystemic shunting is not superior to endoscopic variceal band ligation for prevention
of variceal rebleeding in cirrhotic patients: a randomized, controlled trial. Scand J
Gastroenterol 2002;37(3):338–43.
69. Luca A, D'Amico G, La Galla R, et al. TIPS for prevention of recurrent bleeding in
patients with cirrhosis: meta-analysis of randomized clinical trials. Radiology
1999;212(2):411–21.
70. Papatheodoridis GV, Goulis J, Leandro G, et al. Transjugular intrahepatic portosystemic shunt compared with endoscopic treatment for prevention of variceal
rebleeding: a meta-analysis. Hepatology 1999;30(3):612–22. http://dx.doi.org/
10.1002/hep.510300316.
71. Burroughs AK, Vangeli M. Transjugular intrahepatic portosystemic shunt versus
endoscopic therapy: randomized trials for secondary prophylaxis of variceal
bleeding: an updated meta-analysis. Scand J Gastroenterol 2002;37(3):249–52.
72. Zheng M, Chen Y, Bai J, et al. Transjugular intrahepatic portosystemic shunt
versus endoscopic therapy in the secondary prophylaxis of variceal rebleeding
in cirrhotic patients: meta-analysis update. J Clin Gastroenterol 2008;42(5):
507–16. http://dx.doi.org/10.1097/MCG.0b013e31815576e6.
73. Escorsell A, Banares R, Garcia-Pagan JC, et al. TIPS versus drug therapy in preventing variceal rebleeding in advanced cirrhosis: a randomized controlled trial.
Hepatology 2002;35(2):385–92. http://dx.doi.org/10.1053/jhep.2002.30418.
74. Angermayr B, Cejna M, Koenig F, et al. Survival in patients undergoing transjugular intrahepatic portosystemic shunt: EPTFE-covered stentgrafts versus bare
stents. Hepatology 2003;38(4):1043–50. http://dx.doi.org/10.1053/jhep.2003.
50423.
75. Barrio J, Ripoll C, Banares R, et al. Comparison of transjugular intrahepatic portosystemic shunt dysfunction in PTFE-covered stent-grafts versus bare stents.
Eur J Radiol 2005;55(1):120–4. http://dx.doi.org/10.1016/j.ejrad.2004.10.007.
76. Bureau C, Pagan JC, Layrargues GP, et al. Patency of stents covered with polytetrafluoroethylene in patients treated by transjugular intrahepatic portosystemic
shunts: long-term results of a randomized multicentre study. Liver Int 2007;
27(6):742–7. http://dx.doi.org/10.1111/j.1478-3231.2007.01522.x.
77. Yang Z, Han G, Wu Q, et al. Patency and clinical outcomes of transjugular intrahepatic portosystemic shunt with polytetrafluoroethylene-covered stents versus
bare stents: a meta-analysis. J Gastroenterol Hepatol 2010;25(11):1718–25.
http://dx.doi.org/10.1111/j.1440-1746.2010.06400.x.
78. Rees CJ, Nylander DL, Thompson NP, et al. Do gastric and oesophageal varices
bleed at different portal pressures and is TIPS an effective treatment? Liver
2000;20(3):253–6.
79. Primignani M, Carpinelli L, Preatoni P, et al. Natural history of portal hypertensive
gastropathy in patients with liver cirrhosis. the New Italian Endoscopic Club for
the study and treatment of esophageal varices (NIEC). Gastroenterology 2000;
119(1):181–7.

80. Wong F, Sniderman K, Liu P, et al. The mechanism of the initial natriuresis after transjugular intrahepatic portosystemic shunt. Gastroenterology 1997;112(3): 899–907.

81. Lebrec D, Giuily N, Hadengue A, et al. Transjugular intrahepatic portosystemic shunts: comparison with paracentesis in patients with cirrhosis and refractory ascites: a randomized trial. French Group of Clinicians and a Group of Biologists. J Hepatol 1996;25(2):135–44.

82. Rossle M, Ochs A, Gulberg V, et al. A comparison of paracentesis and transjugular intrahepatic portosystemic shunting in patients with ascites. N Engl J Med 2000;342(23):1701–7. http://dx.doi.org/10.1056/NEJM200006083422303.

83. Saab S, Nieto JM, Ly D, et al. TIPS versus paracentesis for cirrhotic patients with refractory ascites. Cochrane Database Syst Rev 2004;(3):CD004889. http://dx.doi.org/10.1002/14651858.CD004889.

84. Deltenre P, Mathurin P, Dharancy S, et al. Transjugular intrahepatic portosystemic shunt in refractory ascites: a meta-analysis. Liver Int 2005;25(2):349–56. http://dx.doi.org/10.1111/j.1478-3231.2005.01095.x.

85. Salerno F, Camma C, Enea M, et al. Transjugular intrahepatic portosystemic shunt for refractory ascites: a meta-analysis of individual patient data. Gastroenterology 2007;133(3):825–34. http://dx.doi.org/10.1053/j.gastro.2007.06.020.

86. Alberts WM, Salem AJ, Solomon DA, et al. Hepatic hydrothorax. Cause and management. Arch Intern Med 1991;151(12):2383–8.

87. Kiafar C, Gilani N. Hepatic hydrothorax: current concepts of pathophysiology and treatment options. Ann Hepatol 2008;7(4):313–20.

88. Gordon FD, Anastopoulos HT, Crenshaw W, et al. The successful treatment of symptomatic, refractory hepatic hydrothorax with transjugular intrahepatic portosystemic shunt. Hepatology 1997;25(6):1366–9. http://dx.doi.org/10.1002/hep.510250611.

89. Jeffries MA, Kazanjian S, Wilson M, et al. Transjugular intrahepatic portosystemic shunts and liver transplantation in patients with refractory hepatic hydrothorax. Liver Transpl Surg 1998;4(5):416–23.

90. Spencer EB, Cohen DT, Darcy MD. Safety and efficacy of transjugular intrahepatic portosystemic shunt creation for the treatment of hepatic hydrothorax. J Vasc Interv Radiol 2002;13(4):385–90.

91. Testino G, Ferro C, Sumberaz A, et al. Type-2 hepatorenal syndrome and refractory ascites: role of transjugular intrahepatic portosystemic stent-shunt in eighteen patients with advanced cirrhosis awaiting orthotopic liver transplantation. Hepatogastroenterology 2003;50(54):1753–5.

92. Rossle M, Olschewski M, Siegerstetter V, et al. The Budd-Chiari syndrome: outcome after treatment with the transjugular intrahepatic portosystemic shunt. Surgery 2004;135(4):394–403. http://dx.doi.org/10.1016/j.surg.2003.09.005.

93. Fried MW, Connaghan DG, Sharma S, et al. Transjugular intrahepatic portosystemic shunt for the management of severe venoocclusive disease following bone marrow transplantation. Hepatology 1996;24(3):588–91. http://dx.doi.org/10.1002/hep.510240321.

94. Azoulay D, Castaing D, Lemoine A, et al. Transjugular intrahepatic portosystemic shunt (TIPS) for severe veno-occlusive disease of the liver following bone marrow transplantation. Bone Marrow Transplant 2000;25(9):987–92. http://dx.doi.org/10.1038/sj.bmt.1702386.

95. Malinchoc M, Kamath PS, Gordon FD, et al. A model to predict poor survival in patients undergoing transjugular intrahepatic portosystemic shunts. Hepatology 2000;31(4):864–71. http://dx.doi.org/10.1053/he.2000.5852.

96. Ferral H, Vasan R, Speeg KV, et al. Evaluation of a model to predict poor survival in patients undergoing elective TIPS procedures. J Vasc Interv Radiol 2002;13(11): 1103–8.
97. Schepke M, Roth F, Fimmers R, et al. Comparison of MELD, Child-Pugh, and Emory model for the prediction of survival in patients undergoing transjugular intrahepatic portosystemic shunting. Am J Gastroenterol 2003;98(5):1167–74. http://dx.doi.org/10.1111/j.1572-0241.2003.07515.x.
98. Kamath PS, Wiesner RH, Malinchoc M, et al. A model to predict survival in patients with end-stage liver disease. Hepatology 2001;33(2):464–70. http://dx. doi.org/10.1053/jhep.2001.22172.
99. Kovacs A, Schepke M, Heller J, et al. Short-term effects of transjugular intrahepatic shunt on cardiac function assessed by cardiac MRI: preliminary results. Cardiovasc Intervent Radiol 2010;33(2):290–6. http://dx.doi.org/10.1007/s00270-009-9696-2.
100. Salerno F, Merli M, Cazzaniga M, et al. MELD score is better than Child-Pugh score in predicting 3-month survival of patients undergoing transjugular intrahepatic portosystemic shunt. J Hepatol 2002;36(4):494–500.
101. Hausegger KA, Tauss J, Karaic K, et al. Use of the left internal jugular vein approach for transjugular portosystemic shunt. AJR Am J Roentgenol 1998; 171(6):1637–9. http://dx.doi.org/10.2214/ajr.171.6.9843303.
102. Sze DY, Magsamen KE, Frisoli JK. Successful transfemoral creation of an intrahepatic portosystemic shunt with use of the Viatorr device. J Vasc Interv Radiol 2006;17(3):569–72. http://dx.doi.org/10.1097/01.rvi.0000200054.73714.e1.
103. Casado M, Bosch J, Garcia-Pagan JC, et al. Clinical events after transjugular intrahepatic portosystemic shunt: correlation with hemodynamic findings. Gastroenterology 1998;114(6):1296–303.
104. Tesdal IK, Filser T, Weiss C, et al. Transjugular intrahepatic portosystemic shunts: adjunctive embolotherapy of gastroesophageal collateral vessels in the prevention of variceal rebleeding. Radiology 2005;236(1):360–7. http://dx. doi.org/10.1148/radiol.2361040530.
105. Haskal ZJ, Duszak R Jr, Furth EE. Transjugular intrahepatic transcaval portosystemic shunt: the gun-sight approach. J Vasc Interv Radiol 1996;7(1):139–42.
106. Suhocki PV, Smith AD, Tendler DA, et al. Treatment of TIPS/biliary fistula-related endotipsitis with a covered stent. J Vasc Interv Radiol 2008;19(6):937–9. http:// dx.doi.org/10.1016/j.jvir.2008.01.026.
107. Freedman AM, Sanyal AJ, Tisnado J, et al. Complications of transjugular intrahepatic portosystemic shunt: a comprehensive review. Radiographics 1993; 13(6):1185–210. http://dx.doi.org/10.1148/radiographics.13.6.8290720.
108. LaBerge JM, Ring EJ, Gordon RL, et al. Creation of transjugular intrahepatic portosystemic shunts with the wallstent endoprosthesis: results in 100 patients. Radiology 1993;187(2):413–20. http://dx.doi.org/10.1148/radiology.187.2.8475283.
109. LaBerge JM, Ferrell LD, Ring EJ, et al. Histopathologic study of transjugular intrahepatic portosystemic shunts. J Vasc Interv Radiol 1991;2(4):549–56.
110. Bureau C, Garcia-Pagan JC, Otal P, et al. Improved clinical outcome using polytetrafluoroethylene-coated stents for TIPS: results of a randomized study. Gastroenterology 2004;126(2):469–75.
111. Hausegger KA, Karnel F, Georgieva B, et al. Transjugular intrahepatic portosystemic shunt creation with the Viatorr expanded polytetrafluoroethylene-covered stent-graft. J Vasc Interv Radiol 2004;15(3):239–48.
112. Sanyal AJ, Freedman AM, Shiffman ML, et al. Portosystemic encephalopathy after transjugular intrahepatic portosystemic shunt: results of a prospective controlled study. Hepatology 1994;20(1 Pt 1):46–55.

113. Hauenstein KH, Haag K, Ochs A, et al. The reducing stent: treatment for transjugular intrahepatic portosystemic shunt-induced refractory hepatic encephalopathy and liver failure. Radiology 1995;194(1):175–9. http://dx.doi.org/10.1148/radiology.194.1.7997547.

114. Riggio O, Angeloni S, Salvatori FM, et al. Incidence, natural history, and risk factors of hepatic encephalopathy after transjugular intrahepatic portosystemic shunt with polytetrafluoroethylene-covered stent grafts. Am J Gastroenterol 2008;103(11):2738–46. http://dx.doi.org/10.1111/j.1572-0241.2008.02102.x.

115. Maleux G, Perez-Gutierrez NA, Evrard S, et al. Covered stents are better than uncovered stents for transjugular intrahepatic portosystemic shunts in cirrhotic patients with refractory ascites: a retrospective cohort study. Acta Gastroenterol Belg 2010;73(3):336–41.

116. Haskal ZJ, Cope C, Soulen MC, et al. Intentional reversible thrombosis of transjugular intrahepatic portosystemic shunts. Radiology 1995;195(2):485–8. http://dx.doi.org/10.1148/radiology.195.2.7724771.

117. Sanyal AJ, Freedman AM, Purdum PP, et al. The hematologic consequences of transjugular intrahepatic portosystemic shunts. Hepatology 1996;23(1):32–9. http://dx.doi.org/10.1002/hep.510230105.

118. Sanyal AJ, Reddy KR. Vegetative infection of transjugular intrahepatic portosystemic shunts. Gastroenterology 1998;115(1):110–5.

119. Zizka J, Elias P, Krajina A, et al. Value of Doppler sonography in revealing transjugular intrahepatic portosystemic shunt malfunction: a 5-year experience in 216 patients. AJR Am J Roentgenol 2000;175(1):141–8. http://dx.doi.org/10.2214/ajr.175.1.1750141.

Transarterial Chemoembolization and Yittrium-90 for Liver Cancer and Other Lesions

CrossMark

Jeet Minocha, MD[a],*, Riad Salem, MD, MBA[b],
Robert J. Lewandowski, MD[b]

KEYWORDS

- Transarterial chemoembolization (TACE) • Chemoembolization
- Drug-eluting bead (DEB)-TACE • Yittrium 90 (^{90}Y) • Radioembolization
- Liver cancer • Hepatocellular carcinoma (HCC) • Hepatic metastases

KEY POINTS

- Transarterial chemoembolization (TACE) and yittrium 90 (^{90}Y) radioembolization are catheter-based therapies that selectively deliver high-dose anticancer treatments directly to tumor(s) using imaging guidance.
- TACE and ^{90}Y radioembolization have been widely investigated during the past decade for the treatment of primary and metastatic liver tumors and have led to encouraging response, survival, and quality of life outcomes, with reduced toxicity profiles.
- TACE and ^{90}Y radioembolization are applicable in many clinical scenarios and have great potential in combination with other treatments, including ablation and systemic therapies.

INTRODUCTION: NATURE OF THE PROBLEM

Hepatocellular carcinoma (HCC) is a major worldwide health problem. It is the most common primary malignancy of the liver and the third most common cause of cancer-related mortality. The incidence of primary liver cancer is increasing in several developed countries, including the United States, and the increase will likely continue for some decades. Only 10% of patients with HCC are eligible for curative therapies,

Disclosures: none.
[a] Division of Interventional Radiology, Department of Radiology, University of Illinois Hospital & Health Sciences System, 1740 West Taylor Street (MC 931), Chicago, IL 60612, USA; [b] Section of Interventional Radiology, Department of Radiology, Robert H. Lurie Comprehensive Cancer Center, Northwestern Memorial Hospital, 676 North Saint Clair Street, Suite 800, Chicago, IL 60611, USA
* Corresponding author.
E-mail address: jeetminocha@gmail.com

because of late stage presentation, comorbidities, and limited liver transplant donor availability.[1,2]

In 2002, transarterial chemoembolization (TACE) became the standard of care for unresectable HCC, after 2 randomized controlled trials[3,4] reported a significant survival benefit in patients undergoing this procedure versus best supportive care. According to the Barcelona Clinic Liver Cancer (BCLC) staging and treatment system for HCC (**Fig. 1**), TACE is the recommended treatment of intermediate stage (BCLC stage B) disease.[5] Separately, radioembolization has emerged as an alternative treatment of patients with HCC with intermediate stage (BCLC stage B) disease to overcome the shortcomings of external beam radiation in the treatment of liver cancer.[6]

Both TACE and radioembolization are minimally invasive, image-guided procedures performed by interventional radiologists, most commonly in the liver. They are catheter-based therapies, in which high-dose anticancer treatments (eg, chemotherapy [TACE] or radioactive microspheres [radioembolization]) are selectively injected into tumor-feeding arteries to locally target tumors and limit systemic toxicities. Transcatheter intra-arterial therapies are possible because liver tumors nearly exclusively derive their blood supply from the hepatic artery, whereas normal liver parenchyma receives most of its blood supply from the portal vein.[7,8]

TACE and radioembolization have been widely investigated during the past decade for the treatment of HCC and have led to encouraging response, survival, and quality

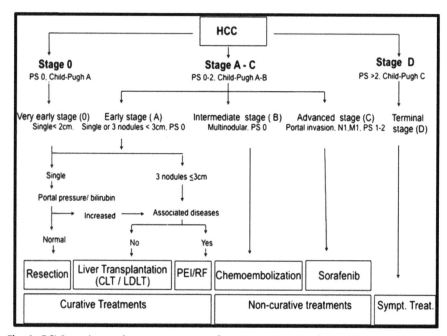

Fig. 1. BCLC staging and treatment system for HCC. Patients with HCC are stratified into 5 stages: very early, early, intermediate, advanced, and end stage, according to tumor burden, liver function, and physical condition. Staging is linked to treatment indication according to evidence-based data. CLT, cadaveric liver transplantation; LDLT, living donor liver transplantation; PEI, percutaneous ethanol injection; RF, radiofrequency ablation. (*From* Forner A, Reig ME, de Lope CR, et al. Current strategy for staging and treatment: the BCLC update and future prospects. Semin Liver Dis 2010;30(1):64; with permission.)

of life outcomes, with reduced toxicity profiles.[1] This finding has led to the use of these therapies in patients with hepatic metastases, most commonly from colorectal cancer (CRC) and neuroendocrine tumors (NET).[9] Occasionally, they are used for patients with other cancers with liver-dominant metastases.

In this article, the current state of the practice of TACE and radioembolization are reviewed and recent scientific data are presented that support their role in the treatment of HCC and hepatic metastatic disease.

INDICATIONS/CONTRAINDICATIONS
Indications

In general, TACE and radioembolization are indicated for treatment of patients with unresectable HCC or hepatic metastases with:

1. Preserved performance status (eg, Eastern Cooperative Oncology Group [ECOG] Performance Status 0–2; **Table 1**)[10]
2. Preserved liver function (eg, serum bilirubin level <2–3 mg/dL, albumin level <3 g/dL, international normalized ratio ≤1.5)
3. Disease burden that is confined or predominantly confined to the liver (ie, liver disease burden is considered to be the dominant source of morbidity and mortality)

Although transcatheter intra-arterial therapies are the recommended treatment of patients with HCC with intermediate stage (BCLC stage B) disease, they play an important therapeutic role across all BCLC stages.[1] These treatments have been effective in maintaining tumor size within Milan criteria for liver transplantation and downsizing previously unresectable disease to curative treatments.[11]

Contraindications

Box 1 lists common contraindications to TACE and radioembolization.

TECHNIQUE/PROCEDURE

This section provides a brief technical overview of TACE and radioembolization. The procedural techniques described have been thoroughly detailed in the medical literature.[3,4,12–14]

Table 1 ECOG performance status	
Grade	**ECOG Definition**
0	Fully active, able to carry on all predisease performance without restriction
1	Restricted in physically strenuous activity but ambulatory and able to carry out work of a light or sedentary nature (eg, light house work, office work)
2	Ambulatory and capable of all self-care but unable to carry out any work activities. Up and about more than 50% of waking hours
3	Capable of only limited self-care, confined to bed or chair more than 50% of waking hours
4	Completely disabled. Cannot carry on any self-care. Totally confined to bed or chair
5	Dead

Data from Oken MM, et al. Toxicity and response criteria of the Eastern Cooperative Oncology Group. Am J Clin Oncol 1982;5(6):649–55.

Box 1
Common contraindications

Absolute

- Poor performance status (eg, ECOG >2)
- Poorly compensated or advanced liver disease (eg, Child-Pugh C)
  - Ascites
  - Encephalopathy
- Active systemic infection
- Large burden of metastatic disease outside liver

Relative

- Poor hepatic reserve
  - Serum bilirubin level greater than 2 mg/dL
  - Lactate dehydrogenase level greater than 425 U/L
  - Aspartate aminotransferase level greater than 100 U/L
- Contraindications to angiography
  - Anaphylactic reaction to radiographic contrast media
  - Uncorrectable coagulopathy
- Contraindications to administration of chemotherapy
  - Thrombocytopenia
  - Leukopenia
  - Cardiac or renal insufficiency (serum creatinine level >2 mg/dL)
- Contraindications to hepatic artery embolization
  - Biliary obstruction (TACE > radioembolization)
  - Portal vein thrombosis (TACE only; radioembolization safe)
  - Uncorrectable flow to the gastrointestinal tract (radioembolization > TACE)
- Significant hepatopulmonary lung shunting (radioembolization > TACE)

Treatment planning for TACE and radioembolization incorporates findings on physical examination (including performance status), serologic values (including liver function and tumor markers when appropriate), and cross-sectional imaging studies.[15] The procedures are most commonly performed under moderate sedation.

TACE

Patients are typically admitted the morning of the TACE procedure for hydration, antibiotics, antiemetics, and narcotic loading.

Conventional TACE

Conventional TACE (cTACE) is defined as the intra-arterial infusion of 1 or more chemotherapeutic agents directly to tumor(s) followed by embolization (hence, chemoembolization).[15] The most commonly used drugs for cTACE include doxorubicin alone or in combination with mitomycin C or cisplatin, because these agents have been shown to be the most active against HCC. After its initial success, the triple-drug combination has been the preferred method in the United States.[16] The vehicle used to deliver chemotherapy in cTACE is lipiodol, a radiopaque oil that carries the chemotherapy to the tumor(s).

cTACE procedure

1. Access common femoral artery after sterile preparation of the groin area
2. Perform diagnostic arteriography, including abdominal aortogram (to exclude collateral tumor blood supply), superior mesenteric arteriogram (to exclude accessory hepatic arteries), and celiac arteriogram
3. Place catheter or coaxial microcatheter into tumor-feeding artery (placement should be proximal enough to treat entire targeted lesion but distal enough to minimize nontarget embolization)
4. Infuse chemotherapy/lipiodol emulsion directly to the targeted tumor under continuous fluoroscopic visualization to avoid/minimize nontarget deposition
5. Embolize with particles such as polyvinyl alcohol, calibrated microspheres, or gelatin sponge to prevent delivered drug washout
6. Remove catheter(s) and groin access and obtain femoral artery hemostasis

Immediately after cTACE, a noncontrast computed tomography (CT) scan could be obtained to show proper targeting of the chemotherapy/lipiodol combination (**Fig. 2**).

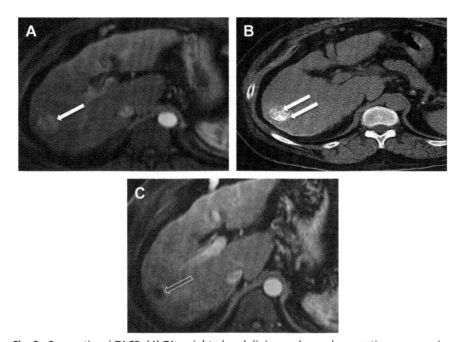

Fig. 2. Conventional TACE. (A) T1-weighted gadolinium-enhanced magnetic resonance imaging shows an enhancing mass (*arrow*) in the right hepatic lobe. After a complete workup, this patient (nonsurgical candidate) underwent cTACE. (B) Noncontrast CT scan performed after cTACE showed proper targeting of the chemotherapy/lipiodol combination within the targeted tumor (*double arrows*). There is some nontarget lipiodol uptake within the noncancerous hepatic parenchyma adjacent to the tumor. (C) Six months after treatment, follow-up T1-weighted gadolinium-enhanced MRI shows complete necrosis (ie, no enhancement) of treated tumor (*open arrow*).

Drug-eluting bead TACE

Drug-eluting bead (DEB) TACE builds on the rationale for cTACE. More specifically, the rationale for using DEBs as opposed to a lipiodol emulsion relies on increased intratumoral retention and decreased bioavailability of chemotherapeutic agent(s) with DEBs, translating into lower toxicity rates when compared with cTACE.[17] Through a drug-loading process, polyvinyl alcohol-based microspheres absorb the chemotherapeutic agent (doxorubicin for HCC and noncolorectal metastases, and irinotecan for metastatic colorectal carcinoma). These unique properties permit release of drug in a controlled and sustained manner.[18]

The procedure itself is similar to cTACE. Instead of a chemotherapy/lipiodol emulsion, the DEBs are delivered to the tumor-feeding artery. In this procedure, the DEBs serve as the vehicle for chemotherapy delivery as well as the embolic microspheres (ie, steps 4–5 are combined into one).

Radioembolization

Radioembolization is defined as the delivery of radioactive microspheres to tumor(s) via hepatic arterial injection in an attempt to achieve cell death by delivering a high dose of focused radiation to the tumor(s) (**Fig. 3**).[19] The most common radionuclide used (yttrium 90 [^{90}Y]) is available in 2 forms:

1. TheraSphere (Nordion for BTG International, Ottawa, Canada) consists of nonbiodegradable glass microspheres, in which ^{90}Y is an integral constituent of the glass. The US Food and Drug Administration (FDA) approved this product in 1999 under a humanitarian device exemption, defined as safe and probably beneficial for the treatment of unresectable HCC with or without portal vein thrombosis, or as a bridge to transplantation in patients who could have appropriately positioned catheters.
2. SIR-Spheres (Sirtex, Lane Cove, Australia) consist of biocompatible resin microspheres containing ^{90}Y. The FDA granted premarket approval for this device in 2002 for the treatment of unresectable metastatic liver tumors from primary CRC with adjuvant intrahepatic artery chemotherapy for floxuridine. This device is also approved in Europe, Australia, and several Asian countries for the treatment of liver neoplasia.

All patients undergo pretreatment (ie, planning) mesenteric angiography and a technetium 99m (Tc 99m)-labeled macroaggregated albumin (MAA) scan approximately

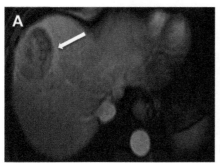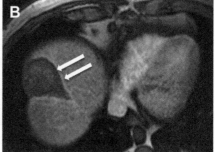

Fig. 3. Radioembolization. (*A*) T1-weighted gadolinium-enhanced magnetic resonance imaging shows a heterogeneously enhancing mass (*arrow*) in the right hepatic lobe. After a complete workup, this patient (not a transplant candidate based on Milan criteria) underwent yttrium 90 radioembolization. (*B*) Six months after treatment, follow-up T1-weighted gadolinium-enhanced MRI shows complete segmental necrosis (ie, no enhancement) (*double arrows*).

1 week before the first planned treatment; this is usually not repeated for subsequent treatments.

Pretreatment procedure

1. Access common femoral artery after sterile preparation of the groin area
2. Perform diagnostic arteriography, including abdominal aortogram (to exclude collateral tumor blood supply), superior mesenteric arteriogram (to exclude accessory hepatic arteries), and celiac arteriogram
3. Identify and coil-embolize vessel(s) that may lead to nontarget deposition of the radioactive microspheres (eg, gastroduodenal or right gastric arteries), if necessary
4. Identify vascular supply of the tumor(s)
5. Place catheter or coaxial microcatheter into tumor-feeding artery
6. Infuse Tc 99m MAA (test beads)
7. Remove catheter(s) and groin access and obtain femoral artery hemostasis

The MAA scan quantifies the lung shunt fraction; this is incorporated into dosimetry calculations to minimize radiation dose to the lungs.

Radioembolization procedure

1. Access common femoral artery after sterile preparation of the groin area
2. Place catheter or coaxial microcatheter into previously identified tumor-feeding artery
3. Inject activity vial of ^{90}Y microspheres
4. Remove catheter(s) and groin access and obtain femoral artery hemostasis

A treatment paradigm that parallels TACE is recommended (ie, lobar or segmental infusions).

COMPLICATIONS AND MANAGEMENT
Side Effects

Side effects after TACE (ie, postembolization syndrome) tend to be more severe than those after radioembolization (ie, postradioembolization syndrome),[20] including abdominal pain/discomfort, nausea and vomiting, fatigue, anorexia, and fever.

Complications

Complications after transcatheter intra-arterial therapies may occur as a result of toxicity to normal liver parenchyma, nontarget embolization (eg, gastrointestinal ulcer), or complications of angiography (eg, groin complication or vessel dissection).[15,19]

Complications related to TACE and radioembolization are summarized in **Table 2**.

POSTPROCEDURE CARE

TACE is performed as an inpatient procedure to manage postembolization syndrome. In contrast, radioembolization is performed as an outpatient procedure, because unlike TACE, the intent of radioembolization is not vessel occlusion. Rather, the radioactive microspheres lodge within tumor arterioles and irradiate surrounding tissue.[21] Consequently, because macroscopic vessel occlusion does not occur, hospitalization is not required (ie, no postembolization syndrome).

Postprocedure Management (TACE)

1. Inpatient symptomatic support (typically 1–3 days): vigorous hydration, pain control (eg, patient-controlled anesthesia), antiemetics, and antibiotics

Table 2
Complications after TACE and radioembolization

Complication	Risk Factor(s)	Frequency If Risk Factor Present (%)	Management/Prevention
Liver failure, death, encephalopathy	Child-Pugh C Bilirubin ≥4 mg/dL Albumin ≤2 mg/dL Poor performance status	5–10 Unknown	Symptomatic support Treatment should be avoided in high-risk patients
Liver abscess	Compromised sphincter of Oddi (eg, biliary-enteric anastomosis); concurrent systemic infection	30–80 (otherwise 2)	Antibiotic therapy with/without percutaneous drainage
Biloma	Compromised sphincter of Oddi (eg, biliary-enteric anastomosis); biliary dilatation	Uncommon	Biloma drainage Percutaneous transhepatic biliary drainage
Nontarget embolization			
Gastrointestinal (GI) ulcer	Aberrant arterial anatomy	<10	Symptomatic support Acid suppression; severe or nonhealing ulcers may require surgery
Cholecystitis	Aberrant arterial anatomy	<10	Symptomatic support (Prophylactic) antibiotics
Pulmonary embolism	Tumor shunting	<1	Symptomatic support
Acute renal failure	Renal insufficiency, diabetes	0.05–5	Hydration, nephroprotectants, minimize contrast before/during procedure

2. Discharge goals: ambulatory after angiography, adequate oral intake, and adequate urine output
3. Discharge medications: 5-day to 7-day antibiotic course, oral pain medications as needed

Postprocedure Management (Radioembolization)

1. Outpatient discharge goals: ambulatory after angiography
2. Discharge medications: 7-day to 10-day proton pump inhibitor course for gastrointestinal ulcer prophylaxis

REPORTING, FOLLOW-UP, AND CLINICAL IMPLICATIONS

Posttherapy imaging is typically obtained 1 month after treatment and then every 3 months (dynamic gadolinium-enhanced magnetic resonance imaging (MRI) or triphasic CT for HCC; CT for metastatic disease). Assessing response can be challenging secondary to posttreatment changes in the tumor and surrounding hepatic parenchyma. This factor is more pronounced with radioembolization, in which the intent is not to embolize the tumor-feeding artery and produce immediate necrosis.

Traditional assessment of therapy response is based on anatomic measurements of tumor size, most commonly using World Health Organization (WHO) and RECIST (Response Evaluation Criteria in Solid Tumors) guidelines. An important feature of transcatheter intra-arterial therapies is the presence of necrosis, defined as a lack of enhancement of the lesion(s) after treatment on contrast-enhanced CT or MRI. Both WHO and RECIST do not consider tissue viability when assessing response. Thus, more recently, guidelines to assess tumor necrosis/viability (eg, European Association for the Study of the Liver [EASL] and modified RECIST [mRECIST] guidelines) have proved useful for evaluating hypervascular tumors such as HCC. Studies have found that the EASL and mRECIST criteria were independent prognostic factors to predict survival for patients with HCC treated with cTACE.[22] Because it may take months after therapy before an anatomic response is realized, functional parameters (eg, tumor markers, diffusion-weighted MRI, positron emission tomography) can be useful. However, these parameters remain adjunctive, given their lack of standardization.

TACE is typically repeated until imaging shows greater than 90% tumor necrosis, the tumor does not respond after at least 2 treatments, or the patient develops a contraindication to therapy. Some repeat this procedure on schedule (eg, every so many months), whereas others perform this procedure on demand (eg, in the setting of progressive disease). Radioembolization is most often repeated if/when progression occurs.

OUTCOMES

TACE and radioembolization have been used to treat numerous types of liver tumors. However, the best current evidence supports their use in unresectable HCC and metastatic CRC. Outcomes from select studies are summarized in **Tables 3** and **4**.

HCC

In 2002, 2 randomized controlled trials reported a significant survival benefit in patients with Child-Pugh A or B with unresectable HCC treated with cTACE compared with best supportive care.[3,4] Lo and colleagues[3] reported the 1-year, 2-year, and 3-year survival in cTACE-treated patients to be 57%, 31%, and 26%, compared with 32%, 11%, and 3%, respectively, in the symptomatic treatment control group. Llovet and colleagues[4] published results from their trial, which was stopped early because cTACE provided a statistically significant survival benefit in the treatment group (1-year and 2-year survival of 82% and 63% for TACE vs 63% and 27% for the supportive care group).

The next generation of TACE (DEB-TACE) has not shown a benefit over cTACE; however, the best available evidence suggests that it may be better tolerated, especially in patients with more advanced liver disease.[17] In a comparative analysis,[6] radioembolization and TACE have shown similar survival times, but radioembolization resulted in longer time to progression and less toxicity than TACE. Although therapy selection is multifactorial and may include institutional expertise and cost-effectiveness, radioembolization may have a niche application in patients with HCC with portal vein thrombosis.[24,25] In addition, quality of life may be increased after radioembolization.[20]

Metastatic CRC

In metastatic CRC, cTACE data are not standardized and impart marginal benefit. However, DEB-TACE with irinotecan may represent a more promising TACE alternative. Fiorentini and colleagues[29] reported a median survival of 22 months after DEB-TACE with

Table 3
cTACE, DEB-TACE, and radioembolization for HCC

Authors, Year	Treatment	Summary
Lo et al,[3] 2002	cTACE	80 patients with unresectable HCC Randomized controlled trial Chemoembolization vs symptomatic treatment Chemoembolization significantly improves survival in select patients
Llovet et al,[4] 2002	cTACE	112 patients with unresectable HCC Randomized controlled trial 3 treatment arms: arterial embolization, chemoembolization, conservative management Chemoembolization improved survival of stringently selected patients
Vogl et al,[17] 2011	DEB-TACE	212 patients with intermediate stage HCC randomized to TACE with DEBs or conventional TACE (PRECISION V trial) Fewer liver toxicities in the DEB-TACE group compared with cTACE group
Salem et al,[23] 2010	Radioembolization	291 patients with HCC treated with ^{90}Y radioembolization Response rates 42% (WHO criteria) and 57% (EASL criteria) Patients with Child-Pugh A disease, with or without portal vein thrombosis, benefited most from radioembolization Time to progression and overall survival varied by tumor stage and liver function
Mazzaferro et al,[24] 2013	Radioembolization	52 patients with intermediate to advanced HCC Prospective, phase II study Median time to progression 11 mo (no difference between portal vein thrombosis vs no portal vein thrombosis) Median overall survival 15 mo Various grades of reduced liver function in 36.5% within 6 mo

irinotecan compared with 15 months for systemic irinotecan, fluorouracil, and leucovorin (FOLFIRI) in patients with hepatic metastases from CRC. Radioembolization has shown encouraging median survival in the salvage setting, with reported median survival of 10.5 months.[32] In addition, there is enthusiasm for combining radioembolization with a standard chemotherapy regimen as first-line therapy in patients with nonresectable CRC liver metastases (eg, SIRFLOX randomized controlled study).

Other Liver Tumors

The role of TACE and radioembolization in other liver tumors, including metastatic NET, seems promising but is still being established.[33–37] In general, these therapies seem to provide local disease control and maintain quality of life.

CURRENT CONTROVERSIES/FUTURE CONSIDERATIONS

TACE and radioembolization are establishing an important role in the treatment of patients with HCC and metastatic liver tumors. Although most of the current data

Table 4
cTACE, DEB-TACE, and radioembolization for metastatic CRC

Authors, Year	Treatment	Summary
Tellez et al,[26] 1998	cTACE	30 patients with metastatic CRC with failure of ≥ 1 systemic treatments 63% radiologic response (defined as decrease in lesion density of 75% or lesion size of 25%) 95% had at least 25% decrease from baseline carcinoembryonic antigen levels 100% experienced postembolization syndrome Chemoembolization is a feasible treatment of patients with metastatic CRC who have failed other systemic treatments
Geschwind et al,[27] 2006	cTACE	Patients with unresectable liver CRC metastases that progress despite systemic chemotherapy can undergo palliative chemoembolization (or radioembolization), with survival benefit
Martin et al,[28] 2011	DEB-TACE	55 patients who received previous systemic chemotherapy underwent 99 DEB-TACE (irinotecan) treatments for metastatic CRC Response rates were 66% at 6 mo and 75% at 12 mo Overall survival was 19%, with progression-free survival 11 mo Adverse events in 28% (median grade of 2)
Fiorentini et al,[29] 2012	DEB-TACE	74 patients with hepatic metastases from CRC Patients randomized to TACE (DEBs with irinotecan; DEBIRI) vs systemic irinotecan, fluorouracil, and leucovorin (FOLFIRI) Significantly longer overall survival, progression-free survival, and quality of life in DEBIRI patients compared with FOLFIRI
Gray et al,[30] 2001	Radioembolization	Phase 3 randomized clinical trial of 74 patients with nonresectable liver metastases from adenocarcinoma of the large bowel Single administration of ^{90}Y microspheres to a regimen of regional hepatic artery chemotherapy vs same chemotherapy alone Median time to progression significantly longer for patients receiving ^{90}Y compared with patients receiving hepatic artery chemotherapy alone 1-y, 2-y, 3-y, and 5-y survival was 72%, 39%, 17%, and 3.5% (^{90}Y) compared with 68%, 29%, 6.5%, and 0% (HAC alone)
Van Hazel et al,[31] 2004	Radioembolization	21 patients with previously untreated advanced CRC liver metastases were randomized to systemic fluorouracil/leucovorin vs same chemotherapy plus single administration of ^{90}Y microspheres Combination treatment significantly increased treatment-related response, time to progression (18.6 vs 3.6 mo) and survival (29.4 vs 12.8 mo) compared with chemotherapy alone
Kennedy et al,[32] 2006	Radioembolization	208 patients with unresectable, chemorefractory CRC liver metastases treated with ^{90}Y microspheres CT partial response rate 35%; positron emission tomography response rate 91% Median survival 10.5 mo for responders but only 4.5 mo in nonresponders No treatment-related procedure deaths or radiation-related venoocclusive liver failures

supporting these therapies have been generated from retrospective studies or prospective registry-type projects, there are numerous ongoing clinical trials that will generate more robust evidence for these treatments.[13]

Ongoing research in this field is aimed at improving drug delivery techniques and developing new, more potent and specific therapies, which can be locally delivered. Transcatheter therapies have great potential in combination with other treatment modalities such as ablation or systemic therapies, such as antiangiogenic or radiosensitizing agents. Results from future studies are expected to further solidify the role of transcatheter intra-arterial therapies in the treatment of primary and metastatic liver tumors.

SUMMARY

- TACE and ^{90}Y radioembolization are catheter-based therapies that selectively deliver high-dose anticancer treatments directly to tumor(s) using imaging guidance.
- TACE and ^{90}Y radioembolization have been widely investigated during the past decade for the treatment of primary and metastatic liver tumors and have led to encouraging response, survival, and quality of life outcomes, with reduced toxicity profiles.
- TACE and ^{90}Y radioembolization are applicable in many clinical scenarios, because they are less limited than systemic treatments by tumor characteristics. Furthermore, they have great potential in combination with other treatments, including ablation and systemic therapies.

REFERENCES

1. Salem R, Lewandowski RJ. Chemoembolization and radioembolization for hepatocellular carcinoma. Clin Gastroenterol Hepatol 2013;11(6):604–11 [quiz: e43–4].
2. Bosch FX, Ribes J, Diaz M, et al. Primary liver cancer: worldwide incidence and trends. Gastroenterology 2004;127(5 Suppl 1):S5–16.
3. Lo CM, Ngan H, Tso WK, et al. Randomized controlled trial of transarterial lipiodol chemoembolization for unresectable hepatocellular carcinoma. Hepatology 2002;35(5):1164–71.
4. Llovet JM, Real MI, Montana X, et al. Arterial embolisation or chemoembolisation versus symptomatic treatment in patients with unresectable hepatocellular carcinoma: a randomised controlled trial. Lancet 2002;359(9319):1734–9.
5. Forner A, Reig ME, de Lope CR, et al. Current strategy for staging and treatment: the BCLC update and future prospects. Semin Liver Dis 2010;30(1):61–74.
6. Salem R, Lewandowski RJ, Kulik L, et al. Radioembolization results in longer time-to-progression and reduced toxicity compared with chemoembolization in patients with hepatocellular carcinoma. Gastroenterology 2011;140(2):497–507.e2.
7. Gyves JW, Ziessman HA, Ensminger WD, et al. Definition of hepatic tumor microcirculation by single photon emission computerized tomography (SPECT). J Nucl Med 1984;25(9):972–7.
8. Bierman HR, Byron RL Jr, Kelley KH, et al. Studies on the blood supply of tumors in man. III. Vascular patterns of the liver by hepatic arteriography in vivo. J Natl Cancer Inst 1951;12(1):107–31.
9. Memon K, Lewandowski RJ, Riaz A, et al. Chemoembolization and radioembolization for metastatic disease to the liver: available data and future studies. Curr Treat Options Oncol 2012;13(3):403–15.

10. Oken MM, Creech RH, Tormey DC, et al. Toxicity and response criteria of the Eastern Cooperative Oncology Group. Am J Clin Oncol 1982;5(6):649–55.
11. Kulik LM, Atassi B, van Holsbeeck L, et al. Yttrium-90 microspheres (Thera-Sphere) treatment of unresectable hepatocellular carcinoma: downstaging to resection, RFA and bridge to transplantation. J Surg Oncol 2006;94(7): 572–86.
12. Lencioni R, de Baere T, Burrel M, et al. Transcatheter treatment of hepatocellular carcinoma with Doxorubicin-loaded DC Bead (DEBDOX): technical recommendations. Cardiovasc Intervent Radiol 2012;35(5):980–5.
13. Lewandowski RJ, Geschwind JF, Liapi E, et al. Transcatheter intraarterial therapies: rationale and overview. Radiology 2011;259(3):641–57.
14. Salem R, Thurston KG. Radioembolization with 90Yttrium microspheres: a state-of-the-art brachytherapy treatment for primary and secondary liver malignancies. Part 1: technical and methodologic considerations. J Vasc Interv Radiol 2006; 17(8):1251–78.
15. Brown DB, Gould JE, Gervais DA, et al. Transcatheter therapy for hepatic malignancy: standardization of terminology and reporting criteria. J Vasc Interv Radiol 2009;20(7 Suppl):S425–34.
16. Solomon B, Soulen MC, Baum RA, et al. Chemoembolization of hepatocellular carcinoma with cisplatin, doxorubicin, mitomycin-C, ethiodol, and polyvinyl alcohol: prospective evaluation of response and survival in a US population. J Vasc Interv Radiol 1999;10(6):793–8.
17. Vogl TJ, Lammer J, Lencioni R, et al. Liver, gastrointestinal, and cardiac toxicity in intermediate hepatocellular carcinoma treated with PRECISION TACE with drug-eluting beads: results from the PRECISION V randomized trial. AJR Am J Roentgenol 2011;197(4):W562–70.
18. Gonzalez MV, Tang Y, Phillips GJ, et al. Doxorubicin eluting beads-2: methods for evaluating drug elution and in-vitro:in-vivo correlation. J Mater Sci Mater Med 2008;19(2):767–75.
19. Salem R, Lewandowski RJ, Gates VL, et al. Research reporting standards for radioembolization of hepatic malignancies. J Vasc Interv Radiol 2011;22(3):265–78.
20. Salem R, Gilbertsen M, Butt Z, et al. Increased quality of life among hepatocellular carcinoma patients treated with radioembolization, compared with chemoembolization. Clin Gastroenterol Hepatol 2013;11(10):1358–65.e1.
21. Sato K, Lewandowski RJ, Bui JT, et al. Treatment of unresectable primary and metastatic liver cancer with yttrium-90 microspheres (TheraSphere): assessment of hepatic arterial embolization. Cardiovasc Intervent Radiol 2006;29(4):522–9.
22. Guo Y, Yaghmai V, Salem R, et al. Imaging tumor response following liver-directed intra-arterial therapy. Abdom Imaging 2013;38(6):1286–99.
23. Salem R, Lewandowski RJ, Mulcahy MF, et al. Radioembolization for hepatocellular carcinoma using yttrium-90 microspheres: a comprehensive report of long-term outcomes. Gastroenterology 2010;138(1):52–64.
24. Mazzaferro V, Sposito C, Bhoori S, et al. Yttrium-90 radioembolization for intermediate-advanced hepatocellular carcinoma: a phase 2 study. Hepatology 2013;57(5):1826–37.
25. Kulik LM, Carr BI, Mulcahy MF, et al. Safety and efficacy of 90Y radiotherapy for hepatocellular carcinoma with and without portal vein thrombosis. Hepatology 2008;47(1):71–81.
26. Tellez C, Benson AB 3rd, Lyster MT, et al. Phase II trial of chemoembolization for the treatment of metastatic colorectal carcinoma to the liver and review of the literature. Cancer 1998;82(7):1250–9.

27. Geschwind J, Hong K, Georgiades C. Utility of transcatheter arterial chemoembolization for liver dominant colorectal metastatic adenocarcinoma in the salvage setting, in American Society of Clinical Oncology Gastrointestinal Cancers Symposium. San Francisco, January 26–28, 2006.

28. Martin RC, Joshi J, Robbins K, et al. Hepatic intra-arterial injection of drug-eluting bead, irinotecan (DEBIRI) in unresectable colorectal liver metastases refractory to systemic chemotherapy: results of multi-institutional study. Ann Surg Oncol 2011;18(1):192–8.

29. Fiorentini G, Aliberti C, Tilli M, et al. Intra-arterial infusion of irinotecan-loaded drug-eluting beads (DEBIRI) versus intravenous therapy (FOLFIRI) for hepatic metastases from colorectal cancer: final results of a phase III study. Anticancer Res 2012; 32(4):1387–95.

30. Gray B, Van Hazel G, Hope M, et al. Randomised trial of SIR-Spheres plus chemotherapy vs. chemotherapy alone for treating patients with liver metastases from primary large bowel cancer. Ann Oncol 2001;12(12):1711–20.

31. Van Hazel G, Blackwell A, Anderson J, et al. Randomised phase 2 trial of SIR-Spheres plus fluorouracil/leucovorin chemotherapy versus fluorouracil/leucovorin chemotherapy alone in advanced colorectal cancer. J Surg Oncol 2004;88(2): 78–85.

32. Kennedy AS, Coldwell D, Nutting C, et al. Resin 90Y-microsphere brachytherapy for unresectable colorectal liver metastases: modern USA experience. Int J Radiat Oncol Biol Phys 2006;65(2):412–25.

33. Roche A, Girish BV, de Baere T, et al. Trans-catheter arterial chemoembolization as first-line treatment for hepatic metastases from endocrine tumors. Eur Radiol 2003;13(1):136–40.

34. Liapi E, Geschwind JF, Vossen JA, et al. Functional MRI evaluation of tumor response in patients with neuroendocrine hepatic metastasis treated with transcatheter arterial chemoembolization. AJR Am J Roentgenol 2008;190(1):67–73.

35. Gaur SK, Friese JL, Sadow CA, et al. Hepatic arterial chemoembolization using drug-eluting beads in gastrointestinal neuroendocrine tumor metastatic to the liver. Cardiovasc Intervent Radiol 2011;34(3):566–72.

36. Rhee TK, Lewandowski RJ, Liu DM, et al. 90Y Radioembolization for metastatic neuroendocrine liver tumors: preliminary results from a multi-institutional experience. Ann Surg 2008;247(6):1029–35.

37. Memon K, Lewandowski RJ, Mulcahy MF, et al. Radioembolization for neuroendocrine liver metastases: safety, imaging, and long-term outcomes. Int J Radiat Oncol Biol Phys 2012;83(3):887–94.

Endoscopic Retrograde Cholangiopancreatography for Cholangiocarcinoma

Todd H. Baron, MD

KEYWORDS

- Cholangiocarcinoma • ERCP • Stents • Plastic • Metal • Palliation

KEY POINTS

- Endoscopic retrograde cholangiopancreatography (ERCP) is technically challenging in hilar cholangiocarcinoma.
- ERCP is used for biliary decompression most often for palliation.
- Preprocedural planning using CT and MRI are important to select areas of drainage.

INTRODUCTION

Cholangiocarcinoma is an increasingly frequent disorder. Patients most often present with obstructive jaundice. Endoscopic retrograde cholangiopancreatography (ERCP) is used primarily for biliary drainage rather than a purely diagnostic procedure.

INDICATIONS/CONTRAINDICATIONS

ERCP is indicated in the presence of biliary obstruction after detailed imaging has been performed. The typical sequence is patient presentation of painless jaundice and weight loss followed by investigation with laboratory testing and transabdominal ultrasound. Once biliary ductal dilation is established by ultrasound, CT or MRI is undertaken. The ultrasound should be able to distinguish between distal (nonhilar) and hilar obstruction based on the level of ductal dilation. MRI is the preferred imaging technique for the evaluation of suspected hilar lesions,[1,2] although 3D-CT cholangiography is also useful.[3]

Based on the imaging studies and operative status, the patient is considered operable or nonoperable (resectable lesion, operable patient). Operable patients should undergo surgery without ERCP, although there are exceptions based on individual patients and surgeon preference.

Disclosure: None.
Division of Gastroenterology & Hepatology, University of North Carolina, Campus Box 7080, Chapel Hill, NC 27599, USA
E-mail address: todd_baron@med.unc.edu

Thus, ERCP is indicated to relieve obstructive jaundice in nonoperable patients and in selected preoperative situations, and to apply therapy (**Box 1**).

ERCP is contraindicated in the setting of ongoing luminal perforation, gastric outlet obstruction, uncontrolled coagulopathy, and inability to obtain consent (see **Box 1**).

TECHNIQUE/PROCEDURE
Preparation

A complete laboratory profile, including international normalized ratio and platelet count, is obtained. Anesthesia assessment and support are needed for most patients, especially those who are American Society of Anesthesiologists physical status classification system 3 or greater. Antithrombotic agents are temporarily discontinued as appropriate, especially if biliary sphincterotomy is anticipated. If the patient is to receive photodynamic therapy, a porphyrin agent is administered 48 hours before the procedure.

Patient Positioning

Before the procedure, the patient is maintained nil per os as per institutional and anesthesia protocol. The procedure is performed with the patient placed on the fluoroscopy table in the ERCP suite in the prone or supine position based on endoscopist preference. Anecdotally, the supine position allows better fluoroscopic imaging of hilar lesions because it opens up the bifurcation and separates the right and left hepatic ducts. A rotatable fluoroscopy allows the bifurcation to be visualized.

Approach

Before the procedure, the endoscopic approach is formulated based on cross-sectional imaging (CT, MRI). If the lesion is below the bifurcation, then a single biliary stent is placed. For hilar lesions, the Bismuth classification (**Fig. 1**) and the presence of liver parenchymal atrophy[4,5] are used to decide whether unilateral or bilateral stents are placed, and which biliary segments to drain. Bile ducts within atrophic segments

---

Box 1
Indications and contraindications for ERCP in hilar cholangiocarcinoma

Indications

- Diagnostic: brush cytology, intraductal biopsies, cholangioscopy. Biliary drainage must be provided at the same time
- Preoperative decompression (selected cases) to relieve obstructive jaundice before surgery in selected patients
- Palliation of obstructive jaundice: stent placement in nonoperable patients. Plastic or metal
- Photodynamic therapy for improvement and/or prolongation of palliation
- Application of intraductal radiofrequency ablation for improvement and/or prolongation of palliation

Contraindications

- Ongoing luminal perforation
- Esophageal/duodenal obstruction with inability to pass endoscope
- Inability to obtain informed consent
- Uncontrolled coagulopathy (if sphincterotomy planned)

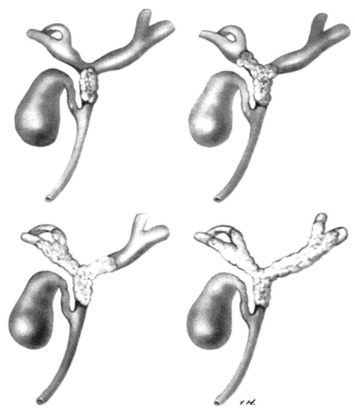

Fig. 1. Bismuth classification for hilar lesions.

of the liver are avoided because introduction of contrast into these segments requires drainage to prevent cholangitis but without providing functional advantage.

Technique/Procedure

- A therapeutic (4.2-mm channel diameter) side-viewing endoscope (duodenoscope) is passed to the level of the major papilla. The bile duct is selectively cannulated using a catheter and guide wire.
- Bismuth Type I Lesions
  - For distal, nonhilar lesions, contrast can be injected as needed to outline the stricture without concern for inadequate drainage after the procedure. A guide wire is used to traverse the lesion. This author prefers to use angled hydrophilic wires.
  - A biliary sphincterotomy is usually performed to prevent post-ERCP pancreatitis, although this is not mandatory because a single stent is placed. In addition, if a short metal stent is placed across the stricture it may not cross the papilla on the distal end and a sphincterotomy is unnecessary.
  - Balloon or bougie dilation of the stricture is usually not necessary. A single 10-Fr plastic stent or self-expandable metal stent is placed across the stricture with the distal end deployed into the duodenum, though it can be left within the bile duct above the papilla. The decision to use plastic or metal is based on projected life-expectancy and health care costs. Self-expandable metal stents

provide prolonged patency compared with plastic stents but are far more expensive. Their cost is offset by a reduced rate of stent occlusion and subsequent need for repeat procedures and/or hospitalization.

- Bismuth Type II Lesions
  - For hilar lesions, the bile duct is cannulated with minimal to no contrast injection. After selective cannulation, contrast is only injected to the point of the obstruction. A guide wire is used to traverse the lesion and to pass selectively into the right or left intrahepatic system, as determined by the preprocedural approach using MRI/MR cholangiopancreatography. A sphincterotomy is performed to accommodate more than one stent if it is planned that they exit the papilla.
  - For unilateral drainage of hilar lesions, the guide wire is advanced into either the right or the left intrahepatic system as determined by imaging. The catheter is passed over the wire and into the intrahepatic system. Contrast is injected and the catheter is withdrawn. Either a single 10-Fr stent or uncovered self-expandable metal stent is placed. Covered metal stents are rarely used for hilar lesions.
  - For bilateral stent placement, the bile duct is recannulated alongside the initial guide wire with a second guide wire. The wire is passed selectively into the opposite intrahepatic system. Balloon dilation of each stricture, usually the right and left hepatic duct and common hepatic duct, is performed sequentially to 6 mm. It may be necessary to dilate the normal narrow distal bile duct below the lesion to accommodate two 10-Fr stents.
  - In patients with atrophy of the left lobe and involvement of the right anterior and right posterior system, it may be necessary to place a stent in each of these segments similar to the patient in whom bilateral hilar stents are placed.
  - If self-expandable metal stents are used, they are passed sequentially and deployed. Self-expandable stents with small-diameter predeployment delivery systems of 6-Fr can be placed side-by-side before deployment and then deployed sequentially.[6] Stents with large diameter interstices (cell-width) can be deployed in a Y (stent-in-stent) configuration.[7] In this scenario, one stent is placed across the bifurcation. A guide wire is passed through the initial stent and out the side through an interstice. The second stent is then deployed. This configuration may provide better anatomic positioning and avoid "stent crowding" as is seen in side-by-side configuration.

COMPLICATIONS AND MANAGEMENT

Box 2 shows the adverse events (complications) that can occur following ERCP for cholangiocarcinoma. Such adverse events can be graded as mild, moderate, and severe.[8] These adverse events are managed as follows (with the exception of sedation complications, which will not be discussed).

Cholangitis

For patients undergoing ERCP for hilar cholangiocarcinoma and anticipated inadequate drainage (Bismuth type II, III, IV), antibiotics are administered preprocedurally to prevent cholangitis. If cholangitis develops and adequate drainage seems assured, then treatment with intravenous or per oral antibiotics is needed, depending on severity. If adequate drainage has not been established endoscopically, then reassessment with drainage is needed. Drainage can be with additional endoscopic manipulation or percutaneously.

> **Box 2**
> **Adverse events (complications) following ERCP for cholangiocarcinoma**
>
> - Cholangitis
> - Pancreatitis
> - Bleeding
> - Perforation
> - Sedation

Pancreatitis

Post-ERCP pancreatitis can be prevented with use of rectally administered nonsteroidal agents in high-risk cases. If pancreatitis develops, it is managed supportively. Patients with clinically severe pancreatitis require management in the intensive care unit.

Bleeding

Bleeding is almost always due to sphincterotomy. Management includes support with fluid resuscitation. In patients with active or ongoing bleeding, endoscopic therapy is required. Uncontrolled sphincterotomy bleeding is managed with angiographic embolization. Rarely, bleeding from the tumor as a direct result of endoscopic manipulation can occur. If clinically significant, then angiography is warranted.

Perforation

Perforation can be at any point of passage of the endoscope in the esophagus, stomach, or duodenum. It can also occur at the sphincterotomy, which can then be retroperitoneal, intraperitoneal, or both. Finally, guide wire perforation can also occur. Management of perforation is beyond the scope of this article and is reviewed by Baron and colleagues.[9]

POSTOPERATIVE CARE

- Diet is reinstituted the same day, assuming no postprocedural adverse events occurred.
- Antibiotics are continued for approximately 1 week in advanced hilar cases.
- Serum bilirubin should be followed serially until it reaches a normal value or plateaus. If it does not decrease by at least 50% by 2 weeks and/or if cholangitis develops early postprocedurally, then reimaging and reassessment to repeat endoscopy and/or percutaneous therapy for drainage are needed.
- In patients in whom plastic stents are placed, removal and replacement are needed on scheduled intervals, usually every 3 months in the presence of 10-Fr stents.

OUTCOMES

Technical success rates for endoscopic stent placement in Bismuth type I lesions should be nearly 100% when performed by experienced endoscopists, and similar to for other distal malignant obstructions (eg, pancreatic cancer). In patients with otherwise healthy hepatic parenchyma, the clinical success (relief of jaundice) should be nearly uniform as well. Limiting factors for technical success are ability to obtain deep cannulation of the bile duct and passage of a guide wire across the stricture.

Technical and clinical success rates for endoscopic stent placement decrease as Bismuth classification increases. In the hands of experienced endoscopists, the technical success remains high. However, as the tumor involves successively more intrahepatic ducts (Bismuth IV), the technical success is approximately 90%. Complete resolution of jaundice may not occur because it is now thought that at least 50% of normal liver needs to be drained to achieve complete resolution of jaundice.[4]

CURRENT CONTROVERSIES/FUTURE CONSIDERATIONS

There remains controversy about routine bilateral stent placement versus unilateral stent placement for hilar cholangiocarcinoma in the absence of hepatic atrophy. In addition, there remains controversy on routine placement of plastic stents or metal stents. Finally, the use of photodynamic therapy and radiofrequency ablation is still not considered standard therapy. The latter has been recently introduced and requires further study.

SUMMARY

ERCP for hilar cholangiocarcinoma is technically difficult, particularly in patients with advanced hilar lesions. In expert centers, the success rates are high and adverse event rates low. Clinical success with complete resolution of jaundice is variable based on Bismuth stage, presence of atrophy, underlying liver disease, and adequacy of stent placement.

REFERENCES

1. Katabathina VS, Dasyam AK, Dasyam N, et al. Adult bile duct strictures: role of MR imaging and MR cholangiopancreatography in characterization. Radiographics 2014;34(3):565–86.
2. Singh A, Mann HS, Thukral CL, et al. Diagnostic accuracy of MRCP as compared to ultrasound/CT in patients with obstructive jaundice. J Clin Diagn Res 2014; 8(3):103–7.
3. Ajiki T, Fukumoto T, Ueno K, et al. Three-dimensional computed tomographic cholangiography as a novel diagnostic tool for evaluation of bile duct invasion of perihilar cholangiocarcinoma. Hepatogastroenterology 2013;60(128):1833–8.
4. Vienne A, Hobeika E, Gouya H, et al. Prediction of drainage effectiveness during endoscopic stenting of malignant hilar strictures: the role of liver volume assessment. Gastrointest Endosc 2010;72(4):728–35.
5. Kozarek RA. Malignant hilar strictures: one stent or two? Plastic versus self-expanding metal stents? The role of liver atrophy and volume assessment as a predictor of survival in patients undergoing endoscopic stent placement. Gastrointest Endosc 2010;72(4):736–8.
6. Law R, Baron TH. Bilateral metal stents for hilar biliary obstruction using a 6Fr delivery system: outcomes following bilateral and side-by-side stent deployment. Dig Dis Sci 2013;58(9):2667–72.
7. Chahal P, Baron TH. Expandable metal stents for endoscopic bilateral stent-within-stent placement for malignant hilar biliary obstruction. Gastrointest Endosc 2010;71(1):195–9.

8. Cotton PB, Eisen GM, Aabakken L, et al. A lexicon for endoscopic adverse events: report of an ASGE workshop. Gastrointest Endosc 2010;71(3):446–54.
9. Baron TH, Wong Kee Song LM, Zielinski MD, et al. A comprehensive approach to the management of acute endoscopic perforations (with videos). Gastrointest Endosc 2012;76(4):838–59.

Endoscopic Retrograde Cholangiopancreatography for Primary Sclerosing Cholangitis

(®) CrossMark

Nirav Thosani, MD, Subhas Banerjee, MD*

KEYWORDS

- Primary sclerosing cholangitis • Bile duct stricture • Dominant stricture • ERCP
- Cholangioscopy • Choledochoscopy • Biliary drainage • Bile duct sampling

KEY POINTS

- The results from several nonrandomized trials indicate clinical improvement and improved 5-year transplant free survival rates after endoscopic interventions in patients with primary sclerosing cholangitis (PSC) with dominant stricture.
- Optimal endoscopic intervention for dominant stricture remains unclear. Based on cumulative evidence from retrospective and small uncontrolled prospective studies, some experts currently recommend endoscopic balloon dilation only for management of dominant stricture in PSC.
- Stent placement is recommended by some experts only for PSC patients with clinically overt cholangitis, and if stricture dilation alone is unsuccessful. A short duration of stenting—as few as 10 days—is also recommended by some experts.
- Despite advances in medical science, the distinction between a benign dominant stricture and cholangiocarcinoma in a PSC patient remains challenging. However, newer endoscopic techniques such as cholangioscopy with biopsy and advanced cytologic techniques such as fluorescence in situ hybridization are likely to improve sensitivity for the diagnosis of cholangiocarcinoma over that achieved by traditional cytology brushing alone.

INTRODUCTION

Primary sclerosing cholangitis (PSC) is an immune-medicated, chronic, cholestatic liver disease characterized by inflammation and fibrosis of both intrahepatic and extra-hepatic bile ducts.[1–3] PSC is a progressive disease and most patients eventually develop cirrhosis, hepatic decompensation, and portal hypertension.[3] PSC must be

Funding Source: None.
Conflict of Interest: None.
Division of Gastroenterology and Hepatology, Stanford University School of Medicine, 300 Pasteur Drive, MC: 5244, Stanford, CA 94305, USA
* Corresponding author.
E-mail address: sbanerje@stanford.edu

differentiated from secondary sclerosing cholangitis, which is characterized by a similar multifocal biliary structuring process that develops secondary to identifiable causes of long-term biliary obstruction with infection and inflammation that can lead to bile duct destruction and secondary biliary cirrhosis.[4] A diagnosis of PSC may be reached based on a cholestatic biochemical profile, characteristic bile duct changes with multifocal strictures on cholangiography, and after exclusion of secondary sclerosing cholangitis. Traditionally, endoscopic retrograde cholangiography (ERC) was considered the gold standard in diagnosing PSC[5,6]; however, over the last 2 decades, the role of ERC has changed dramatically and it is now mainly considered a therapeutic rather than a diagnostic procedure.[7] This article discusses the current role of ERC and cholangioscopy in diagnosis of PSC, management of complications of PSC including bile duct strictures, biliary infections, choledocholithiasis and cholangiocarcinoma (CCA) in patients with PSC.

DIAGNOSIS OF PSC: ERC OR MAGNETIC RESONANCE CHOLANGIOGRAPHY?

The clinical presentation of PSC is varied and many patients with PSC are asymptomatic at the time of initial diagnosis. PSC is frequently diagnosed after the workup of incidentally discovered abnormal cholestatic liver function tests.[2] Typical symptoms of PSC that develop later in the course of the disease include right upper quadrant abdominal discomfort, fatigue, pruritus, and weight loss.[8] Fever and chills owing to cholangitis are extremely rare features at initial presentation, in the absence of prior biliary surgery or instrumentation such as ERC.[5] The most frequent liver function test abnormality in PSC is an elevation of serum alkaline phosphatase levels.[3,8,9]

The cholangiographic finding of multifocal, short, annular strictures alternating with normal or slightly dilated biliary segments resulting in a "beaded" pattern is characteristic of PSC. Both ERC and magnetic resonance cholangiography (MRC) have relatively comparable diagnostic accuracies, and are recommended as gold standard tests for the diagnosis of PSC by the American Association for the Study of Liver Diseases.[2] Compared with ERC, the sensitivity and specificity of MRC are 80% or greater and 87% or greater, respectively, for the diagnosis of PSC.[10–14] However, MRC offers the advantages of a safe, noninvasive test with no radiation exposure, whereas ERC is an invasive procedure with potentially serious complications, including bacterial cholangitis and pancreatitis. Hospitalization rates of up to 10% have been reported after ERC procedures in PSC patients.[15] Given the invasive nature of ERC and the potential for complications, MRC has now become the initial diagnostic test of choice when PSC is suspected. However, early changes of PSC may not be detected by MRC, and in certain patients visualization of the bile duct is less than optimal with MRC.[10] In these situations, ERC still has a useful role in the initial diagnosis of PSC.

DOMINANT STRICTURE IN PSC

A dominant stricture has been defined as a stenosis with a diameter of 1.5 mm or less in the common bile duct or 1 mm or less in the hepatic ducts.[16,17] PSC patients with fibrosing inflammation on liver histology (stages 2–4) are frequently noted to develop dominant strictures on long-term follow-up.[17] Over a 13-year follow-up period, Stiehl and colleagues[17] showed that 50% of these patients developed a dominant stricture. Similarly, several other studies also indicate that over long-term follow-up, dominant strictures develop in 36% to 58% of PSC patients.[3,16–20]

The progressive stricturing of the biliary tree results in inhibition of bile flow and increased biliary back pressure, resulting in obstructive symptoms and eventually in decompensation of liver function. PSC patients with dominant biliary strictures are also prone to developing bacterial cholangitis.[21,22] Up to 15% to 20% of PSC patients experience obstruction from discrete areas of narrowing within the extrahepatic biliary tree[10,15] which may be amenable to therapeutic intervention. In general, patients with symptoms from dominant strictures, including jaundice, pruritus, cholangitis, right upper quadrant pain, or worsening biochemical indices, are considered appropriate candidates for therapeutic intervention to relieve the biliary obstruction.[2]

NONENDOSCOPIC VERSUS ENDOSCOPIC MANAGEMENT OF DOMINANT STRICTURE
Nonendoscopic Management of Dominant Stricture
Medical management of PSC and dominant stricture
Medical therapy with ursodeoxycholic acid (UDCA) has been investigated in the prevention of disease progression and of complications of PSC. Several small initial pilot studies indicated biochemical and histologic improvement in PSC patients with use of UDCA.[23–26] A subsequent double-blind, placebo-controlled trial also indicated an improvement in liver function tests in PSC patients treated with UDCA at dose of 13 to 15 mg/kg.[27] Stiehl and colleagues[28] prospectively studied the efficacy of UDCA combined with endoscopic dilation of dominant strictures in PSC patients over a period of 8 years. They found that UDCA did not prevent or mitigate major bile duct obstruction and that, within 8 years, 35% of the patients either continued to have a preexisting dominant stricture or had developed a new dominant stricture.[28] Subsequently, a multicenter clinical trial using UDCA at a dose of 28 to 30 mg/kg indicated an increased risk of death or liver transplantation and serious adverse events in patients randomized to receive UDCA.[29] Recently, another randomized trial found no difference in long-term survival between patients with PSC treated with either UDCA or placebo for 5 years.[30] Owing to a lack of clear benefits and the potential for harm, UDCA use is not recommended as medical therapy for PSC.[2,31,32]

Percutaneous management of dominant strictures
Initial nonsurgical techniques to manage dominant biliary strictures in PSC patients were developed by interventional radiologists, who pioneered biliary dilation via the percutaneous route.[33] Biliary access was obtained either via a T tube or by a percutaneous transhepatic approach.[33] Dominant strictures were dilated and percutaneous drains were placed for up to 3 months.[33] Stricture dilation resulted in significant reduction in the frequency of cholangitis and also a reduction in serum bilirubin levels.[33] After initial clinical improvement, a recurrence of the stricture was observed in 33% of patients over 6 to 18 months of follow-up.[33] In a retrospective study, 19 patients were treated with percutaneous balloon dilation with stent placement, 34 were endoscopic balloon dilation alone, and 14 with endoscopic dilation and stent placement. Percutaneous dilation and stent placement was associated with a significantly higher complication rate compared with endoscopic balloon dilation with or without stent placement.[34] A total of 23 different complications were noted, including cholangitis, sepsis, pancreatitis, bile duct perforation, bile leak, bleeding, choledochoduodenal fistula, and tube site infections in the 19 patients who underwent percutaneous dilation with stent placement.[34]

Owing to the overall high rate of complications, need for frequent reinterventions, and lack of patient acceptance of external drainage, endoscopic management evolved to be the preferred choice over the percutaneous approach over last 2 decades. For high-grade strictures located more proximally in the biliary tree, beyond 2 cm from the bifurcation,[17] endoscopic treatment options are limited; these strictures may be more amenable to percutaneous management.

Surgical management of dominant stricture

Nontransplant surgical management options for dominant strictures include biliary bypass by cholangioenterostomy or resection of the bile duct and extrahepatic biliary stricture with creation of a Roux-en-Y hepaticojejunostomy.[35–37] Because dominant strictures are typically close to the bifurcation and because the intrahepatic ducts are invariably involved, biliary bypass is performed infrequently.[36] Elevated bilirubin levels greater than 2 mg/dL and cirrhosis are associated with decreased survival, limiting the option of extrahepatic bile duct resection and Roux-en-Y hepaticojejunostomy to only a few carefully selected, noncirrhotic patients.[35] Also, none of these surgical options have been shown to affect the natural history or disease progression in PSC[2] and thus are rarely utilized.

Endoscopic Management of Dominant Stricture

The goal of endoscopic treatment is to relieve biliary obstruction and to reduce the serum alkaline phosphatase level to below 1.5 times the upper limit of normal.[2,38] Improvement in serum alkaline phosphatase level to normal or below 1.5 times the upper limit of normal has been shown to be associated with improved survival and a reduced risk of CCA in patients with PSC.[30,39] Although to date there are no randomized trials attesting to the efficacy of endoscopic management of dominant strictures, the results from several nonrandomized trials indicate clinical improvement and improved 5-year transplant-free survival rates after endoscopic interventions.[17,19,40,41] Owing to a lack of head to head clinical trials, the optimal endoscopic approach is still debatable and several different endoscopic interventions continue to be utilized either alone or in combination, including sphincterotomy, catheter or balloon dilation, and stent placement.

Endoscopic sphincterotomy

The biliary sphincter of Oddi may be involved by the sclerosing process and can contribute to biliary obstruction.[2] In a report of an open series of various endoscopic interventions performed at single center, biliary sphincterotomy alone was performed in small subset of patients in whom stent placement was unsuccessful.[42] In this small uncontrolled group, improvements in bilirubin and serum alkaline phosphatase values were noted after biliary sphincterotomy alone. However, biliary sphincterotomy is seldom utilized as a solitary endoscopic intervention. It is typically performed to facilitate subsequent endopscopic interventions, including balloon dilation, stent placement, and stone extractions. Because complete biliary sphincterotomy may theoretically increase the risk of ascending bile duct infection, one current expert opinion is to perform a small biliary sphincterotomy.[7] However, this expert opinion is not based on scientific evidence. One might equally argue that a complete biliary sphincterotomy will facilitate complete drainage of contrast and bile, and may thereby prevent the development of biliary infection.

Endoscopic stricture dilation

Endoscopic stricture dilation with or without stent placement has been utilized for the management of biliary obstruction in PSC. In a prospective, single-center, uncontrolled study, 96 patients with dominant stricture were treated with endoscopic interventions, predominantly balloon dilation.[40] A total of 500 balloon dilations were performed in 96 patients over a study period extending over 20 years.[40] In 5 patients with cholangitis and severe cholestasis, a short-term stent was also placed for 1 to 2 weeks in addition to balloon dilation. Repeated endoscopic balloon dilation allowed preservation of a functioning common bile duct and of at least 1 hepatic duct up to 2 cm above the bifurcation in all patients.[40] At 5 years after the first dilation of the dominant stricture, the survival free of liver transplantation rate was 81%; at 10 years, it was 52%.[40]

The ideal goal of dilation is to dilate the main hepatic ducts up to 2 cm proximal to the bifurcation up to 18F.[17] However, there is no consensus regarding the ideal dilation strategy in terms of coaxial rigid dilators versus balloon dilators. Some experts recommend initial rigid dilation of tight dominant strictures from 5F to 7F to allow for the introduction of balloon dilators for subsequent dilation up to 18F to 24F (6–8 mm).[7] At our center, we routinely perform balloon dilation only, starting with a 4-mm dilating balloon and sequentially increasing to 6 and 8 mm, depending on the maximum diameter of bile duct above and below the stricture.

Endoscopic stent placement

Endoscopic stent placement was initially attempted almost 3 decades ago by Grijm and colleagues[43] for the treatment of dominant strictures in PSC. A subsequent small retrospective study evaluating endoscopic stent therapy on 25 PSC patients indicated that endoscopic stent therapy was technically successful in 21 patients (84%) and resulted in sustained clinical and biochemical improvement in 12 patients (57%) over a median follow-up of 29 months (range, 2–120).[44] In this study 7F or 10F stents were placed, then either removed or exchanged during ERC performed electively at 2- to 3-month intervals.[44] However, almost one third of the follow-up ERCPs in this study were performed nonelectively owing to development of icterus or cholangitis attributed to early stent occlusion.[44] In PSC patients, early stent occlusion is thought to be related to inflammatory material, mainly cellular debris, which is shed from bile ducts.[44]

Owing to the problem of early stent occlusion, subsequent studies focused on a strategy of short-term stent placement and found it to be safe and effective for the management of symptomatic dominant strictures in PSC.[45,46] Ponsioen and colleagues[45] prospectively treated 32 patients with dominant strictures with insertion of 7F or 10F polyethylene stents across the stricture. The stents were kept for only a short period of time with a mean stenting duration of 11 days (range, 1–23).[45] Cholestatic complaints including pruritus, fatigue, and right upper quadrant abdominal pain improved in 83% of patients after 2 months.[45] Serum bilirubin levels returned to normal in 12 of the 14 patients (86%) who were initially jaundiced, and 60% of patients did not require any further interventions over 3 years of follow-up.[45] In another small study, 16 patients with symptomatic dominant strictures were treated with short-term stent placement (median duration, 9 days).[46] Over a median follow-up of 19 months, 13 patients (81%) were asymptomatic and no patients had a recurrence of symptoms.[46]

Although stent placement has the advantage of maintaining the effect of dilation and prevention of rapid reocclusion of the stenosed bile duct, one of the major disadvantages of stent placement is the need to repeat ERC for stent removal. Also, stent occlusion, should it occur, can lead to worsening of cholestasis and the development of cholangitis. Stent placement may also potentially lead to increased bacterial translocation and colonization of biliary tree. Indeed, microbiological studies of bile from PSC patients undergoing liver transplantation report a 58% positive culture rate, with an inverse relationship between infection rate and time from the last ERCP.[22] Rates of bacterobilia as high as 98% are observed in patients with a biliary stent in situ compared with 55% in those without a stent.[47] Moreover, for patients with a dominant stenosis close to the bifurcation, stent placement in 1 hepatic duct can hinder the bile flow from the other hepatic duct. These limitations with conventional "Amsterdam"-type tubular polyethylene stents may potentially be successfully overcome by the newly designed biliary Wing stent (ViaDuct, GI Supply, Camp Hill, PA, USA) that lacks a lumen, has a star-shaped cross-section and is designed to allow bile to flow along grooves on the outer surface of the stent.[48] It has been postulated that the winged stent design with a lack of central lumen obviates the risk of luminal occlusion and that the risk of occlusion, given the presence of multiple external drainage channels, is smaller.[48] However, although our anecdotal experience with the biliary Wing stent in a small number of PSC patients has been good with no episodes of occlusion or infection, this stent has not been studied prospectively in PSC patients and additional studies are needed to determine its long-term safety and efficacy in this patient group.

Outcomes after endoscopic balloon dilation versus balloon dilation with stent placement have not been compared in randomized, controlled trials. However, a retrospective, single-center study compared endoscopic balloon dilation with either percutaneous or endoscopic dilation with stent placement in a total of 71 patients. In this study, 34 patients were treated with endoscopic balloon dilation alone, 19 patients were treated with percutaneous balloon dilation with stent placement, 14 with endoscopic balloon dilation and stent placement, and 4 with both percutaneous and endoscopic dilation and stent placement. Although there was no difference with regard to improving cholestasis between the balloon dilation and dilation with stent groups, the number of intervention-related complications and the incidence of acute cholangitis were higher in the dilation with stent group compared with balloon dilation alone group. The authors concluded that there was no additional benefit from stenting after balloon dilation and recommended against routine stent placement.[34] However, a subgroup analysis revealed that there were more complications related to percutaneous stent placement than with endoscopic stent placement (23 vs 7; $P = .001$).[34] Also, it is important to note that this was a retrospective study, which is likely prone to bias. Thus, although both treatment groups were comparable based on clinical indication and biochemical profile, it is possible that patients with more severe structuring disease and/or multifocal strictures were selected for stent placement, thereby explaining the higher complication rate in the dilation with stent placement group.

Based on cumulative evidence from retrospective and small, uncontrolled, prospective studies, some experts currently recommend endoscopic balloon dilation only for management of dominant stricture in PSC.[2,7] Stent placement is recommended by some experts only for PSC patients with clinically overt cholangitis and if stricture dilation alone is unsuccessful. A short duration of stenting—for as few as 10 days—is also recommended by some experts.[7,38] Optimal endoscopic intervention however remains unclear. A multicenter European trial is currently ongoing (www.clinicaltrials.gov, NCT01398917) evaluating short-term stenting versus balloon dilation for dominant strictures in PSC. The trial aims to recruit 100 patients and recruitment is expected to be complete by May 2015. This prospective, randomized study seeks to resolve this important issue.

EFFICACY OF ENDOSCOPIC MANAGEMENT IN PSC

Although there are no randomized, controlled trials assessing the efficacy of ERCP, there is already substantial indirect evidence that can be drawn from large retrospective studies attesting to the effectiveness of ERCP in clinical improvement and in prolonging survival (**Figs. 1** and **2**). Baluyut and colleagues[41] reported that PSC patients with dominant stricture undergoing ERCP had a significantly better 5-year survival rate than that predicted by the Mayo Risk Score (83% vs 65%; $P = .027$). Similarly, Gluck and colleagues[19] reported that PSC patients undergoing ERCP therapy had a significantly higher survival than that predicted by the Mayo Risk Score at 3 years (86.8% vs 76.3%; $P = .021$) and at 4 years (82.8% vs 71.3%; $P = .021$).

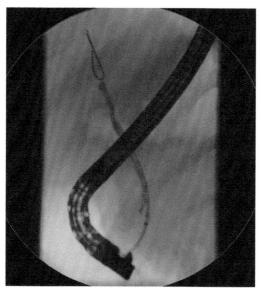

Fig. 1. Cholangiogram depicting a short, tight common hepatic duct stricture in a patient with PSC, with no progress of contrast through the stricture.

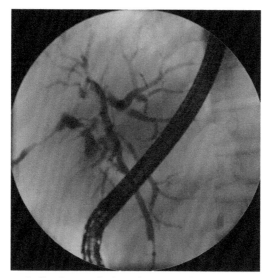

Fig. 2. Cholangiogram indicating resolution of common hepatic duct stenosis after dilation and stenting.

Complications of ERCP in PSC Patients

All therapeutic procedures carry a risk of complications. In large series of patients with PSC undergoing ERCP, the rate of complications directly attributed to ERCP ranged from 7.3% to 20%.[19,41] Gluck and colleagues[19] reported a complication rate of 7.3% among 317 procedures performed on 117 patients over a mean follow-up duration of 8 years (range, 2–20). In this study, the most common complication was pancreatitis

(3.8%); other complications, such as cholangitis, sepsis, duct perforation, post sphincterotomy bleeding, and liver abscess, were each reported in fewer than 1% of patients.[19] In contrast, Baluyut and colleagues[41] reported a complication rate of 20% among 63 consecutive patients with PSC undergoing ERCP. In this study, the most common complication was bile duct perforation (16%) followed by pancreatitis (3%) and delayed cholangitis (1%).[41] These complications were managed conservatively, except in 1 patient who developed severe necrotizing pancreatitis that required surgical debridement.[41]

BACTERIAL COLONIZATION, CHOLANGITIS, AND ANTIBIOTIC PROPHYLAXIS

Dominant strictures can induce stagnation of bile resulting in bacterial colonization and subsequent cholangitis. A population-based study from Canada reported that 6.1% of PSC patients had cholangitis at initial presentation.[49] A study of 22 PSC patients undergoing ERCP and bile aspirate culture reported positive bile cultures in 25% of naïve PSC patients undergoing ERCP for first time (3/12) compared with positive bile cultures in 60% of PSC patients with history of prior ERCP (6/10).[50] In this study, 75% of the positive bile cultures were Gram-positive isolates, mainly alpha-hemolytic Streptococci and 25% were enteric bacteria.[50] In contrast, another similar study found enteric bacteria in 40% of PSC patients with a dominant stricture but in none of 13 controls with PSC without a dominant stricture.[51] In this study, a 1-week course of ciprofloxacin after ERCP was not effective in eradicating bacteria from the bile ducts of PSC patients with dominant strictures.[51] Current guidelines from the American Association for the Study of Liver Diseases recommend antimicrobial therapy with correction of bile duct obstruction in PSC patients with dominant strictures.[2] Because PSC patients have multifocal biliary strictures and complete drainage may not be achieved during ERCP, current guidelines from the American Society of Gastrointestinal Endoscopy recommend routine antimicrobial prophylaxis for PSC patients undergoing ERCP.[52]

DIFFERENTIATING BENIGN STENOSIS VERSUS CCA

CCA develops in 10% to 15% of patients with PSC and early diagnosis may be difficult in this disease where benign strictures coexist.[53] CCA in PSC frequently presents as a stenotic ductal lesion in the perihilar region and it is imperative to distinguish CCA from benign stenotic lesions. Because dominant strictures are seen in up to 58% of PSC patients, stenotic lesions are far more often benign than malignant. Duration of PSC is not a risk factor for development of CCA[54] and in fact, in approximately one half of patients with PSC with CCA, the malignancy is detected at the time of diagnosis or within the first year after diagnosis.[55] Despite advances in medical science, the distinction between a benign dominant stricture and CCA in a PSC patient remains challenging.

In symptomatic patients with PSC, a serum carbohydrate antigen 19-9 (CA 19-9) cutoff value of 130 U/mL (normal, <55) has a sensitivity of 79% and specificity of 98% for the diagnosis of CCA.[56–60] However, the value of serum CA 19-9 test as a screening modality in asymptomatic PSC populations has not been studied. Also, CA 19-9 is frequently elevated in patients with cholestasis and bacterial cholangitis.[61] In addition, CA 19-9 is virtually undetectable in 7% of the normal population who are negative for the Lewis antigen.[61] Neither computed tomography nor magnetic resonance imaging studies are able to differentiate between benign stenosis and CCA in PSC patients. In a large study, ultrasonography, computed tomography, and magnetic resonance imaging studies were all shown to have overall limited positive predictive values of 48%, 38%, and 40%, respectively, in identifying CCA in patients with PSC.[59]

Similarly, direct cholangiography by ERCP also has a very low positive predictive value of only 23% for detecting CCA in PSC.[59] Conventional brush cytology obtained by ERCP has an excellent specificity of 100% for CCA, but large studies indicate sensitivities ranging between only 18% to 40%.[59,60,62] A recent study demonstrated that polysomy (duplication of 2 or more chromosomes) in 5 or more cells by fluorescent in situ hybridization of cytologic specimens has a sensitivity of 41% and a specificity of 98% for the diagnosis of CCA in PSC.[62] In this study, a positive fluorescent in situ hybridization test doubled the sensitivity of conventional cytology. In another small study of 61 patients, the finding of high-grade dysplasia was highly sensitive for the diagnosis of CCA, with an overall sensitivity of 73% and specificity of 95%.[63] However, the fluorescent in situ hybridization-based and dysplasia-based approaches have not been widely validated by additional studies.

ROLE OF CHOLANGIOSCOPY IN PSC

Cholangioscopy allows direct visualization of the bile duct during ERCP. The cholangioscope is advanced through the working channel of a duodenoscope, then advanced into the bile duct over a guidewire.[64] A major advance in the field of cholangioscopy was the introduction of a single operator cholangioscope in 2007. The single operator cholangioscope allows superior 4-way tip deflection, greater irrigation capability, and has dedicated accessories including mini biopsy forceps.[64]

In PSC patients, cholangioscopy is frequently used to evaluate indeterminate strictures by direct visualization and targeted biopsies. In non-PSC patients, fiberoptic cholangioscopy has been shown to have a sensitivity of 92% and specificity of 93% in identifying malignant strictures.[65,66] In addition to the evaluation of indeterminate strictures, in our experience cholangioscopy has been extremely helpful in navigating the guidewire across long and tortuous dominant strictures that have been difficult to traverse using standard techniques. Cholangioscopy may also be useful in performing lithotripsy to assist in extraction of bile duct stones present proximal to dominant strictures.

SUMMARY

Although there are no randomized, controlled trials evaluating the efficacy of ERC in PSC patients, there is substantial indirect evidence supporting the effectiveness of ERC in symptomatic PSC patients with a dominant stricture. Currently, cumulative evidence from retrospective and prospective case series with small numbers of patients supports the role of ERC with endoscopic dilation with or without additional short-term stent placement for symptomatic PSC patients with a dominant stricture. Differentiating benign dominant strictures from CCA remains difficult; however, newer endoscopic techniques such as cholangioscopy with biopsy and advanced cytologic techniques such as fluorescence in situ hybridization are likely to improve sensitivity for the diagnosis of CCA over that achieved by traditional cytology brushing alone.

REFERENCES

1. Maggs JR, Chapman RW. An update on primary sclerosing cholangitis. Curr Opin Gastroenterol 2008;24(3):377–83.
2. Chapman R, Fevery J, Kalloo A, et al. Diagnosis and management of primary sclerosing cholangitis. Hepatology 2010;51(2):660–78.
3. Tischendorf JJ, Hecker H, Kruger M, et al. Characterization, outcome, and prognosis in 273 patients with primary sclerosing cholangitis: a single center study. Am J Gastroenterol 2007;102(1):107–14.

4. Abdalian R, Heathcote EJ. Sclerosing cholangitis: a focus on secondary causes. Hepatology 2006;44(5):1063–74.
5. Lee YM, Kaplan MM. Primary sclerosing cholangitis. N Engl J Med 1995;332(14): 924–33.
6. MacCarty RL, LaRusso NF, Wiesner RH, et al. Primary sclerosing cholangitis: findings on cholangiography and pancreatography. Radiology 1983;149(1): 39–44.
7. Gotthardt D, Stiehl A. Endoscopic retrograde cholangiopancreatography in diagnosis and treatment of primary sclerosing cholangitis. Clin Liver Dis 2010; 14(2):349–58.
8. Broome U, Olsson R, Loof L, et al. Natural history and prognostic factors in 305 Swedish patients with primary sclerosing cholangitis. Gut 1996;38(4):610–5.
9. Chapman RW, Arborgh BA, Rhodes JM, et al. Primary sclerosing cholangitis: a review of its clinical features, cholangiography, and hepatic histology. Gut 1980; 21(10):870–7.
10. Berstad AE, Aabakken L, Smith HJ, et al. Diagnostic accuracy of magnetic resonance and endoscopic retrograde cholangiography in primary sclerosing cholangitis. Clin Gastroenterol Hepatol 2006;4(4):514–20.
11. Weber C, Kuhlencordt R, Grotelueschen R, et al. Magnetic resonance cholangiopancreatography in the diagnosis of primary sclerosing cholangitis. Endoscopy 2008;40(9):739–45.
12. Textor HJ, Flacke S, Pauleit D, et al. Three-dimensional magnetic resonance cholangiopancreatography with respiratory triggering in the diagnosis of primary sclerosing cholangitis: comparison with endoscopic retrograde cholangiography. Endoscopy 2002;34(12):984–90.
13. Fulcher AS, Turner MA, Franklin KJ, et al. Primary sclerosing cholangitis: evaluation with MR cholangiography-a case-control study. Radiology 2000;215(1):71–80.
14. Angulo P, Pearce DH, Johnson CD, et al. Magnetic resonance cholangiography in patients with biliary disease: its role in primary sclerosing cholangitis. J Hepatol 2000;33(4):520–7.
15. Bangarulingam SY, Gossard AA, Petersen BT, et al. Complications of endoscopic retrograde cholangiopancreatography in primary sclerosing cholangitis. Am J Gastroenterol 2009;104(4):855–60.
16. Bjornsson E, Lindqvist-Ottosson J, Asztely M, et al. Dominant strictures in patients with primary sclerosing cholangitis. Am J Gastroenterol 2004;99(3): 502–8.
17. Stiehl A, Rudolph G, Kloters-Plachky P, et al. Development of dominant bile duct stenoses in patients with primary sclerosing cholangitis treated with ursodeoxycholic acid: outcome after endoscopic treatment. J Hepatol 2002;36(2):151–6.
18. Okolicsanyi L, Fabris L, Viaggi S, et al. Primary sclerosing cholangitis: clinical presentation, natural history and prognostic variables: an Italian multicentre study. The Italian PSC Study Group. Eur J Gastroenterol Hepatol 1996;8(7): 685–91.
19. Gluck M, Cantone NR, Brandabur JJ, et al. A twenty-year experience with endoscopic therapy for symptomatic primary sclerosing cholangitis. J Clin Gastroenterol 2008;42(9):1032–9.
20. Rudolph G, Gotthardt D, Kloters-Plachky P, et al. Influence of dominant bile duct stenoses and biliary infections on outcome in primary sclerosing cholangitis. J Hepatol 2009;51(1):149–55.
21. Wiesner RH, Grambsch PM, Dickson ER, et al. Primary sclerosing cholangitis: natural history, prognostic factors and survival analysis. Hepatology 1989;10(4):430–6.

22. Olsson R, Bjornsson E, Backman L, et al. Bile duct bacterial isolates in primary sclerosing cholangitis: a study of explanted livers. J Hepatol 1998; 28(3):426–32.

23. Beuers U, Spengler U, Kruis W, et al. Ursodeoxycholic acid for treatment of primary sclerosing cholangitis: a placebo-controlled trial. Hepatology 1992;16(3): 707–14.

24. Chazouilleres O, Poupon R, Capron JP, et al. Ursodeoxycholic acid for primary sclerosing cholangitis. J Hepatol 1990;11(1):120–3.

25. O'Brien CB, Senior JR, Arora-Mirchandani R, et al. Ursodeoxycholic acid for the treatment of primary sclerosing cholangitis: a 30-month pilot study. Hepatology 1991;14(5):838–47.

26. Stiehl A. Ursodeoxycholic acid therapy in treatment of primary sclerosing cholangitis. Scand J Gastroenterol Suppl 1994;204:59–61.

27. Lindor KD. Ursodiol for primary sclerosing cholangitis. Mayo Primary Sclerosing Cholangitis-Ursodeoxycholic Acid Study Group. N Engl J Med 1997;336(10): 691–5.

28. Stiehl A, Rudolph G, Sauer P, et al. Efficacy of ursodeoxycholic acid treatment and endoscopic dilation of major duct stenoses in primary sclerosing cholangitis. An 8-year prospective study. J Hepatol 1997;26(3):560–6.

29. Lindor KD, Kowdley KV, Luketic VA, et al. High-dose ursodeoxycholic acid for the treatment of primary sclerosing cholangitis. Hepatology 2009;50(3): 808–14.

30. Lindstrom L, Hultcrantz R, Boberg KM, et al. Association between reduced levels of alkaline phosphatase and survival times of patients with primary sclerosing cholangitis. Clin Gastroenterol Hepatol 2013;11(7):841–6.

31. Imam MH, Sinakos E, Gossard AA, et al. High-dose ursodeoxycholic acid increases risk of adverse outcomes in patients with early stage primary sclerosing cholangitis. Aliment Pharmacol Ther 2011;34(10):1185–92.

32. Eaton JE, Silveira MG, Pardi DS, et al. High-dose ursodeoxycholic acid is associated with the development of colorectal neoplasia in patients with ulcerative colitis and primary sclerosing cholangitis. Am J Gastroenterol 2011;106(9):1638–45.

33. May GR, Bender CE, LaRusso NF, et al. Nonoperative dilatation of dominant strictures in primary sclerosing cholangitis. AJR Am J Roentgenol 1985;145(5):1061–4.

34. Kaya M, Petersen BT, Angulo P, et al. Balloon dilation compared to stenting of dominant strictures in primary sclerosing cholangitis. Am J Gastroenterol 2001;96(4):1059–66.

35. Ahrendt SA, Pitt HA, Kalloo AN, et al. Primary sclerosing cholangitis: resect, dilate, or transplant? Ann Surg 1998;227(3):412–23.

36. Myburgh JA. Surgical biliary drainage in primary sclerosing cholangitis. The role of the Hepp-Couinaud approach. Arch Surg 1994;129(10):1057–62.

37. Cameron JL, Pitt HA, Zinner MJ, et al. Resection of hepatic duct bifurcation and transhepatic stenting for sclerosing cholangitis. Ann Surg 1988;207(5):614–22.

38. Baron TH Sr, Davee T. Endoscopic management of benign bile duct strictures. Gastrointest Endosc Clin N Am 2013;23(2):295–311.

39. Al Mamari S, Djordjevic J, Halliday JS, et al. Improvement of serum alkaline phosphatase to <1.5 upper limit of normal predicts better outcome and reduced risk of cholangiocarcinoma in primary sclerosing cholangitis. J Hepatol 2013;58(2): 329–34.

40. Gotthardt DN, Rudolph G, Kloters-Plachky P, et al. Endoscopic dilation of dominant stenoses in primary sclerosing cholangitis: outcome after long-term treatment. Gastrointest Endosc 2010;71(3):527–34.

41. Baluyut AR, Sherman S, Lehman GA, et al. Impact of endoscopic therapy on the survival of patients with primary sclerosing cholangitis. Gastrointest Endosc 2001;53(3):308–12.

42. Gaing AA, Geders JM, Cohen SA, et al. Endoscopic management of primary sclerosing cholangitis: review, and report of an open series. Am J Gastroenterol 1993;88(12):2000–8.

43. Grijm R, Huibregtse K, Bartelsman J, et al. Therapeutic investigations in primary sclerosing cholangitis. Dig Dis Sci 1986;31(8):792–8.

44. van Milligen de Wit AW, van Bracht J, Rauws EA, et al. Endoscopic stent therapy for dominant extrahepatic bile duct strictures in primary sclerosing cholangitis. Gastrointest Endosc 1996;44(3):293–9.

45. Ponsioen CY, Lam K, van Milligen de Wit AW, et al. Four years experience with short term stenting in primary sclerosing cholangitis. Am J Gastroenterol 1999; 94(9):2403–7.

46. van Milligen de Wit AW, Rauws EA, van Bracht J, et al. Lack of complications following short-term stent therapy for extrahepatic bile duct strictures in primary sclerosing cholangitis. Gastrointest Endosc 1997;46(4):344–7.

47. Rerknimitr R, Fogel EL, Kalayci C, et al. Microbiology of bile in patients with cholangitis or cholestasis with and without plastic biliary endoprosthesis. Gastrointest Endosc 2002;56(6):885–9.

48. Raju GS, Sud R, Elfert AA, et al. Biliary drainage by using stents without a central lumen: a pilot study. Gastrointest Endosc 2006;63(2):317–20.

49. Kaplan GG, Laupland KB, Butzner D, et al. The burden of large and small duct primary sclerosing cholangitis in adults and children: a population-based analysis. Am J Gastroenterol 2007;102(5):1042–9.

50. Bjornsson ES, Kilander AF, Olsson RG. Bile duct bacterial isolates in primary sclerosing cholangitis and certain other forms of cholestasis–a study of bile cultures from ERCP. Hepatogastroenterology 2000;47(36):1504–8.

51. Pohl J, Ring A, Stremmel W, et al. The role of dominant stenoses in bacterial infections of bile ducts in primary sclerosing cholangitis. Eur J Gastroenterol Hepatol 2006;18(1):69–74.

52. Banerjee S, Shen B, Baron TH, et al. Antibiotic prophylaxis for GI endoscopy. Gastrointest Endosc 2008;67(6):791–8.

53. Bergquist A, Ekbom A, Olsson R, et al. Hepatic and extrahepatic malignancies in primary sclerosing cholangitis. J Hepatol 2002;36(3):321–7.

54. Lazaridis KN, Gores GJ. Primary sclerosing cholangitis and cholangiocarcinoma. Semin Liver Dis 2006;26(1):42–51.

55. Fevery J, Verslype C, Lai G, et al. Incidence, diagnosis, and therapy of cholangiocarcinoma in patients with primary sclerosing cholangitis. Dig Dis Sci 2007; 52(11):3123–35.

56. Levy C, Lymp J, Angulo P, et al. The value of serum CA 19-9 in predicting cholangiocarcinomas in patients with primary sclerosing cholangitis. Dig Dis Sci 2005;50(9):1734–40.

57. Nichols JC, Gores GJ, LaRusso NF, et al. Diagnostic role of serum CA 19-9 for cholangiocarcinoma in patients with primary sclerosing cholangitis. Mayo Clin Proc 1993;68(9):874–9.

58. Chalasani N, Baluyut A, Ismail A, et al. Cholangiocarcinoma in patients with primary sclerosing cholangitis: a multicenter case-control study. Hepatology 2000;31(1):7–11.

59. Charatcharoenwitthaya P, Enders FB, Halling KC, et al. Utility of serum tumor markers, imaging, and biliary cytology for detecting cholangiocarcinoma in primary sclerosing cholangitis. Hepatology 2008;48(4):1106–17.

60. Siqueira E, Schoen RE, Silverman W, et al. Detecting cholangiocarcinoma in patients with primary sclerosing cholangitis. Gastrointest Endosc 2002;56(1):40–7.
61. Steinberg W. The clinical utility of the CA 19-9 tumor-associated antigen. Am J Gastroenterol 1990;85(4):350–5.
62. Moreno Luna LE, Kipp B, Halling KC, et al. Advanced cytologic techniques for the detection of malignant pancreatobiliary strictures. Gastroenterology 2006;131(4): 1064–72.
63. Boberg KM, Jebsen P, Clausen OP, et al. Diagnostic benefit of biliary brush cytology in cholangiocarcinoma in primary sclerosing cholangitis. J Hepatol 2006;45(4): 568–74.
64. Shah RJ, Adler DG, Conway JD, et al. Cholangiopancreatoscopy. Gastrointest Endosc 2008;68(3):411–21.
65. Shah RJ, Langer DA, Antillon MR, et al. Cholangioscopy and cholangioscopic forceps biopsy in patients with indeterminate pancreaticobiliary pathology. Clin Gastroenterol Hepatol 2006;4(2):219–25.
66. Tischendorf JJ, Kruger M, Trautwein C, et al. Cholangioscopic characterization of dominant bile duct stenoses in patients with primary sclerosing cholangitis. Endoscopy 2006;38(7):665–9.

Endoscopic Retrograde Cholangiography for Biliary Anastomotic Strictures After Liver Transplantation

Alejandro Fernández-Simon, MD[a], Alvaro Díaz-Gonzalez, MD[a],
Paul J. Thuluvath, MD, FRCP[b], Andrés Cárdenas, MD, MMSc, AGAF[a],*

KEYWORDS

- ERCP • Anastomotic biliary stricture • Liver transplantation • Biliary dilatation
- Biliary stents • Self-expanding metal stents

KEY POINTS

- When an anastomotic stricture (AS) is suspected, a magnetic resonance cholangiopancreatography (MRCP) is recommended before performing endoscopic retrograde cholangiography (ERC). In cases in which the availability of MRCP is limited and there is a high suspicion of AS, ERC can be safely performed.
- Standard treatment for AS includes therapeutic ERC with balloon dilation and plastic stent placement every 3 months with up to 4 to 5 sessions.
- Early strictures (<1 month post-LT) usually present good response to a single endoscopic therapy session. Late strictures are usually related to ischemic injury of the bile duct anastomosis and need longer treatments.
- Endoscopic therapy with dilation and maximal plastic stent therapy is associated with success in 70% to 100% of cases.
- To date, the use of fully covered self-expandable metallic stents (SEMS) does not seem to confer a better resolution of AS when compared with maximal plastic stent therapy strategy.

Biliary complications are an important cause of mortality and morbidity after liver transplantation (LT) and they occur in 10% to 40% of LT recipients. Bile duct strictures (anastomotic [AS] and nonanastomotic [NAS]) are the most common type of complications, accounting for approximately 60% of all biliary complications after LT.[1–7] In most

Disclosure: None.
[a] GI/Endoscopy Unit, Institut de Malalties Digestives i Metaboliques, Hospital Clinic, University of Barcelona, Villarroel 170, Esc 3-2, Barcelona 08036, Spain; [b] Medical Director, Institute for Digestive Health & Liver Disease, Mercy Medical Center, 301 Street, Paul Place, Baltimore, MD 21202, USA
* Corresponding author.
E-mail addresses: acardena@clinic.ub.es; acv69@hotmail.com

cases, the anastomosis of the bile duct is performed as a duct-to-duct reconstruction, which makes endoscopic therapy with endoscopic retrograde cholangiography (ERC) feasible in most patients. Patients who undergo a Roux-en-Y choledochojejunostomy can also develop strictures at the anastomosis with the bowel and in most cases percutaneous therapy by interventional radiology is performed. In high-volume LT centers with experienced endoscopists, ERC can be successfully performed in patients with a Roux-en-Y choledochojejunostomy with small bowel enteroscopy; however, this topic is out of the scope of this review and is discussed elsewhere.[8–12] In this review, we discuss the diagnostic approach and the management of biliary anastomotic strictures after LT because this type of complication accounts for most of the interventional procedures performed in the biliary tract of LT recipients.

TYPES OF BILIARY STRICTURES

Depending on the location of the stricture, these lesions are classified as AS or NAS. ASs are defined as a dominant short narrowing at the anastomotic site without free or effective passage of contrast material as demonstrated by cholangiography (**Fig. 1**). Most ASs occur within the first 12 months after LT.[13] AS identified within 6 months after LT usually have good response to short-term stenting (3–6 months of treatment), whereas late strictures are more difficult to treat.[14] NASs are usually referred to as ischemic strictures and they usually occur before AS. NAS can occur proximal to the anastomosis, mainly in the intrahepatic bile duct. There may be multiple strictures involving the hilum and intrahepatic ducts causing a cholangiographic appearance that resembles primary sclerosing cholangitis. NASs are more difficult to treat than ASs, with outcomes that are not as favorable as those with AS and will not be discussed in this review. Strictures also are classified according to the time in which they occur; early strictures are those that appear in the first month after LT, whereas late strictures occur after the first month post-LT. In some patients, a transient

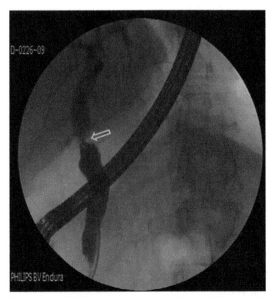

Fig. 1. ASs are defined as a dominant short narrowing at the anastomotic site (*arrow*) without free or effective passage of contrast material as demonstrated by cholangiography.

narrowing of the anastomosis may become evident within the first 1 to 2 months after LT due to postoperative edema and inflammation.[15]

RISK FACTORS

There are several known risk factors for the development of biliary AS after LT (**Box 1**). The most common risk factor is the development of hepatic artery thrombosis (HAT). The biliary system receives blood supply solely via the hepatic artery; thus, HAT can lead to complex anastomotic and hilar strictures. Hepatic artery stenosis can also lead to both AS and NAS, particularly when associated with long cold ischemia time.[16] T-tube placement in LT is controversial. Originally T-tubes were routinely placed as a prophylactic measure for AS development. The results of several comparative studies, systematic reviews, and meta-analyses have favored the actual trend toward the abandonment of the use of T-tubes after LT. A meta-analysis that included more than 1000 patients showed that, although patients with T-tube in general presented superior results in terms of biliary strictures, the overall complication rate was superior compared with patients without T-tube.[17] A second meta-analysis of 5 randomized controlled trials indicated that patients with T-tube had significantly fewer ASs, but there were no differences in the overall rate of complications.[18] Despite these results, some investigators still defend the role of T-tube in LT. In a recent randomized single-center prospective trial that evaluated 188 LTs, the use of T-tubes resulted in fewer ASs (n = 2, 2.1%) compared with the non–T-tube group (n = 13, 14.1%; P = .002).[19] Other well-described risk factors include bile leak after T-tube removal, technical factors during surgery (tight anastomosis, excessive dissection and electrocautery during the reconstruction, redundant bile duct), mismatched size between donor and recipient bile ducts, ischemia/reperfusion injury, presence of cytomegalovirus infection, donation after cardiac death, ABO blood group mismatch, older age of donor, graft steatosis, prolonged cold and warm ischemia times, and primary sclerosing cholangitis.[16,20–31]

DIAGNOSTIC APPROACH

Occasionally patients will present with nonspecific symptoms (fever and anorexia), abdominal pain (especially if associated with bile leaks), pruritus, or jaundice, but in most cases, a biliary stricture is usually suspected in asymptomatic LT recipients

Box 1
Risk factors for biliary anastomotic strictures after LT
Hepatic artery thrombosis
Hepatic artery stenosis
Bile leak
Technical factors
ABO mismatch
Ischemia/reperfusion injury
Cytomegalovirus infection
Donation after cardiac death
Primary sclerosing cholangitis
Ischemia
Age

with persistent elevations of serum bilirubin, alkaline phosphatase, transaminases, and/or gamma-glutamyl transferase (GGT) levels. Absence of abdominal pain does not exclude the presence of biliary obstruction, as pain may be absent in the transplant setting because of hepatic denervation in some patients.[14,20,32] The challenge for the LT team is to tease out between obstructive jaundice from one of the many other causes of cholestasis in patients after LT, such as acute rejection, chronic rejection, recurrence of primary disease, fibrosing cholestatic hepatitis C, or drug-induced cholestasis.

The initial evaluation should include an abdominal ultrasound with a Doppler evaluation of the hepatic vessels to rule out hepatic artery thrombosis or stenosis and/or portal or hepatic vein occlusion. Unfortunately, abdominal ultrasound may not be sufficiently sensitive (sensitivity 40%–66%) to detect biliary obstruction in many LT recipients.[33] Thus, the absence of bile duct dilation on ultrasound should not preclude further evaluation with more sensitive tests if there is clinical suspicion of a biliary stricture. In such a case, magnetic resonance cholangiopancreatography (MRCP) is considered an optimal noninvasive diagnostic tool for the assessment of the biliary complications in patients after LT.[9] Although ERC or percutaneous transhepatic cholangiography remains the gold standard, MRCP has gained acceptance as the most reliable noninvasive study for the evaluation of the bile ducts in patients after LT (sensitivity 96%, specificity 94%).[34] Our approach is to order an MRCP first in any patient with a suspicion of biliary obstruction. That said, proceeding with a diagnostic invasive procedure, such as ERC, without detailed imaging (ie, MRCP) can be an acceptable clinical strategy in some patients because of the high likelihood that a therapeutic intervention will be required.[35] An algorithm depicting the diagnostic approach for patients with suspected AS is shown in **Fig. 2**.

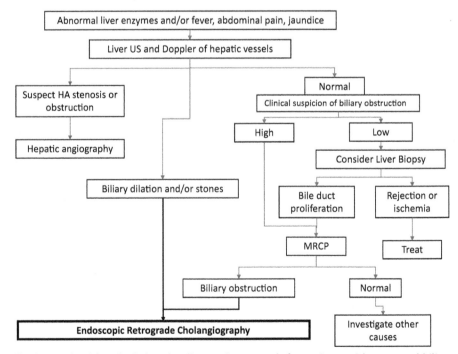

Fig. 2. An algorithm depicting the diagnostic approach for patients with suspected biliary anastomotic strictures. HA, hepatic artery; US, ultrasound.

TREATMENT STRATEGIES
Dilation and Plastic Stent Placement

Most patients with AS require ongoing ERC sessions every 3 months with balloon dilation and long-term stenting (for 12–24 months). This technique consists of placing a guidewire across the stricture (**Fig. 3**), followed by a dilation of the AS using balloon diameters of 6 to 8 mm, and finally placing 8.0-Fr to 11.5-Fr plastic stents with an increasing diameter and number if possible in each session (**Fig. 4**). The standard technique requires sphincterotomy of the papilla before stent placement. However, similar success rates and remission rates of the AS have been reported in patients without sphincterotomy, placing the stent above the intact sphincter of Oddi.[36] Plastic stents need to be exchanged every 3 months to avoid occlusion and bacterial cholangitis. This approach has been reported to be more effective than dilation alone.[37] Increasing the number of stents in each session improves success rates and, thus, placing the maximal amount of stents possible in each session is recommended, in general up to 4 or 5 stents are needed (see **Fig. 4**). In a retrospective study of 83 LT recipients with AS, treatment success was associated with the number of stents placed (8.0 in the success group vs 3.5 in those whose treatment failed).[38] This approach usually requires several interventional sessions (mean of 3–5 sessions per patient) to achieve long-term success rates of 70% to 100%.[3,14,37,39–43] **Table 1** describes the findings of different studies, including our own experience (Andrés Cárdenas, MD, MMSc, AGAF and colleagues, unpublished data, 2014), evaluating the outcome of dilation and plastic stent placement of biliary AS.

Self-Expandable Metal Stents

Some studies have reported promising results using self-expandable metal stents (SEMS) for AS in LT recipients.[49–53] Uncovered SEMS have an important drawback, and that is the inevitable reactive hyperplasia that may cause difficulty in the stent removal, especially once it has been in place for more than 3 months[54]; thus, these stents should not be placed in LT recipients. Fully covered SEMS are a more feasible

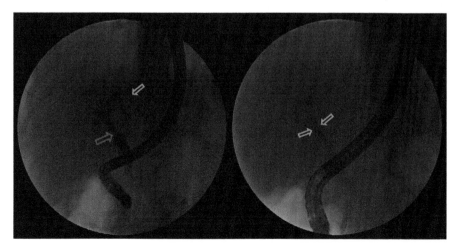

Fig. 3. (*Left*) A guidewire (*green arrow*) is pushed across the anastomotic stricture (*red arrow*). (*Right*) The guidewire allowed the dilation of the stricture and afterward, the placement of 2 plastic stents (*green arrows*) across the stricture. Once placed, the stents permitted the proper drainage of bile and contrast.

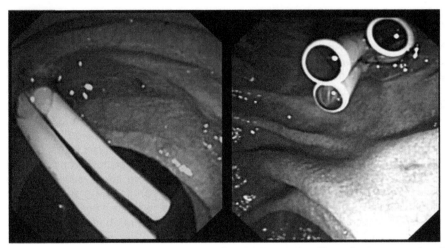

Fig. 4. Endoscopic view of the distal end of multiple transpapillary plastic stents placed across the anastomotic stricture.

option, as they can be easily removed even after a longer period of time (**Fig. 5**). The main concern with fully covered SEMS is migration and the risk of occluding secondary branch ducts (particularly in living donor LT [LDLT] recipients) or the pancreatic duct, complications that could lead to cholangitis and pancreatitis, respectively.[55] That said, this approach offers the advantage of not requiring dilation of the AS and obviating the need for repeated stent exchanges. In a systematic review that included 200 patients treated with covered SEMS, AS resolution rate was 80% to 95% when the stent duration was 3 months or longer. By comparison, the stricture resolution rate with dilation and plastic stents was 94% to 100% for patients who were treated for 12 months or more. Another drawback was SEMS migration, which occurred in 16% of the patients.[56] In fact, migration is the most important limitation, especially if a fully covered SEMS migrates proximally. In this scenario, if ERC is not successful in extracting the migrated stent, surgery or retransplantation may be needed. A small randomized, prospective but underpowered study that compared the use of fully covered SEMS and plastic stents showed similar resolution and recurrence rates and a reduced number of procedures needed, which could lead to the conclusion that this strategy may be cost-effective due to the reduced number of ERCs in the SEMS group.[57] However, a recent prospective study that included 42 LT recipients with AS treated with fully covered SEMS reported a resolution rate of only 68%, with a significant complication rate (38%) mainly due to cholangitis.[58] Therefore, there is not enough data to support the systematic use of SEMS over plastic stents in the treatment of AS. The use of SEMS may be beneficial in patients who fail therapy with plastic stents and dilatation; however, data are scarce and migration rates in this setting are also high.[58] Finally, there are also encouraging data on the use of drug-eluting stents. A prospective study that included 13 patients with AS after LT analyzed the use of paclitaxel-eluting stents; 12 of 13 patients achieved sustained clinical success, meaning that they did not need any further intervention, and most needed only one intervention.[59]

Limitations of Endoscopic Therapy

In 4% to 17% of the cases it is not possible to pass a guidewire through the AS, which precludes any further endoscopic therapy.[14,41,42,60,61] Previous bile leaks and high

Table 1
Studies in liver transplant recipients treated with stricture dilation and multiple plastic stents

Investigators, Year, Country (Number of Patients Who Underwent ERC After LT)	Number of Patients with AS	Age (mean)	Time to Diagnosis of AS (mo)	Technical Success Rate (%)	Number of Stents (mean)	Number of Procedures Per Patient (mean)	Follow-Up in Months (mean)	Resolution, n (%)	AS Recurrence	Recurrence Treatment
Rerknimitr et al,[3] 2002, USA (n = 121)	43	36.5	8.3	43/43 (100)	3.6	3.7	39.6	43/43 (100)	0	0
Morelli et al,[41] 2003, USA (n = 25)	25	48	4.5*	24/25 (96)	3	3*	54	22/25 (88)	2/22 (9)	1 ERCP
Alazmi et al,[44] 2006, USA (n = 148)	148	—	2.1	143/148 (97)	2–4	3	28	131/148 (89)	24/131 (18)	1–4 ERCP
Pasha et al,[40] 2007, USA (n = 25)	25	46.7	2*	25/25 (100)	2–3	3.5*	21.5*	18/25 (72)	4/18 (22)	2 ERCP 2 Surgery
Holt et al,[42] 2007, UK (n = 53)	53	48.5	30.5*	49/53 (92)	3	3*	18*	34/53 (64)	1/34 (3)	1 ERCP
Morelli et al,[45] 2008, USA (n = 38)	38	52.6	2.9	38/38 (100)	0.5	3.45	12	33/38 (89)	5/33 (15)	4 ERCP 1 Surgery
Tabibian et al,[38] 2010, USA (n = 83)	69	52.5	20	69/69 (100)	3 max.	4.2 ± 2.8	11*	65/69 (94)	2/65 (3)	ERCP
Sanna et al,[46] 2011, Italy (n = 94)	45	—	—	34/34 (100)	—	2.5 ± 1.2	88.8*	22/34 (65)	6/34 (18)	Surgery
Hsieh et al,[47] 2013, USA (n = 38)	32	—	2.1	32/32 (100)	3	4	74.2	32/32 (100)	8 (21)	8 ERCP
Poley et al,[48] 2013, Netherlands (NA)	63	61	—	31/31 (80.6)	4	5	28	25/31 (80.6)	6 (19.4)	1 ERCP (SEMS) 5 Surgery
Cardenas et al, Hospital Clinic, 2014, Spain (n = 50)/[unpublished data]	42	52.5	16.5	42/42 (100)	3.12	3.12	41.48	37/42 (88)	3/37 (8.2)	3 ERCP

Abbreviations: ERCP, endoscopic retrograde cholangiopancreatography; NA, not available; SEMS, self-expandable metallic stents.
* median value

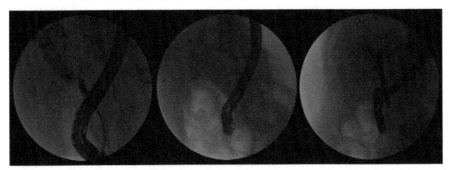

Fig. 5. (*Left*) Fluoroscopic view of an anastomotic stricture; (*center*) a self-expandable metal stent was placed across the stricture; (*right*) resolution of the stricture after stent removal, confirmed with an occlusion cholangiography.

blood transfusion requirements during surgery are risk factors for initial ERC failure in LT recipients with AS.[62] Most of these patients will need surgery for definitive therapy; however, in some instances, biliary recanalization of the difficult-to-traverse AS can be achieved using a needle-knife catheter.[63,64] When ERC fails, the alternatives are either percutaneous transhepatic cholangiogram (PTC) or surgical repair/conversion. The most suitable technique in each case depends on the type of biliary reconstruction after LT, the likelihood of intervention, and the available expertise.[12]

Recurrence

Patients require long-term surveillance because strictures often recur. The recurrence rate of AS after an initial successful endoscopic treatment ranges between 18% and 34%, depending on the series.[41,42,44] In a recent study that evaluated risk factors for recurrence in AS after LT, the occurrence of AS 6 weeks or more after LT was a significant predictor of AS recurrence after endoscopic therapy. The recurrence rate after endoscopic treatment was 34%, with a mean time to recurrence of 14.5 months.[7] Interestingly, when AS recurrence was again treated with ERC (mean time of follow-up of 151 weeks), long-term resolution rate of the AS was 95.7%. These data suggest that long-term follow-up of late biliary strictures, with repeated endoscopic therapy if recurrence is detected, is essential to achieve high rates of resolution.[13]

LDLT AND BILIARY STRICTURES

LDLT has been associated with a higher rate of biliary complications and the incidence of AS is reported to be as high as 40%.[65,66] Aside from the previously mentioned risk factors, known risk factors for AS after LDLT are a long duration of surgery, donor age older than 50, and Model for End-Stage Liver Disease score greater than 35.[67,68] Also, a biliary leak can predict the occurrence of a biliary stricture. In a retrospective study of a predominantly living donor liver transplant center, of a series of 338 transplants, 17 patients developed biliary leaks and received endoscopic treatment. After resolution of the leak, 10 of the 17 patients developed biliary stricture.[69] The reconstruction of the biliary anastomosis in LDLT is technically challenging, as the duct size is smaller and often multiple reconstructions are required.[70] It is not clear if Roux-en-Y reconstruction has less incidence of biliary complications than duct-to-duct anastomosis in this setting; however, most centers prefer duct-to-duct anastomosis because normal bilioenteric integrity is maintained and future endoscopic access to the bile duct is possible.[66,71,72] Right lobe graft recipients develop biliary complications more frequently compared with left lobe grafts, particularly if a duct-to-duct anastomosis has been used involving small-sized duct. Some investigators argue that if duct size is smaller than 4 mm in diameter, a hepaticojejunostomy is preferred.[73]

Endoscopic treatment in LDLT is often more complex. Patients usually are treated in similar fashion as deceased donor LT recipients, but require smaller-diameter stents (7.0–8.5 Fr) and balloon dilation. Resolution rates range between 75% and 80%, but recurrence rate after initial endoscopic therapy can occur in up to 30%, especially when stenting duration is short.[74] Maximal stent therapy has been evaluated for the treatment of AS in patients after LDLT. In a report of 110 patients, 38 of whom developed AS, ERC was attempted as initial therapy in all patients. Thirty-two were managed entirely with endoscopic therapy, whereas 6 underwent PTC to traverse the stricture and proceed with ERC thereafter. Resolution rate was 79%, recurrent strictures were reported in 21% of the patients, and all of them were successfully treated with repeated endoscopic sessions.[47] Recipients of liver from donors after cardiac death also have a high incidence of biliary complications (up to 33%), especially diffuse ischemic cholangiopathy. Focal strictures in this type of donor livers can be treated successfully with endoscopic therapy, whereas diffuse strictures usually require retransplantation.[75]

CHOLANGIOSCOPY

Single-operator cholangioscopy is a technique that can provide direct imaging of the bile duct mucosa, and can be useful in the management of biliary strictures after LT. In a prospective study of 16 patients who developed biliary complications after LT, single-operator cholangioscopy (SOC) was performed and was feasible and tissue was obtained in all cases. Twelve patients presented AS, among them 2 distinct visual patterns were easily identified with SOC; one was mild erythema and the other showed significant edema, ulceration, and sloughing. Those with the latter pattern required a longer period of stenting than patients with only mild erythema and scarring (457 vs 167 days). In addition, in patients with mild erythema, resolution of strictures with endoscopic therapy was better than those with an edema, ulceration, and sloughing pattern (66% vs 33%). This distinction may help to predict outcomes of endoscopic therapy[76]; however more studies are need in this area.

COMPLICATIONS OF ERC

Although ERC is associated with significant complications, the rate of these complications does not seem to differ from that of the general population. There is up to 9% complication rate per procedure.[4,5,77,78] The most common complications are pancreatitis, cholangitis, and postsphincterotomy bleeding. Other complications include bile leak, subcapsular hematoma, perforation, and stent migration. Biliary sphincterotomy, renal failure, repeated pancreatic duct injections, and therapy with mammalian target of rapamycin inhibitors may place patients at risk for complications after ERC.[78,79]

SUMMARY

Biliary ASs are common in recipients of deceased donor and live donor liver transplants. Clinicians should have a high index of suspicion and promptly order an abdominal ultrasound. In those patients in whom there is a strong clinical suspicion of biliary obstruction, an ERC should be done, whereas an MRCP may be preferred if the index of suspicion for bile obstruction is lower. ERC is the preferred treatment for the management of most biliary AS. The combination of stricture dilation and plastic stent placement every 3 months is the best approach. Fully covered SEMS should not be placed as first-line therapy, and their use should be considered on a case-by-case basis. The recurrence rate after therapy can be as high as 30%, but most patients respond to repeat endoscopic therapy.

REFERENCES

1. Stratta RJ, Wood RP, Langnas AN, et al. Diagnosis and treatment of biliary tract complications after orthotopic liver transplantation. Surgery 1989;106:675–83 [discussion: 683–4].
2. Greif F, Bronsther OL, Van Thiel DH, et al. The incidence, timing, and management of biliary tract complications after orthotopic liver transplantation. Ann Surg 1994;219:40–5.
3. Rerknimitr R, Sherman S, Fogel EL, et al. Biliary tract complications after orthotopic liver transplantation with choledochocholedochostomy anastomosis: endoscopic findings and results of therapy. Gastrointest Endosc 2002;55:224–31.
4. Pfau PR, Kochman ML, Lewis JD, et al. Endoscopic management of postoperative biliary complications in orthotopic liver transplantation. Gastrointest Endosc 2000; 52:55–63.
5. Thuluvath PJ, Atassi T, Lee J. An endoscopic approach to biliary complications following orthotopic liver transplantation. Liver Int 2003;23:156–62.
6. Thethy S, Thomson BN, Pleass H, et al. Management of biliary tract complications after orthotopic liver transplantation. Clin Transplant 2004;18:647–53.
7. Zimmerman MA, Baker T, Goodrich NP, et al. Development, management, and resolution of biliary complications after living and deceased donor liver transplantation: a report from the adult-to-adult living donor liver transplantation cohort study consortium. Liver Transpl 2013;19:259–67.
8. Azeem N, Tabibian JH, Baron TH, et al. Use of a single-balloon enteroscope compared with variable-stiffness colonoscopes for endoscopic retrograde cholangiography in liver transplant patients with Roux-en-Y biliary anastomosis. Gastrointest Endosc 2013;77:568–77.
9. Arain MA, Attam R, Freeman ML. Advances in endoscopic management of biliary tract complications after liver transplantation. Liver Transpl 2013;19:482–98.
10. Chua TJ, Kaffes AJ. Balloon-assisted enteroscopy in patients with surgically altered anatomy: a liver transplant center experience (with video). Gastrointest Endosc 2012;76:887–91.
11. Kawano Y, Mizuta K, Hishikawa S, et al. Rendezvous penetration method using double-balloon endoscopy for complete anastomosis obstruction of hepaticojejunostomy after pediatric living donor liver transplantation. Liver Transpl 2008; 14:385–7.
12. Chahal P, Baron TH, Poterucha JJ, et al. Endoscopic retrograde cholangiography in post-orthotopic liver transplant population with Roux-en-Y biliary reconstruction. Liver Transpl 2007;13:1168–73.
13. Albert JG, Filmann N, Elsner J, et al. Long-term follow-up of endoscopic therapy for stenosis of the biliobiliary anastomosis associated with orthotopic liver transplantation. Liver Transpl 2013;19:586–93.
14. Verdonk RC, Buis CI, Porte RJ, et al. Anastomotic biliary strictures after liver transplantation: causes and consequences. Liver Transpl 2006;12:726–35.
15. Verdonk RC, Buis CI, Porte RJ, et al. Biliary complications after liver transplantation: a review. Scand J Gastroenterol Suppl 2006;89–101.

16. Dacha S, Barad A, Martin J, et al. Association of hepatic artery stenosis and biliary strictures in liver transplant recipients. Liver Transpl 2011;17:849–54.
17. Sotiropoulos GC, Sgourakis G, Radtke A, et al. Orthotopic liver transplantation: T-tube or not T-tube? Systematic review and meta-analysis of results. Transplantation 2009;87:1672–80.
18. Riediger C, Müller MW, Michalski CW, et al. T-Tube or no T-tube in the reconstruction of the biliary tract during orthotopic liver transplantation: systematic review and meta-analysis. Liver Transpl 2010;16:705–17.
19. López-Andújar R, Orón EM, Carregnato AF, et al. T-tube or No T-tube in cadaveric orthotopic liver transplantation: the eternal dilemma: results of a prospective and randomized clinical trial. Ann Surg 2013;258:21–9.
20. Pascher A, Neuhaus P. Biliary complications after deceased-donor orthotopic liver transplantation. J Hepatobiliary Pancreat Surg 2006;13:487–96.
21. Sanchez-Urdazpal L, Gores GJ, Ward EM, et al. Ischemic-type biliary complications after orthotopic liver transplantation. Hepatology 1992;16:49–53.
22. Sanchez-Urdazpal L, Gores GJ, Ward EM, et al. Diagnostic features and clinical outcome of ischemic-type biliary complications after liver transplantation. Hepatology 1993;17:605–9.
23. Busquets J, Figueras J, Serrano T, et al. Postreperfusion biopsies are useful in predicting complications after liver transplantation. Liver Transpl 2001;7:432–5.
24. Sanchez-Urdazpal L, Batts KP, Gores GJ, et al. Increased bile duct complications in liver transplantation across the ABO barrier. Ann Surg 1993;218:152–8.
25. Ludwig J, Wiesner RH, Batts KP, et al. The acute vanishing bile duct syndrome (acute irreversible rejection) after orthotopic liver transplantation. Hepatology 1987;7:476–83.
26. Graziadei IW. Recurrence of primary sclerosing cholangitis after liver transplantation. Liver Transpl 2002;8:575–81.
27. Maheshwari A, Maley W, Li Z, et al. Biliary complications and outcomes of liver transplantation from donors after cardiac death. Liver Transpl 2007;13:1645–53.
28. Fung JJ, Eghtesad B, Patel-Tom K. Using livers from donation after cardiac death donors—a proposal to protect the true Achilles heel. Liver Transpl 2007;13:1633–6.
29. Welling TH, Heidt DG, Englesbe MJ, et al. Biliary complications following liver transplantation in the model for end-stage liver disease era: effect of donor, recipient, and technical factors. Liver Transpl 2008;14:73–80.
30. Jay CL, Lyuksemburg V, Ladner DP, et al. Ischemic cholangiopathy after controlled donation after cardiac death liver transplantation: a meta-analysis. Ann Surg 2011;253:259–64.
31. Brunner SM, Junger H, Ruemmele P, et al. Bile duct damage after cold storage of deceased donor livers predicts biliary complications after liver transplantation. J Hepatol 2013;58:1133–9.
32. Thuluvath PJ, Pfau PR, Kimmey MB, et al. Biliary complications after liver transplantation: the role of endoscopy. Endoscopy 2005;37:857–63.
33. Sharma S, Gurakar A, Jabbour N. Biliary strictures following liver transplantation: past, present and preventive strategies. Liver Transpl 2008;14:759–69.
34. Jorgensen JE, Waljee AK, Volk ML, et al. Is MRCP equivalent to ERCP for diagnosing biliary obstruction in orthotopic liver transplant recipients? A meta-analysis. Gastrointest Endosc 2011;73:955–62.
35. Elmunzer BJ, Debenedet AT, Volk ML, et al. Clinical yield of diagnostic endoscopic retrograde cholangiopancreatography in orthotopic liver transplant recipients with suspected biliary complications. Liver Transpl 2012;18:1479–84.

36. Kurita A, Kodama Y, Minami R, et al. Endoscopic stent placement above the intact sphincter of Oddi for biliary strictures after living donor liver transplantation. J Gastroenterol 2013;48:1097–104.
37. Zoepf T, Maldonado-Lopez EJ, Hilgard P, et al. Balloon dilatation vs. balloon dilatation plus bile duct endoprostheses for treatment of anastomotic biliary strictures after liver transplantation. Liver Transpl 2006;12:88–94.
38. Tabibian JH, Asham EH, Han S, et al. Endoscopic treatment of postorthotopic liver transplantation anastomotic biliary strictures with maximal stent therapy (with video). Gastrointest Endosc 2010;71:505–12.
39. Graziadei IW, Schwaighofer H, Koch R, et al. Long-term outcome of endoscopic treatment of biliary strictures after liver transplantation. Liver Transpl 2006;12:718–25.
40. Pasha SF, Harrison ME, Das A, et al. Endoscopic treatment of anastomotic biliary strictures after deceased donor liver transplantation: outcomes after maximal stent therapy. Gastrointest Endosc 2007;66:44–51.
41. Morelli J, Mulcahy HE, Willner IR, et al. Long-term outcomes for patients with post-liver transplant anastomotic biliary strictures treated by endoscopic stent placement. Gastrointest Endosc 2003;58:374–9.
42. Holt AP, Thorburn D, Mirza D, et al. A prospective study of standardized nonsurgical therapy in the management of biliary anastomotic strictures complicating liver transplantation. Transplantation 2007;84:857–63.
43. Kulaksiz H, Weiss KH, Gotthardt D, et al. Is stenting necessary after balloon dilation of post-transplantation biliary strictures? Results of a prospective comparative study. Endoscopy 2008;40:746–51.
44. Alazmi WM, Fogel EL, Watkins JL, et al. Recurrence rate of anastomotic biliary strictures in patients who have had previous successful endoscopic therapy for anastomotic narrowing after orthotopic liver transplantation. Endoscopy 2006;38:571–4.
45. Morelli G, Fazel A, Judah J, et al. Rapid-sequence endoscopic management of posttransplant anastomotic biliary strictures. Gastrointest Endosc 2008;67:879–85.
46. Sanna C, Giordanino C, Giono I, et al. Safety and efficacy of endoscopic retrograde cholangiopancreatography in patients with post-liver transplant biliary complications: results of a cohort study with long-term follow-up. Gut Liver 2011;5:328–34.
47. Hsieh TH, Mekeel KL, Crowell MD, et al. Endoscopic treatment of anastomotic biliary strictures after living donor liver transplantation: outcomes after maximal stent therapy. Gastrointest Endosc 2013;77:47–54.
48. Poley JW, Lekkerkerker MN, Metselaar HJ, et al. Clinical outcome of progressive stenting in patients with anastomotic strictures after orthotopic liver transplantation. Endoscopy 2013;45:567–70.
49. Sauer P, Chahoud F, Gotthardt D, et al. Temporary placement of fully covered self-expandable metal stents in biliary complications after liver transplantation. Endoscopy 2012;44:536–8.
50. Traina M, Tarantino I, Barresi L, et al. Efficacy and safety of fully covered self-expandable metallic stents in biliary complications after liver transplantation: a preliminary study. Liver Transpl 2009;15:1493–8.
51. Tarantino I, Traina M, Mocciaro F, et al. Fully covered metallic stents in biliary stenosis after orthotopic liver transplantation. Endoscopy 2012;44:246–50.
52. Cerecedo-Rodriguez J, Phillips M, Figueroa-Barojas P, et al. Self expandable metal stents for anastomotic stricture following liver transplant. Dig Dis Sci 2013;58:2661–6.

53. Chaput U, Scatton O, Bichard P, et al. Temporary placement of partially covered self-expandable metal stents for anastomotic biliary strictures after liver transplantation: a prospective, multicenter study. Gastrointest Endosc 2010;72:1167–74.
54. Larghi A, Tringali A, Lecca PG, et al. Management of hilar biliary strictures. Am J Gastroenterol 2008;103:458–73.
55. Luigiano C, Bassi M, Ferrara F, et al. Placement of a new fully covered self-expanding metal stent for postoperative biliary strictures and leaks not responding to plastic stenting. Surg Laparosc Endosc Percutan Tech 2013;23:159–62.
56. Kao D, Zepeda-Gomez S, Tandon P, et al. Managing the post-liver transplantation anastomotic biliary stricture: multiple plastic versus metal stents: a systematic review. Gastrointest Endosc 2013;77:679–91.
57. Kaffes A, Griffin S, Vaughan R, et al. A randomized trial of a fully covered self-expandable metallic stent versus plastic stents in anastomotic biliary strictures after liver transplantation. Therap Adv Gastroenterol 2014;7:64–71.
58. Devière J, Nageshwar Reddy D, Püspök A, et al. Successful management of benign biliary strictures with fully covered self-expanding metal stents. Gastroenterology 2014;147:385–95.
59. Kabar I, Cicinnati VR, Beckebaum S, et al. Use of paclitaxel-eluting balloons for endotherapy of anastomotic strictures following liver transplantation. Endoscopy 2012;44:1158–60.
60. Barriga J, Thompson R, Shokouh-Amiri H, et al. Biliary strictures after liver transplantation. Predictive factors for response to endoscopic management and long-term outcome. Am J Med Sci 2008;335:439–43.
61. Weber A, Prinz C, Gerngross C, et al. Long-term outcome of endoscopic and/or percutaneous transhepatic therapy in patients with biliary stricture after orthotopic liver transplantation. J Gastroenterol 2009;44:1195–202.
62. Balderramo D, Sendino O, Burrel M, et al. Risk factors and outcomes of failed endoscopic retrograde cholangiopancreatography in liver transplant recipients with anastomotic biliary strictures: a case-control study. Liver Transpl 2012;18:482–9.
63. Gupta K, Aparicio D, Freeman ML, et al. Endoscopic biliary recanalization by using a needle catheter in patients with complete ligation or stricture of the bile duct: safety and feasibility of a novel technique (with videos). Gastrointest Endosc 2011;74:423–8.
64. Martins FP, De Paulo GA, Macedo EP, et al. Endoscopic biliary recanalization with a needle-knife in post liver-transplant complete anastomotic stricture. Endoscopy 2012;44(Suppl 2):E304–5.
65. Takatsuki M, Eguchi S, Kawashita Y, et al. Biliary complications in recipients of living-donor liver transplantation. J Hepatobiliary Pancreat Surg 2006;13:497–501.
66. Wang SF, Huang ZY, Chen XP. Biliary complications after living donor liver transplantation. Liver Transpl 2011;17:1127–36.
67. Shah SA, Grant DR, McGilvray ID, et al. Biliary strictures in 130 consecutive right lobe living donor liver transplant recipients: results of a Western center. Am J Transplant 2007;7:161–7.
68. Liu CL, Lo CM, Chan SC, et al. Safety of duct-to-duct biliary reconstruction in right-lobe live-donor liver transplantation without biliary drainage. Transplantation 2004;77:726–32.
69. Wadhawan M, Kumar A, Gupta S, et al. Post-transplant biliary complications: an analysis from a predominantly living donor liver transplant center. J Gastroenterol Hepatol 2013;28:1056–60.

70. Gondolesi GE, Varotti G, Florman SS, et al. Biliary complications in 96 consecutive right lobe living donor transplant recipients. Transplantation 2004;77: 1842–8.
71. Freise CE, Gillespie BW, Koffron AJ, et al. Recipient morbidity after living and deceased donor liver transplantation: findings from the A2ALL Retrospective Cohort Study. Am J Transplant 2008;8:2569–79.
72. Soejima Y, Taketomi A, Yoshizumi T, et al. Biliary strictures in living donor liver transplantation: incidence, management, and technical evolution. Liver Transpl 2006;12:979–86.
73. Hwang S, Lee SG, Sung KB, et al. Long-term incidence, risk factors, and management of biliary complications after adult living donor liver transplantation. Liver Transpl 2006;12:831–8.
74. Seo JK, Ryu JK, Lee SH, et al. Endoscopic treatment for biliary stricture after adult living donor liver transplantation. Liver Transpl 2009;15:369–80.
75. Croome KP, McAlister V, Adams P, et al. Endoscopic management of biliary complications following liver transplantation after donation from cardiac death donors. Can J Gastroenterol 2012;26:607–10.
76. Balderramo D, Sendino O, Miquel R, et al. Prospective evaluation of single-operator peroral cholangioscopy in liver transplant recipients requiring an evaluation of the biliary tract. Liver Transpl 2013;19:199–206.
77. Rizk RS, McVicar JP, Emond MJ, et al. Endoscopic management of biliary strictures in liver transplant recipients: effect on patient and graft survival. Gastrointest Endosc 1998;47:128–35.
78. Balderramo D, Bordas JM, Sendino O, et al. Complications after ERCP in liver transplant recipients. Gastrointest Endosc 2011;74:285–94.
79. Balderramo D, Navasa M, Cardenas A. Current management of biliary complications after liver transplantation: emphasis on endoscopic therapy. Gastroenterol Hepatol 2011;34:107–15.

Cholangioscopy in Liver Disease

 CrossMark

Brian C. Brauer, MD*, Raj J. Shah, MD

KEYWORDS

- Cholangioscopy • ERCP • Biliary stricture • Biliary tract neoplasms • Biliary stones

KEY POINTS

- Cholangioscopy is an adjunct to endoscopic retrograde cholangiopancreatography (ERCP) and can be used for the diagnosis and therapy of a variety of biliary diseases.
- Cholangioscopy is effective in the management of difficult biliary stones and aids in the diagnosis of biliary tumors.
- Cholangioscopy provides direct visualization to guide selective biliary access and the delivery of other therapies. Multiple cholangioscope platforms exist.
- Cholangisocopy may be associated with a higher complication rate than conventional ERCP.

INTRODUCTION: NATURE OF THE PROBLEM

Miniature endoscopes and catheters have been developed that permit direct visualization of the bile ducts, referred to as cholangioscopes or choledochoscopes. For the purpose of this article, these devices are referred to as cholangioscopes, and the procedure as cholangioscopy. Cholangioscopes are usually passed through the working channel of a standard therapeutic duodenoscope during endoscopic retrograde cholangiopancreatography (ERCP).

The first cholangioscope was described in 1941,[1] and the per oral approach was subsequently introduced in the early 1970s.[2,3] Further improvements in the technology have resulted in smaller diameter cholangioscopes that include a working channel, the ability to deflect the tip of the scope,[4–6] disposable catheter-based delivery systems with a reusable optical fiber,[7] and direct cholangioscopy using slim gastroscopes without the use of a duodenoscope.[8]

Disclosures: No relevant disclosures to report (B.C. Brauer); Medical Advisory Board – Boston Scientific, Inc, Unrestricted educational grant – Boston Scientific, Inc and Olympus America, Inc (R.J. Shah).
Division of Gastroenterology and Hepatology, University of Colorado Anschutz Medical Campus, 1635 Aurora Court, Mailstop F-735, Room 2.031, Aurora, CO 80045, USA
* Corresponding author.
E-mail address: Brian.brauer@ucdenver.edu

This article reviews cholangioscopy performed during ERCP and provides a brief overview of direct cholangioscopy utilizing slim gastroscopes.

INDICATIONS AND CONTRAINDICATIONS

Cholangioscopy is most established for and used primarily for the treatment of difficult bile duct stones using electrohydraulic or laser lithotripsy probes and for the evaluation of indeterminate biliary strictures. These are strictures in which a diagnosis was not certain after ERCP with sampling techniques such as brush cytology or forceps biopsy.[6–19] Cholangioscopy can be used to directly visualize and sample lesions seen on cholangiography, either with direct biopsy through the cholangioscope's working channel, or to target areas for fluoroscopic biopsy through the duodenoscope (eg, cholangioscopy-assisted biopsy).[12] It can also be used to evaluate equivocal fluoroscopy findings on cholangiography, assess the extent of biliary tumors before surgery, identify stones not seen by conventional cholangiography, assess for clearance of stones during ERCP, and for surveillance of primary sclerosing cholangitis (PSC).[13,14] It may also be used to guide advanced imaging with biliary confocal microscopy and selective ductal access, such as cystic duct or difficult to negotiate intrahepatic segments.

Most available cholangioscopes range from 3.1 to 3.4 mm in diameter; thus, the bile duct must be of sufficient caliber to allow passage (**Table 1**).[6] Downstream strictures may require balloon dilation to permit passage of the cholangioscope. Because in 1 study cholangioscopy may be associated with a higher rate of cholangitis than ERCP alone, it should be avoided in patients with active cholangitis.[20] A more recent study did not confirm this increased risk, however (see **Table 1**).[21]

PREPARATION

Before ERCP, patients typically take no food by mouth for 4 to 8 hours and sometimes longer if there is known or suspected delayed gastric emptying.[22] Alternatively, clear liquids can be taken up to 2 hours before elective procedures requiring general anesthesia or sedation/analgesia (American Society of Anesthesiologists guidelines).[23]

Most medications can be continued up to the time of endoscopy and are usually taken with a small sip of water. Some medications may need to be adjusted before upper endoscopy, such as medications for diabetes, owing to decreased oral intake

Table 1 Indications and contraindications to cholangioscopy	
Indications	**Contraindications**
Therapy of difficult bile duct stones	Surgically altered anatomy making bile duct inaccessible
Indeterminate biliary strictures	Ascending cholangitis
Evaluation of equivocal findings during endoscopic retrograde cholangiopancreatography	Small duct <5 mm in diameter
Assessment of biliary tumor extent before surgery	
Assess for residual stones in dilated bile ducts not seen on cholangiography	
Surveillance of dominant stenoses in primary sclerosing cholangitis	

around the time of the procedure. Most blood pressure medications should be maintained, with the exception of angiotensin-converting enzyme inhibitors and angiotensin receptor blockers if patients are undergoing general anesthesia, because these agents can cause significant hypotension during general anesthesia.

Management of Anticoagulants

Decisions regarding the management of antiplatelet agents or anticoagulants must account for the risk of bleeding rendered by maintaining the patient on the agent through the procedure and the risk of a thromboembolic event if the agent is discontinued in the periprocedural period. Many patients undergoing cholangioscopy will require a sphincterotomy. The overall risk of post-sphincterotomy bleeding (immediate or delayed) is less than 2%. Discontinuation of aspirin or nonsteroidal antiinflammatory drugs, up to 1 week before the procedure does not reduce the risk of bleeding. However, anticoagulation with warfarin or heparin within 3 days of sphincterotomy can increase risk of post-sphincterotomy bleeding. Therefore, aspirin and warfarin can be continued before sphincterotomy, but warfarin and heparin should be held before the procedure.[24]

Antibiotic Prophylaxis

Guidelines regarding the use of antibiotics in patients undergoing endoscopic procedures do not specifically address antibiotic prophylaxis for cholangioscopy. However, preprocedural antibiotic prophylaxis has generally been recommended for all patients owing to a potentially higher rate of cholangitis compared with those patients undergoing ERCP without cholangioscopy.[20] The antibiotic regimens used are the same as those used for other patients undergoing ERCP who require antibiotic prophylaxis and are generally broad spectrum delivered intravenously.[25] Further, in the setting of leaks or intrahepatic strictures, we favor a short 5- to7-day course of post-procedure oral antibiotics to further reduce the risk of delayed cholangitis.

Patient Positioning

Patients undergoing cholangioscopy are positioned in a semiprone ERCP position. In our opinion, this allows the most stable scope position for ERCP and reduces stress on the patient's neck compared with the fully prone or supine position. If cardiopulmonary status does not allow for prone positioning, or if the anesthesia provider is not comfortable with a prone position, a supine position or left lateral position can also be used.

Sedation

We recommend general anesthesia for all patients undergoing cholangioscopy, because the procedure times are longer, patient cooperation is essential for optimizing successful visualization, and fluid irrigation used to enhance intraductal visualization and clear intraductal debris can lead to reflux of fluids and pooling within the stomach, increasing the risk of aspiration.[19]

APPROACH
Equipment

Systems available in the United States for cholangioscopy include endoscope-based systems, commonly referred to as "mother–daughter" systems (Olympus America, Center Valley, PA; Pentax, Montvale, NJ) and a catheter-based system (SpyGlass Direct Visualization System, Boston Scientific Endoscopy, Marlboro, MA). In addition, cholangioscopy can be performed using a slim (4.9- to 5.9-mm outer diameter) gastroscope or even standard gastroscope in patients with a dilated common bile duct.[8]

"Mother–Daughter" Systems

These systems are dual operator and composed of a "mother" duodenoscope and a "daughter" cholangioscope, each with its respective control handles. The cholangioscope is inserted through the accessory channel of the duodenoscope. Two endoscopists, or an endoscopist with a trained assistant, are necessary. Cholangioscopes range in diameter from 3.1 to 3.4 mm, with a working channel of 1.2 mm and up–down tip deflection.[16] Commercially available cholangioscopes are fiberoptic, although digital video cholangioscope prototypes are being investigated. The 1.2-mm working channel permits passage of miniature biopsy forceps and intraductal lithotripsy fibers.[7,18]

Catheter-Based System

The catheter-based system is single operator, because it attaches to the duodenoscope, allowing manipulation of both control dials by 1 endoscopist.[7] The system includes a reusable, 0.77-mm optical probe that is passed through a 4-lumen, 3.4-mm in diameter catheter. In addition to a lumen for the optical probe, the catheter includes a 1.2-mm working channel and 2 dedicated 0.6-mm irrigation channels. The tip of the catheter can be deflected in 4 directions (up–down and left–right; **Table 2**).

Slim gastroscopes can be used in patients with dilated common bile ducts generally greater than 10 mm in diameter.[8,16,26–29] Slim gastroscopes have diameters of 5 to 6 mm, and thus can only be used in patients with dilated common bile ducts. If a gastroscope is being used, insufflation with sterile saline, water or CO_2 is preferable, because air insufflation has been associated with air embolism.[29] A single report of CO_2 insufflation causing fatal air embolism in the setting of endoscopic pseudocyst debridement exists; therefore, the use of water or saline is recommended, CO_2 should be used cautiously.[30] The advantages of a slim gastroscope is that it is single operator, video image quality is superior that may include narrow-band imaging (NBI) capability, and the larger working channel accommodates argon plasma coagulation probes, larger biopsy forceps, and lithotripsy fibers.

TECHNIQUE
Scope Insertion

Cholangioscopy is carried out during ERCP. Fluoroscopically visible lesions and suspicious areas can be mapped with spot radiographs to aid with subsequent cholangioscopic localization. A long (450 cm; 0.035") guidewire is advanced to the intrahepatics and the cholangioscope advanced over the guidewire through a

Table 2		
Commercially available cholangioscopes in the United States and specifications		
Endoscope	Tip OD (mm)	Accessory Channel (mm)
SpyGlass (Boston Scientific, Natick, MA)	3.4	1.2
CHF-BP 30 (Olympus, Center Valley, PA)	3.1	1.2
FCP-9P (Pentax, Montvale, NJ)	3.1	1.2

standard therapeutic duodenoscope during "back tension" on the wire exiting the cholangioscope. For endoscope-based systems, a "transfer tube" is placed into the biopsy port to allow wire exit from the working channel. Sphincterotomy and/or stricture dilation are performed, as needed, to facilitate scope passage.[19] The size of most cholangioscopes requires a sphincterotomy unless the major papilla is patulous, such as seen with intraductal papillary biliary neoplasms. Care must be taken to minimize elevator use while advancing the cholangioscope, especially in endoscope-based platforms, which are vulnerable to damage at its bending portion and to optical fibers. If a slim gastroscope is being used, it may be inserted into the duct over a guidewire placed during ERCP or by way of a free-hand technique.[8] Pediatric forceps may be used to gently grasp intraductal mucosa or prototype anchoring balloons to permit advancement of the slim gastroscope to the intrahepatics.[8,28]

Once the cholangioscope is advanced to the desired location within the duct, the guidewire is removed to enhance visualization and to permit use of the working channel.

Narrow ducts diameters or tight strictures complicate or prohibit scope passage. Circumferential visualization may also be compromised in the evaluation of a markedly dilated duct (**Fig. 1**).

Intraductal Lithotripsy

Electrohydraulic lithotripsy (EHL) can be used to treat large bile duct stones. Cholangioscopic visualization during intraductal lithotripsy helps to avoid duct injury. The EHL fiber contains 2 coaxially insulated electrodes ending at an open tip. During water immersion, sparks are generated that produce high-amplitude hydraulic pressure waves for stone fragmentation.[31] A generator produces a series of high-voltage electrical impulses at a frequency of 1 to 20 per second, with power settings ranging from 50 to 100. The tip of the EHL fiber should protrude no more than 2 or 3 mm from the scope and be positioned en face with the stone while the generator's foot pedal is depressed to deliver energy.[19] An alternative to EHL is pulsed laser lithotripsy. During laser lithotripsy, a laser beam is transmitted via a flexible quartz fiber through the working channel of the cholangioscope. The application of repetitive pulses of laser energy to the stone leads to the formation of a gaseous collection of ions and free electrons of high kinetic energy (eg, plasma). Absorption of the laser energy rapidly expands and collapses the plasma inducing a spherical, mechanical shockwave between the laser fiber and stone, leading to stone fragmentation.[32]

Intraductal Biopsy

Two methods can be used to obtain targeted biopsies from the bile duct: cholangioscopy-directed biopsy and cholangioscopy-assisted biopsy. Cholangioscopy-directed biopsy is performed by passing a miniature cholangioscope biopsy forceps through the working channel under direct endoscopic visualization. For cholangioscopy-assisted biopsy, the target biopsy site is localized using cholangioscopic visualization and fluoroscopic spot films of the cholangioscope tip positioned at the lesion. After removing the cholangioscope, a conventional biopsy forceps is then passed through the working channel of the duodenoscope alongside the guidewire to obtain tissue samples under fluoroscopic guidance.[12] The guidewire, along with fluoroscopy view, provides the axis orientation for the forceps during passage. A variety of forceps ranging from standard or pediatric endoscopic biopsy forceps or specialized biliary forceps may be used.

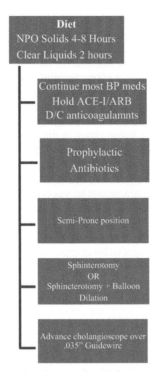

Fig. 1. Preparation, approach, and technique for cholangioscopy.

OUTCOMES
Bile Duct Stones

Cholangioscopy with EHL is associated with a high rate of success for removal of extrahepatic biliary stones that have failed extraction with conventional ERCP techniques. Clearance rates of 83% to 100% have been reported.[10,11,31]

- A retrospective series of 94 patients with difficult biliary stones reported that 90% achieved stone clearance after 1 or 2 EHL sessions.[11] Failure of stone clearance occurred in 11 patients. Reasons for failure included difficult stone location (4 patients), stricturing below the stones (2 patients), poor patient health status precluding additional interventions (1 patient), failure of stone clearance requiring common bile duct exploration (1 patient), and failure to remove a stone owing to a broken cholangioscope. Five of the patients with failed stone clearance had stones in the common hepatic or intrahepatic ducts. Complications were seen in 17% of patients and included cholangitis and/or jaundice, hemobilia, pancreatitis, bile leaks, and bradycardia.
- A 100% clearance rate with no complications was reported in a study that included 26 patients who underwent EHL.[33] Twelve of the patients had had a prior attempt at mechanical lithotripsy. In the remaining 14, mechanical lithotripsy had not been attempted because the stones were intrahepatic (4 patients), a stricture was present (6 patients), the stones were in the cystic duct (2 patients), or the stones were impacted in the common bile duct (2 patients). Mechanical lithotripsy was not reattempted at the referral center according to the study protocol, which may explain the high clearance rate compared with other series.

- An abstract from our group included retrospective analysis of 211 patients with primarily extrahepatic stones. Patients underwent large papillary balloon dilation, mechanical lithotripsy, or cholangioscopy with EHL or laser lithotripsy. Complete clearance was achieved in 99%, 79% at index ERCP and 20% at subsequent ERCP. Large papillary balloon dilation had an higher rate of success at index ERCP, but patients in the cholangioscopy lithotripsy group had significantly larger stones and were likely selected for cholangioscopy for this reason.[34]
- In a study of 60 patients who underwent catheter-based cholangioscopy and laser lithotripsy for biliary stones,[35] 50 of 60 (83.3%) had complete clearance in 1 session; the remainder obtained complete clearance after 2 sessions. However, 34 patients had no prior therapy but were deemed to be difficult extractions owing to impacted stones, Mirrizzi's syndrome, or the presence of casts, which may account for the high rate of clearance in a single session. Complications occurred in 8 patients (13.3%); however, all were minor and included transient fever, mild abdominal pain, and development of a stricture in 1 patient.

Limited and older studies have compared EHL or laser lithotripsy with extracorporeal shock wave lithotripsy (ESWL), in which stones are fragmented using shock waves that are directed through the body onto the stone(s). With the increased availability of cholangioscopy, ESWL for biliary stones is not utilized as ERCP is still required to remove stone fragments.

- A nonrandomized comparison of 118 patients who underwent ESWL or per oral cholangioscopy with EHL revealed similar stone clearance rates in the ESWL and EHL groups (79 vs 74%; $P>.1$).[36] The disadvantage in the ESWL group was the necessity to perform ERCP to extract stone fragments. Cross-over treatments resulted in successful duct clearance in 94% of patients.
- In a randomized, prospective study of 60 patients, cholangioscopy-guided laser lithotripsy demonstrated a significantly higher rate of duct clearance (97 vs 73%) and a lower number of lithotripsy sessions (1.2 vs 3) compared with ESWL.[37] After cross-over therapy, 59 of 60 patients (98%) achieved duct clearance (**Box 1**).

Intrahepatic bile duct stones (seen in the setting of recurrent pyogenic cholangitis) require more intensive endotherapy than extrahepatic stones. One study reported 36 consecutive patients with hepatolithiasis treated with per oral cholangioscopy-directed EHL or laser lithotripsy.[38] Despite a mean of 4.5 cholangioscopy sessions and adjunctive ESWL in one third of the patients, ductal clearance was achieved in only 75% (64% complete, 11% partial). After a mean of 7.8 years of follow-up, symptomatic recurrence developed in 22% and 25% of those with complete and partial clearance, respectively. In general, effective treatment of hepatolithiasis may require combined per oral and percutaneous approaches or surgical resection.[39]

The use of direct cholangioscopy using larger scopes in stone therapy and to confirm stone clearance is a concept that has gained momentum in recent years given that the endoscopes are readily available in most units and carry better image resolution.

- Lee and colleagues[40] reported 48 patients in whom direct cholangioscopy was used to look for residual stones after mechanical lithotripsy and complete clearance of stones confirmed by balloon occlusion cholangiography in patients with dilated ducts greater than 10 mm. Direct cholangioscopy was then performed using an endoscope with an outer diameter of 5 to 5.4 mm. In 48

Box 1
Outcomes of cholangioscopy

Biliary stones

- 90% clearance rate for EHL in 1–2 sessions[9]
- 100% clearance rate for EHL in 26 patients[33]
- 100% clearance after 2 sessions for LL[35]
- ESWL similar to EHL in stone clearance, additional session required to remove stone fragments after ESWL[35]
- LL higher clearance and fewer sessions than ESWL[36]

Biliary tumors

- 92% diagnosis of malignancy by visualization alone[68]
- Cholangioscopy-directed biopsy 88% sensitivity and 94% specificity[70]
- Sensitivity and specificity of ERCP, cholangioscopic visualization, and cholangioscopy-directed tissue biopsies for detecting malignancy were 51 and 54%, 78 and 82%, and 49 and 98% in multicenter study[72]
- In PSC, direct visualization increased yield over cholangiography alone[77]

Abbreviations: EHL, electrohydraulic lithotripsy; ERCP, endoscopic retrograde cholangiopancreatography; ESWL, extracorporeal shock wave lithotripsy; LL, laser lithotripsy; PSC, primary sclerosing cholangitis.

---

attempted cases, direct cholangioscopy was successful in 46. Thirteen of 46 patients (28.3%) had residual stones despite negative cholangiography, indicating that cholangioscopy might have a role in confirmation of stone clearance in dilated ducts.

Suspected Biliary Malignancies

In patients with indeterminate strictures or filling defects at cholangiography, cholangioscopy permits direct inspection of the epithelium for subtle abnormalities or to obtain biopsies. However, stent-associated changes and trauma related to stricture dilation may alter the mucosal appearance, making visual diagnosis more challenging.

The sensitivity of conventional brush cytology or biopsy during ERCP for detecting malignancy in most series ranges from 30% to 88%.[41–71] Cholangioscopic visualization may enhance diagnosis by detecting "tumor vessels" (irregularly dilated and tortuous blood vessels) in the setting of malignancy; however, consensus on the degree of dilatation or tortuosity of vessels should be to constitute suspected malignancy is lacking. In addition, the presence of intraductal nodules or masses, infiltrative or ulcerated strictures, or papillary or villous mucosal projections may indicate malignancy and should prompt biopsies (**Figs. 2** and **3**).[65] A combination of tumor vessels plus percutaneous biopsy diagnosed 96% of cancers in 1 study.[66] Tumor vessels were not present in histologically benign strictures, as determined by 1-year follow-up (**Fig. 4**).

Prospective, single-center case series using either endoscope-based or catheter-based systems have shown that cholangioscopic visualization with or without biopsy has a sensitivity of 89% to 100% and a specificity of 79% to 96% for detecting biliary malignancies.[12,15,67–69] Manta and colleagues[70] reported a prospective study of 52 patients undergoing catheter-based cholangioscopy for indeterminate biliary

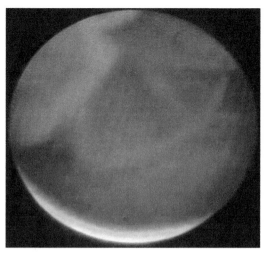

Fig. 2. Catheter-based cholangioscopy showing a papillary/villous-appearing lesion.

strictures. Seven patients were found to have benign lesions by cholangioscopic examination. Biopsies were successful in 43 of the remaining 45. Cholangioscopy-directed biopsies agreed with final surgical diagnosis in 90%; overall sensitivity was 88% and specificity 94%.

In a prospective study of 26 patients comparing cholangioscopy-directed biopsies with brush cytology and standard forceps biopsy, technical success was achieved in all. The sensitivity, accuracy, and negative predictive values were 5.9%, 38.5%, and 36%, respectively, for standard cytology brushings; 29.4%, 53.8%, and 42.8%, respectively, for standard forceps biopsies; and 76.5%, 84.6%, and 69.2%, respectively, for mini-forceps biopsies. Sensitivity and overall accuracy were significantly better versus brush cytology (P<.0001) and standard forceps biopsy (P = .0215) alone,[71] although an explanation for the remarkably low sensitivity with brush cytology was not provided by the authors.

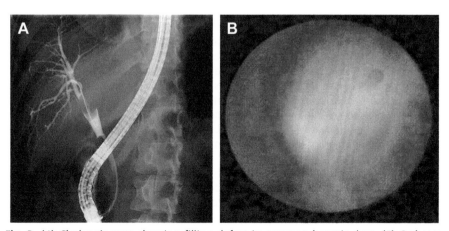

Fig. 3. (A) Cholangiogram showing filling defect in common hepatic duct. (B) Catheter-based cholangioscopy showing a nodular lesion. Biopsies revealed spindle cell lesion, final pathology after surgical resection was consistent with a cystadenoma.

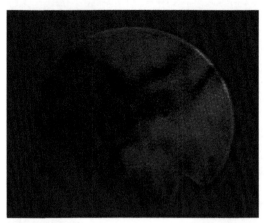

Fig. 4. Fiberoptic cholangioscope (CHF-BP30) demonstrating tumor vessels.

When biopsies are obtained during cholangioscopy, tissue confirmation for malignancy is achieved in 57% to 90% of patients with a final diagnosis of malignancy (based on surgical resection or clinical follow-up).[12,15,45,66–71]

In an international, multicenter, observational series of catheter-based cholangioscopy for indeterminate pancreaticobiliary pathology and difficult stone disease, 226 patients underwent cholangioscopic inspection; 86 had at least 1 prior ERCP. In the group, 140 underwent cholangioscopy-directed biopsies.[72] Complete ERCP, cholangioscopic, and biopsy data were available for 95 patients. The sensitivities and specificities of ERCP, cholangioscopic visualization, and cholangioscopy-directed tissue biopsies for detecting malignancy were 51% and 54%, 78% and 82%, and 49% and 98%, respectively, demonstrating that cholangioscopy with or without biopsy has a much greater sensitivity and specificity than cholangiography alone. However, although this was a highly select referral center population with prior nondiagnostic sampling, the operating characteristics of cholangioscopic visualization alone were somewhat disappointing, possibly owing to a lack of consistent terminology and interpretation of findings among even expert users (see **Box 1**).

Confirming malignancy in the sclerotic type of cholangiocarcinoma can be difficult because malignant cells are often absent on superficial mucosal biopsies as the result of a fibrotic reaction to the tumor and expansion into the subepithelial layers. In a prospective, multicenter study of 87 patients who underwent video cholangioscopy, the investigators were able to distinguish malignant from benign biliary lesions in 92% by visualization alone.[69] Although not commercially available, video cholangioscopy has been combined with NBI at select referral centers in Japan and the United States, and the addition of this technology may enhance mucosal and tumor vessel visualization (**Fig. 5**).[73,74]

With respect to comparing the yield of cholangioscopy with EUS, our group published a retrospective series of a highly select cohort of 66 patients with indeterminate biliary strictures who had undergone both cholangioscopy or pancreatoscopy and endoscopic ultrasonography (EUS) within 3 months. We found a higher diagnostic yield for patients undergoing both EUS and cholangiopancreatoscopy compared with either modality alone, with a combined sensitivity and specificity of 66.7% and 96.3%, respectively.[75]

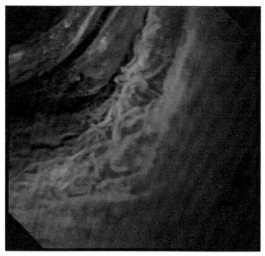

Fig. 5. Video cholangioscopy with narrow-band imaging demonstrating tumor vessels.

A recent prospective study of 39 patients in which EUS-fine needle aspiration biopsy performed first in patients with biliary strictures and negative brushings, and catheter-based cholangioscopy reserved only for negative EUS significantly decreased the number of cholangioscopies required. The need for cholangioscopy was avoided in 24 patients, and an estimated cost savings of US$110,000 was realized. EUS-fine needle aspiration biopsy was diagnostic in 23 patients (58%). The authors of this study advocate an EUS-first approach in these patients.[76] Our group tends to utilize EUS before cholangioscopy and often arrange both procedures at the same endoscopic session proceeding with cholangioscopy if EUS is unremarkable.

PSC

The diagnosis of malignancy in PSC is difficult using only cholangiography or tissue sampling. In a prospective study of 53 patients with PSC, adding direct visualization with cholangioscopy increased the diagnostic yield compared with ERCP alone.[77] Twelve patients (23%) had cancer, and 41 (77%) had benign disease. Compared with cholangiography, cholangioscopy had better sensitivity (92% vs 66%), specificity (93% vs 51%), and negative predictive value (97% vs 84%). However, this yield has not been duplicated by other centers; features traditionally classified as malignant on cholangioscopy, such as nodular and infiltrative strictures, may be present in benign PSC.[13] Cholangioscopy may be useful in detecting and treating stones associated with PSC that may be missed on cholangioscopy.[14]

The addition of NBI to cholangioscopy could be beneficial in the detection of malignant in this population. A series of 30 patients with PSC revealed that NBI allowed improved detection of tumor margins over cholangiography alone and there was an increased detection of suspicious-appearing lesions with more biopsies were taken. However, this did not translate to an improvement of detection of dysplasia and there was overlap in benign and malignant cholangioscopic findings as described.[13] We have found limited value of utilizing cholangioscopy for diagnostic purposes in the PSC population owing to narrower ducts and the difficulty in distinguishing benign from malignant intraductal lesions.

COMPLICATIONS AND MANAGEMENT

Complications associated with per oral cholangioscopy are often associated with specific maneuvers performed during ERCP (eg, sphincterotomy). Complications specific to the performance of cholangiopancreatoscopy include cholangitis, which is related to intraductal fluid irrigation and, uncommonly, hemobilia and bile leaks attributable to intraductal lithotripsy.[6,11,20] Our center retrospectively assessed patients undergoing ERCP with or without cholangiopancreatoscopy and found that ERCP with cholangiopancreatoscopy may be associated with a significantly higher rate of procedure-related complications than ERCP alone.[20] This increased risk was observed in overall complications (7.0% vs 2.9%), consensus complications (pancreatitis, perforation, cholangitis, or bleeding; 4.2% vs 2.2%), and specifically with post-procedural cholangitis (1.0% vs 0.2%). A recent publication of 169 single-operator cholangioscopy procedures that included a multivariate analysis did not show cholangioscopy was associated with an increased complication rate including pancreatitis, infection, bleeding, and perforation.[21]

POST-PROCEDURE CARE

Post-procedure care is the same as for standard ERCP. Electrocardiogram, blood pressure, and pulse oximetry should be monitored until the patient is fully awake. Patients may be monitored in a postoperative unit or a same-day observation unit. Most cholangioscopy procedures are performed on an outpatient basis. Given the possibility of an increased complication rate associated with cholangioscopy, post-procedural pain should raise concern for pancreatitis or perforation, and strong consideration should be given to hospital admission, and appropriate imaging and laboratory workup if pain persists. Patients with post-procedure fever should be presumed to have cholangitis and receive antibiotics regardless of the indication for cholangioscopy. Patients with biliary strictures and incomplete drainage at the conclusion or ERCP such as hilar strictures and PSC should have antibiotics continued after ERCP.[25]

REPORTING, FOLLOW-UP, AND CLINICAL IMPLICATIONS (IF PROCEDURE IS USED FOR DIAGNOSTIC PURPOSES)

Cholangioscopy findings are reported in the ERCP report. It is our practice to include a separate paragraph with cholangioscopy findings and their interpretation. Pathologic and cytologic findings are reported by the pathology department in the usual fashion. Follow-up after cholangioscopy is highly variable depending on indication and therapy performed. In the appropriate clinical setting, even in the absence of confirmatory tissue, if cholangioscopy visualization of tumor vessels or other malignant features are identified then surgical resection may be recommended if autoimmune cholangiopathy or pancreatitis has been sufficiently excluded.[78] In patients undergoing therapy for stones with complete clearance, if no stent is placed, then a follow-up procedure is not required. If stone clearance is incomplete, a stent to the level upstream of the most proximal stone is placed and a follow-up procedure is usually performed in 4 to 8 weeks. Likewise, if cholangioscopy is performed for stricture sampling, if stents are placed to treat a stricture, a follow-up procedure is performed based on stent size and location, usually 4 to 8 weeks unless surgical resection is planned.

CURRENT CONTROVERSIES AND FUTURE CONSIDERATIONS

Cholangioscopy is currently widely available in both referral and community centers; however, expertise in its performance and interpretation is limited mostly to select referral centers. The capital expense of equipment, technical complexity of performing the procedure, fragility of endoscope-based cholangioscopes, and infrequent need for the procedure contribute to the limited expertise with this procedure. The introduction of the catheter-based cholangioscopy system has led to increased interest in performing the procedure. A lower initial capital investment and better durability owing to a disposable delivery catheter has piqued interest. This brings about an additional question regarding the level of training necessary to reliably perform cholangioscopy.

Another point is the likely reduced need for cholangioscopy for large biliary stones as interest has reemerged with the use of large-diameter balloon papillary dilation preceded by a small sphincterotomy to facilitate removal of large stones. Many studies have shown the technique to be safe and highly effective, although earlier studies raised concern about high rates of pancreatitis. A report of 298 patients showed a 91.6% stone clearance rate and a 10.1% pancreatitis rate, with only 1 perforation.[79] A majority of the patients who developed pancreatitis had contrast injection of the pancreatic duct. The advantage to this approach is that the equipment needed is readily available in most endoscopy units, thus obviating the need for referral to tertiary centers. The technique is being perfected, but it is likely that it will remain a viable alternative for the management of large stones. However, cholangioscopy and EHL or laser lithotripsy will still be required for impacted or cuboidal-shaped stones, or those with associated downstream stenoses that cannot be sufficiently dilated to permit extraction.

Inferior optics remain as the major drawback of commercially available mother–daughter cholangioscopy systems. All still rely on fiber-optics, which pale in comparison to the high-definition video we are accustomed to with standard endoscopes. Poor image quality and inadequate light in dilated ducts make visualization difficult at times. A prototype of a video and NBI endoscope-based cholangioscope is available; however, fragility of the instrument and costly repairs have thus far prevented commercial production. Likewise, improvements in the catheter-based system incorporating video chip technology are also under development and are eagerly anticipated.

SUMMARY

Miniature endoscopes and catheters have been developed that permit direct visualization of the bile ducts. These endoscopes and catheters are passed through the working channel of a standard therapeutic duodenoscope during ERCP. Cholangioscopy with intraductal lithotripsy has become an established modality in the treatment of difficult biliary stones. When used to evaluate indeterminate biliary strictures or suspected biliary malignancies, it has an improved sensitivity and specificity over cholangiography alone, with or without biopsy. It also improves the diagnostic yield when performed in conjunction with EUS. Direct cholangioscopy with slim gastroscopes is also a single operator system and has improved visualization, but scope stabilization remains problematic, and traversing malignant strictures is difficult to impossible. Complications specific to the performance of cholangiopancreatoscopy include cholangitis, which is related to intraductal fluid irrigation, and, uncommonly, hemobilia and bile leaks attributable to intraductal lithotripsy. Improvements in the durability of current prototype video cholangioscopes and optics for disposable catheter systems are on the horizon.

REFERENCES

1. McIver MA. An instrument for visualizing the interior of the common duct at operation. Surgery 1941;9:112.

2. Kawai K, Nakajima M, Akasaka Y, et al. A new endoscopic method: the peroral choledocho-pancreatoscopy (author's transl). Leber Magen Darm 1976;6:121–4 [in German].

3. Vennes JA, Silvis SE. Endoscopic visualization of bile and pancreatic ducts. Gastrointest Endosc 1972;18:149–52.

4. Urakami Y, Seifert E, Butke H. Peroral direct cholangioscopy (PDCS) using routine straight-view endoscope: first report. Endoscopy 1977;9:27–30.

5. Soda K, Shitou K, Yoshida Y, et al. Peroral cholangioscopy using new fine-caliber flexible scope for detailed examination without papillotomy. Gastrointest Endosc 1996;43:233–8.

6. ASGE Technology Committee, Shah RJ, Adler DG, et al. Cholangiopancreatoscopy. Gastrointest Endosc 2008;68:411–21.

7. Chen YK, Pleskow DK. SpyGlass single-operator peroral cholangiopancreatoscopy system for the diagnosis and therapy of bile-duct disorders: a clinical feasibility study (with video). Gastrointest Endosc 2007;65:832–41.

8. Brauer BC, Chen YK, Shah RJ. Single-step direct cholangioscopy by Freehand Intubation using standard endoscopes for diagnosis and therapy of biliary diseases. Am J Gastroenterol 2012;107:1030–5.

9. Ponchon T, Chavaillon A, Ayela P, et al. Retrograde biliary ultrathin endoscopy enhances biopsy of stenoses and lithotripsy. Gastrointest Endosc 1989;35:292–7.

10. Piraka C, Shah RJ, Awadallah NS, et al. Transpapillary cholangioscopy-directed lithotripsy in patients with difficult bile duct stones. Clin Gastroenterol Hepatol 2007;5:1333–8.

11. Arya N, Nelles SE, Haber GB, et al. Electrohydraulic lithotripsy in 111 patients: a safe and effective therapy for difficult bile duct stones. Am J Gastroenterol 2004; 99:2330–4.

12. Shah RJ, Langer DA, Antillon MR, et al. Cholangioscopy and cholangioscopic forceps biopsy in patients with indeterminate pancreaticobiliary pathology. Clin Gastroenterol Hepatol 2006;4:219–25.

13. Azeem N, Gostout CJ, Knipschield M, et al. Cholangioscopy with narrow-band imaging in patients with primary sclerosing cholangitis undergoing ERCP. Gastrointest Endosc 2014;79(5):773–9.

14. Awadallah NS, Chen YK, Piraka C, et al. Is there a role for cholangioscopy in patients with primary sclerosing cholangitis? Am J Gastroenterol 2006;101:284–91.

15. Fukuda Y, Tsuyuguchi T, Sakai Y, et al. Diagnostic utility of peroral cholangioscopy for various bile-duct lesions. Gastrointest Endosc 2005;62:374–82.

16. Nguyen NQ, Binmoeller KF, Shah JN. Cholangioscopy and pancreatoscopy (with videos). Gastrointest Endosc 2009;70:1200–10.

17. Jung M, Zipf A, Schoonbroodt D, et al. Is pancreatoscopy of any benefit in clarifying the diagnosis of pancreatic duct lesions? Endoscopy 1998;30:273–80.

18. Iqbal S, Stevens PD. Cholangiopancreatoscopy for targeted biopsies of the bile and pancreatic ducts. Gastrointest Endosc Clin N Am 2009;19:567–77.

19. Shah RJ, Chen YK. Transpapillary and percutaneous choledochoscopy in the evaluation and management of biliary strictures and stones. Tech Gastrointest Endosc 2007;9:161–8.

20. Sethi A, Chen YK, Austin GL, et al. ERCP with cholangiopancreatoscopy may be associated with higher rates of complications than ERCP alone: a single-center experience. Gastrointest Endosc 2011;73:251–6.

21. Hammerle CW, Haider S, Chung M, et al. Endoscopic retrograde cholangiopancreatography complications in the era of cholangioscopy: is there an increased risk? Dig Liver Dis 2012;44(9):754–8.

22. Faigel DO, Eisen GM, Baron TH, et al. Preparation of patients for GI endoscopy. Gastrointest Endosc 2003;57:446–50.
23. American Society of Anesthesiologists Committee. Practice guidelines for pre-operative fasting and the use of pharmacologic agents to reduce the risk of pulmonary aspiration: application to healthy patients undergoing elective procedures: an updated report by the American Society of Anesthesiologists Committee on Standards and Practice Parameters. Anesthesiology 2011;114: 495–511.
24. Anderson MA, Ben-Menachem T, Gan IS, et al. Management of antithrombotic agents for endoscopic procedures. Gastrointest Endosc 2009;70:1062–70.
25. Banerjee S, Shen B, Baron TH, et al. Antibiotic prophylaxis in GI endoscopy. Gastrointest Endosc 2008;67:791–8.
26. Larghi A, Waxman I. Endoscopic direct cholangioscopy by using an ultra-slim upper endoscope: a feasibility study. Gastrointest Endosc 2006;63:853–7.
27. Choi HJ, Moon JH, Ko BM. Overtube-balloon–assisted direct peroral cholangioscopy by using an ultra-slim upper endoscope (with videos). Gastrointest Endosc 2009;69:935–40.
28. Moon JH, Ko BM, Choi HJ, et al. Intraductal balloon-guided direct peroral cholangioscopy with an ultraslim upper endoscope (with videos). Gastrointest Endosc 2009;70:297–302.
29. Albert JG, Friedrich-Rust M, Elhendawy M, et al. Peroral cholangioscopy for diagnosis and therapy of biliary tract disease using an ultra-slim gastroscope. Endoscopy 2011;43:1004–9.
30. Bonnot B, Nion-Larmurier I, Desaint B, et al. Fatal gas embolism after endoscopic transgastric necrosectomy for infected necrotizing pancreatitis. Am J Gastroenterol 2014;109:607–8.
31. Sievert CE Jr, Silvis SE. Evaluation of electrohydraulic lithotripsy as a means of gallstone fragmentation in a canine model. Gastrointest Endosc 1987;33:233–5.
32. Hochberger J, Gruber E, Wirtz P, et al. Lithotripsy of gallstones by means of a quality-switched giant-pulse neodymium:yttrium-aluminum-garnet laser. Basic in vitro studies using a highly flexible fiber system. Gastroenterology 1991; 101:1391–8.
33. Farrell JJ, Bounds BC, Al-Shalabi S, et al. Single-operator duodenoscope-assisted cholangioscopy is an effective alternative in the management of choledocholithiasis not removed by conventional methods, including mechanical lithotripsy. Endoscopy 2005;37:542–7.
34. Camilo J, Nordstrom E, Brown NG, et al. Per oral cholangioscopy (POC) with intraductal lithotripsy, mechanical lithotripsy (ML), and large balloon papillary dilation (LBPD) for extraction of complex biliary stones: a 12-year single academic center experience in 222 patients. Gastrointest Endosc 2013;77:AB313.
35. Maydeo A, Kwek BE, Bhandari S, et al. Single-operator cholangioscopy-guided laser lithotripsy in patients with difficult biliary and pancreatic ductal stones (with videos). Gastrointest Endosc 2011;74(6):1308–14.
36. Adamek HE, Maier M, Jakobs R, et al. Management of retained bile duct stones: a prospective open trial comparing extracorporeal and intracorporeal lithotripsy. Gastrointest Endosc 1996;44:40–7.
37. Neuhaus H, Zillinger C, Born P, et al. Randomized study of intracorporeal laser lithotripsy versus extracorporeal shock-wave lithotripsy for difficult bile duct stones. Gastrointest Endosc 1998;47:327–34.
38. Okugawa T, Tsuyuguchi T, Sudhamshu KC, et al. Peroral cholangioscopic treatment of hepatolithiasis: long-term results. Gastrointest Endosc 2002;56:366–71.

39. Lee SK, Seo DW, Myung SJ, et al. Percutaneous transhepatic cholangioscopic treatment for hepatolithiasis: an evaluation of long-term results and risk factors for recurrence. Gastrointest Endosc 2001;53:318–23.

40. Lee YN, Moon JH, Choi HJ, et al. Direct peroral cholangioscopy using an ultra-slim upper endoscope for management of residual stones after mechanical lithotripsy for retained common bile duct stones. Endoscopy 2012;44:819–24.

41. Howell DA, Parsons WG, Jones MA, et al. Complete tissue sampling of biliary strictures at ERCP using a new device. Gastrointest Endosc 1996;43:498–502.

42. De Bellis M, Sherman S, Fogel EL, et al. Tissue sampling at ERCP in suspected malignant biliary strictures (Part 1). Gastrointest Endosc 2002;56:552–60.

43. Hartman DJ, Slivka A, Giusto DA, et al. Tissue yield and diagnostic efficacy of fluoroscopic and cholangioscopic techniques to assess indeterminate biliary strictures. Clin Gastroenterol Hepatol 2012;10:1042–6.

44. Kurzawinski TR, Deery A, Dooley JS, et al. A prospective study of biliary cytology in 100 patients with bile duct strictures. Hepatology 1993;18:1399–403.

45. Schöfl R. Diagnostic endoscopic retrograde cholangiopancreatography. Endoscopy 2001;33:147–57.

46. Trent V, Khurana KK, Pisharodi LR. Diagnostic accuracy and clinical utility of endoscopic bile duct brushing in the evaluation of biliary strictures. Arch Pathol Lab Med 1999;123:712–5.

47. Lee JG, Leung JW, Baillie J, et al. Benign, dysplastic, or malignant–making sense of endoscopic bile duct brush cytology: results in 149 consecutive patients. Am J Gastroenterol 1995;90:722–6.

48. Logrono R, Kurtycz DF, Molina CP, et al. Analysis of false-negative diagnoses on endoscopic brush cytology of biliary and pancreatic duct strictures: the experience at 2 university hospitals. Arch Pathol Lab Med 2000;124:387–92.

49. Rumalla A, Baron TH, Leontovich O, et al. Improved diagnostic yield of endoscopic biliary brush cytology by digital image analysis. Mayo Clin Proc 2001;76:29–33.

50. Pugliese V, Antonelli G, Vincenti M, et al. Endoductal tissue sampling of biliary strictures through endoscopic retrograde cholangiopancreatography (ERCP). Tumori 1997;83:698–702.

51. Schoefl R, Haefner M, Wrba F, et al. Forceps biopsy and brush cytology during endoscopic retrograde cholangiopancreatography for the diagnosis of biliary stenoses. Scand J Gastroenterol 1997;32:363–8.

52. Parasher VK, Huibregtse K. Endoscopic retrograde wire-guided cytology of malignant biliary strictures using a novel scraping brush. Gastrointest Endosc 1998;48:288–90.

53. Fogel EL, Sherman S. How to improve the accuracy of diagnosis of malignant biliary strictures. Endoscopy 1999;31:758–60.

54. Foutch PG. Diagnosis of cancer by cytologic methods performed during ERCP. Gastrointest Endosc 1994;40:249–52.

55. Howell DA, Beveridge RP, Bosco J, et al. Endoscopic needle aspiration biopsy at ERCP in the diagnosis of biliary strictures. Gastrointest Endosc 1992;38:531–5.

56. Mohandas KM, Swaroop VS, Gullar SU, et al. Diagnosis of malignant obstructive jaundice by bile cytology: results improved by dilating the bile duct strictures. Gastrointest Endosc 1994;40:150–4.

57. Ponsioen CY, Vrouenraets SM, van Milligen de Wit AW, et al. Value of brush cytology for dominant strictures in primary sclerosing cholangitis. Endoscopy 1999;31:305–9.

58. Stewart CJ, Burke GM. Value of p53 immunostaining in pancreatico-biliary brush cytology specimens. Diagn Cytopathol 2000;23:308–13.
59. Ryan ME, Baldauf MC. Comparison of flow cytometry for DNA content and brush cytology for detection of malignancy in pancreaticobiliary strictures. Gastrointest Endosc 1994;40:133–9.
60. Tamada K, Sugano K. Diagnosis and non-surgical treatment of bile duct carcinoma: developments in the past decade. J Gastroenterol 2000;35:319–25.
61. Rumalla A, Petersen BT. Diagnosis and therapy of biliary tract malignancy. Semin Gastrointest Dis 2000;11:168–73.
62. Bain VG, Abraham N, Jhangri GS, et al. Prospective study of biliary strictures to determine the predictors of malignancy. Can J Gastroenterol 2000;14:397–402.
63. Pugliese V, Conio M, Nicolò G, et al. Endoscopic retrograde forceps biopsy and brush cytology of biliary strictures: a prospective study. Gastrointest Endosc 1995;42:520–6.
64. Sugiyama M, Atomi Y, Wada N, et al. Endoscopic transpapillary bile duct biopsy without sphincterotomy for diagnosing biliary strictures: a prospective comparative study with bile and brush cytology. Am J Gastroenterol 1996;91:465–7.
65. Seo DW, Lee SK, Yoo KS, et al. Cholangioscopic findings in bile duct tumors. Gastrointest Endosc 2000;52:630–4.
66. Kim HJ, Kim MH, Lee SK, et al. Tumor vessel: a valuable cholangioscopic clue of malignant biliary stricture. Gastrointest Endosc 2000;52:635–8.
67. Ramchandani M, Reddy DN, Gupta R, et al. Role of single-operator peroral cholangioscopy in the diagnosis of indeterminate biliary lesions: a single-center, prospective study. Gastrointest Endosc 2011;74:511–9.
68. Siddiqui AA, Mehendiratta V, Jackson W, et al. Identification of cholangiocarcinoma by using the Spyglass Spyscope system for peroral cholangioscopy and biopsy collection. Clin Gastroenterol Hepatol 2012;10:466–71.
69. Osanai M, Itoi T, Igarashi Y, et al. Peroral video cholangioscopy to evaluate indeterminate bile duct lesions and preoperative mucosal cancerous extension: a prospective multicenter study. Endoscopy 2013;45:635–42.
70. Manta R, Frazzoni M, Conigliaro R, et al. SpyGlass single-operator peroral cholangioscopy in the evaluation of indeterminate biliary lesions: a single-center, prospective, cohort study. Surg Endosc 2013;27(5):1569–72.
71. Draganov PV, Chauhan S, Wagh MS, et al. Diagnostic accuracy of conventional and cholangioscopy-guided sampling of indeterminate biliary lesions at the time of ERCP: a prospective, long-term follow-up study. Gastrointest Endosc 2012;75:347–53.
72. Chen YK, Parsi MA, Binmoeller KF, et al. Single-operator cholangioscopy in patients requiring evaluation of bile duct disease or therapy of biliary stones (with videos). Gastrointest Endosc 2011;74:805–14.
73. Itoi T, Sofuni A, Itokawa F, et al. Peroral cholangioscopic diagnosis of biliary-tract diseases by using narrow-band imaging (with videos). Gastrointest Endosc 2007;66:730–6.
74. Shah RJ, Chen YK. Video cholangiopancreatoscopy with narrow band imaging (NBI): spectrum of mucosal and vascular patterns in patients with pancreaticobiliary pathology. Gastrointest Endosc 2009;69:AB117.
75. Khan AH, Austin GL, Fukami N, et al. Cholangiopancreatoscopy and endoscopic ultrasound for indeterminate pancreaticobiliary pathology. Dig Dis Sci 2013;58:1110–5.

76. Nguyen NQ, Schoeman MN, Ruszkiewicz A. Clinical utility of EUS before chol-angioscopy in the evaluation of difficult biliary strictures. Gastrointest Endosc 2013;78:868–74.

77. Tischendorf JJ, Krüger M, Trautwein C, et al. Cholangioscopic characterization of dominant bile duct stenoses in patients with primary sclerosing cholangitis. Endoscopy 2006;38:665–9.

78. Asbun HJ, Conlon K, Fernandez-Cruz L, et al. When to perform a pancrea-toduodenectomy in the absence of positive histology? A consensus state-ment by the International Study Group of Pancreatic Surgery. Surgery 2014;155(5):887–92.

79. Kuo CM, Chiu YC, Changchien CS, et al. Endoscopic papillary balloon dilation for removal of bile duct stones: evaluation of outcomes and complications in 298 patients. J Clin Gastroenterol 2012;46(10):860–4.

Molecular Adsorbent Recirculating System and Bioartificial Devices for Liver Failure

Rafael Bañares, MD, PhD[a,b,c], María-Vega Catalina, MD[a,b], Javier Vaquero, MD, PhD[a,b,*]

KEYWORDS

- Albumin dialysis • Acute liver failure • Acute-on-chronic liver failure
- Extracorporeal liver assist device • Hepatic encephalopathy

KEY POINTS

- Substitution of the detoxification, synthetic, and regulatory functions of the failing liver is the rationale for the use of extracorporeal liver support systems in patients with liver failure.
- In contrast to artificial liver support systems, bioartificial systems incorporate a module containing living cells/hepatocytes to provide synthetic functions.
- Artificial and bioartificial liver support devices have shown certain detoxification capabilities and improvement of intermediate endpoints in patients with liver failure, but their effects on survival remain inconclusive.
- Identification of target populations and adequate endpoints, optimization of therapy delivery, and improvement of current prototypes seem essential steps for extracorporeal liver support devices to achieve their long-desired goals.

INTRODUCTION: WHY ARE LIVER SUPPORT DEVICES NECESSARY?

Liver failure may occur in a person without preexisting liver disease (acute liver failure [ALF]) or in a patient with chronic liver disease that suffers an acute decompensation (acute-on-chronic liver failure [ACLF]). In both cases, the sudden impairment of liver

Disclosures: Dr Rafael Bañares has served as advisor and has received an unrestricted grant from Gambro.

[a] Gastroenterology and Hepatology Department, Hospital General Universitario Gregorio Marañón, IiSGM, Madrid, Spain; [b] Centro de investigación en red de enfermedades hepáticas y digestivas (CIBEREHD), Barcelona, Spain; [c] School of Medicine, Universidad Complutense de Madrid (UCM), Madrid, Spain

* Corresponding author. Laboratorio de investigación en Hepatología y Gastroenterología del Hospital General Universitario Gregorio Marañón – IiSGM – CIBERehd, c/ Maiquez 9, Madrid 28009, Spain.

E-mail address: javier.vaquero@iisgm.com

Clin Liver Dis 18 (2014) 945–956
http://dx.doi.org/10.1016/j.cld.2014.07.011
1089-3261/14/$ – see front matter © 2014 Elsevier Inc. All rights reserved.

function leads to characteristic clinical manifestations such as hepatic encephalopathy, jaundice, coagulation disturbances, increased susceptibility to infections, hemodynamic instability, hepatorenal syndrome, and eventually multiorgan failure. Despite recent improvements in its clinical management, the morbidity and mortality of liver failure remains unacceptably high.[1,2] Liver transplantation remains the only therapy with a well-proven beneficial effect on survival,[3] but this procedure is not applicable to all patients because of the shortage of donor organs and the frequent presence of contraindications. In this scenario, the development of extracorporeal liver support devices would be important for maintaining the patient's condition until the spontaneous recovery of liver function occurs or until a donor organ becomes available.

The aim of this review is to summarize the current state of liver support devices in the clinical management of liver failure.

TECHNICAL CHARACTERISTICS OF EXTRACORPOREAL LIVER SUPPORT SYSTEMS

A full description of the types and characteristics of liver support systems is out of the scope of this review, but an understanding of some technical aspects is important.

The extracorporeal liver support systems that have been tested clinically belong to one of the following 2 categories:

1. Artificial Liver Support (ALS) systems, also known as nonbiological or cell-free techniques. The ALS systems are based on the principles of adsorption and filtration and are aimed at removing circulating toxins by using a variety of membranes and adsorbents.
2. Bioartificial Liver Support systems are hybrid devices that incorporate liver cells/hepatocytes to improve the detoxification capacity and to support the failing synthetic liver function.[4]

Overall, most liver support systems combine diverse therapeutic units, ranging from conventional hemodialysis or hemofiltration modules, to specific adsorption systems. In the case of bioartificial systems, the extracorporeal circuit includes bioreactors loaded with liver cells.[5] A summary of devices is provided in **Table 1** and a comparison of pros and cons is provided in **Fig. 1**.

RATIONALE FOR THE USE OF LIVER SUPPORT SYSTEMS IN LIVER FAILURE

From a theoretic perspective, an effective extracorporeal liver support system should replace 3 major functions of the liver: detoxification, biosynthesis, and regulation. In liver failure, the main goals would be to remove putative toxins preventing further aggravation of liver failure, to stimulate liver regeneration, and to improve the pathophysiologic features of liver failure.[6,7] None of the devices currently available, however, fulfill these requirements completely.

Elimination of Toxins

The deterioration of liver function leads to the accumulation of toxic substances such as bilirubin, bile acids, ammonia, protein breakdown products (aromatic amino acids, phenol, mercaptans), lactate, glutamine, mediators of oxidative stress, free fatty acids, endogenous benzodiazepines, inflammatory cytokines, and others. Many of these toxins play key roles in the pathogenesis of liver failure and result in a toxic state that alters the functional capacities of serum albumin,[8] increases the susceptibility to infections, and induces circulatory disturbances and end-organ dysfunction.[9] Secondary liver damage occurs as a consequence of the vicious circle that results from the release of inflammatory mediators, oxidative stress, and sinusoidal endothelial cell damage.

Table 1
Summary of the main artificial and bioartificial liver support devices

Type of Device	Main Mechanism of Action
ALS based on Conventional Extracorporeal Procedures	
Hemodialysis	Exchange diffusion across a semipermeable membrane
Hemofiltration	Continuous convective solute removal across a semipermeable membrane
Hemodiafiltration	Convection (large molecules) and diffusion (small molecules) removal across a semipermeable membrane
Plasmapheresis and high-volume plasmapheresis/plasma exchange with or without hemodiafiltration	Exchange of variable amount of plasma volumes combined or not with hemodiafiltration
Hemodiabsorption	Dialysis against a combination of charcoal and ion exchanger
ALS using albumin dialysis	
MARS	Removal of protein-bound and water-soluble substances across a specialized membrane against albumin-enriched dialysate that recirculates in an intermediate circuit
Single Pass Albumin dialysis (SPAD)	Removal of protein-bound and water-soluble substances across a membrane against albumin enriched dialysate
Fractionated plasma separation and adsorption FPSA (Prometheus)	Hemodiafiltration using albumin dialysate
Bioartificial liver support systems	
ELAD	Large aggregates of C3a Hepatoma line cells. No additional detox devices
HepatAssist	Irregular aggregates of porcine, cryopreserved cells. Charcoal column previous to bioreactor
Bioartificial liver support system	Collagen entrapped porcine, freshly isolated cells. No additional detox devices
TECA Hybrid Artificial Liver Support System	Porcine, freshly isolated cells Charcoal column previous to bioreactor

The assumption that decreasing the load of these toxins may reverse the progression of liver dysfunction and improve the capacity for liver regeneration provides a major rationale for developing liver support systems.[10,11]

Several studies have found that the Molecular Adsorbent Recirculating System (MARS) and Prometheus devices remove significant amounts of toxins in patients with ALF and ACLF,[12,13] but this does not seem to result in improvements of the functional capacities of the patients' albumin.[8]

Improvement of Portal and Systemic Hemodynamics

Hemodynamic instability, characterized by reduced systemic vascular resistance and mean arterial pressure, is common in patients with liver failure irrespective of the etiology, and it plays a major role in the development of multiorgan dysfunction. An increase

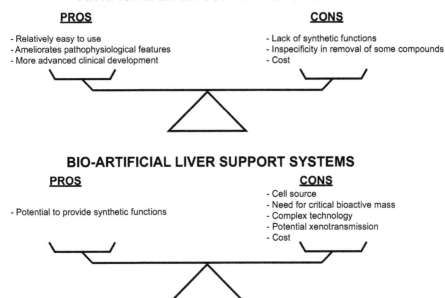

Fig. 1. Main advantages and disadvantages of artificial and bioartificial liver support systems.

in portal pressure[14] and the presence of endothelial dysfunction[15] may further compromise the splanchnic circulation. Importantly, extracorporeal liver support systems were consistently found to remove vasoactive substances and to improve systemic (increase in mean arterial pressure) and splanchnic (decrease in portal pressure) hemodynamics in several clinical studies.[11,16–18]

Improvement of Liver Regeneration

Improving the capacity of the liver to regenerate during liver failure may allow spontaneous recovery from ALF or ACLF[11]; therefore, the final outcome of these patients may be improved. Alternatively, the aim of liver support systems would be to support the patient's condition until a suitable organ is available for transplantation[10] in those cases in which the regeneration capacity of the liver is null.

CLINICAL EFFICACY

Despite the difficulties in performing well-designed clinical trials in these complex medical conditions, many studies have evaluated the use of liver support systems in ALF and in ACLF (**Table 2**).

Bioartificial Liver Support Systems in ALF

Most studies that have assessed the applicability and efficacy of bioartificial support systems in ALF have included a small number of patients.

The extracorporeal liver assist device (ELAD), which incorporates cells derived from human hepatoblastoma, has been tested in 2 small studies.[19,20] In a pilot-controlled trial,[19] 24 patients were stratified by the absence (group I, n = 17 patients; expected mortality, 50%) or presence (group II, n = 7 patients; expected mortality, 90%) of liver transplantation criteria. As positive outcomes, arterial ammonia decreased marginally, and worsening of encephalopathy was less frequent in patients treated with ELAD, whereas the increase in serum bilirubin was more pronounced in the controls. However, these effects were not translated into an improved survival (78% vs 75% in group I and 33% vs 25% in group II).

In the second study, Millis and colleagues[20] reported a phase I trial with a modified ELAD system, in which the device used patient's ultrafiltrate instead of whole blood, and oxygen and glucose consumption were frequently monitored to ensure metabolic activity of the cells in the cartridges. Five ALF patients were treated with the ELAD, which was well tolerated. The patients' clinical courses appeared to stabilize while connected to the ELAD, and all of them were successfully bridged to liver transplantation. Four of the 5 patients survived to the 30-day endpoint of the study. No biomechanical problems were observed.

Another bioartificial device that incorporates porcine-purified hepatocytes (HepatAssist) has been evaluated in a large-scale, randomized, multicenter clinical trial.[21] This study included 171 patients with ALF or with primary nonfunction after liver transplantation that were randomly assigned to receive standard medical treatment (SMT) or SMT plus support with the HepatAssist system. The endpoint of the study was survival, which was assessed as a crude indicator (30-day survival with or without liver transplantation) or adjusted by confounding factors in a multivariate model. The number of HepatAssist treatments ranged from 1 to 9 (mean, 2.9) per patient. Overall, 30-day survival was similar in both arms (71% in the HepatAssist group and 62% in the SMT group). Even though the trial was prematurely stopped because of futility in the predetermined safety interim analysis, the multivariate model that adjusted for the impact of liver transplantation and for the etiology of the disease suggested that HepatAssist therapy was associated with a 44% reduction in the risk of death in patients with ALF (excluding patients with primary nonfunction).

Artificial Liver Support Systems in ALF

Several experimental and nonrandomized studies using MARS in ALF have shown reduction in bilirubin levels, improvement in encephalopathy and cerebral edema,[22,23] and amelioration of systemic hemodynamics and renal function.[24–26] Furthermore, a study suggests that the use of MARS in patients with ALF awaiting emergency liver transplantation could prompt the spontaneous recovery of liver function, ultimately avoiding the necessity of liver transplantation.[27]

The most robust evidence in this field, however, is a recently published randomized, controlled trial performed in 16 French liver transplantation centers (FULMAR study).[28] This study compared the impact of MARS plus SMT versus SMT alone in patients with ALF fulfilling criteria for liver transplantation. Fifty-three patients received MARS treatment, whereas 49 had SMT. A nonstatistically significant trend for improved 6-month survival (84.9% vs 75.5%) was observed in the MARS group, a trend that was stronger among patients with paracetamol-induced ALF (85% vs 68.4%). However, a major confounder was that the median listing-to-transplant time was only 16.2 hours, and 75% of enrolled patients underwent transplant within 24 hours.

Artificial Liver Support Systems in ACLF

The impact of artificial devices in patients with ACLF has been explored in several randomized trials[29–33] (aimed to evaluate different aspects of ACLF) and in meta-analyses,[34,35] and most of them have involved the MARS system.

Table 2
Summary of major randomized, controlled clinical trials of artificial and bioartificial liver support systems in ALF and ACLF

ALS Device	n	Study Population	Design of the Trial	Clinical Results	Study
Liver dialysis	56	ACLF ALF	Liver dialysis vs SMT	Improved neurologic status and hemodynamic profile. Increased bleeding in patients with DIC.	Ash[41]
MARS	70	HE grade 3 or 4	MARS + SMT vs SMT	More frequent and earlier improvement of HE.	Hassanein et al[30]
	18	ACLF in severe AAH (9 MARS, 9 control)	MARS + SMT vs SMT	Improvement of HE. No hemodynamic changes. No changes in plasma cytokines and ammonia levels.	Sen et al[13]
	27	Hypoxic liver failure after cardiogenic shock (bil >8 mg/dL)	MARS vs SMT	Improved survival. Further appropriately sized studies are needed.	El Banayosy et al[42]
	18	ACLF in severe AAH	MARS + SMT vs Prometheus + SMT or SMT alone (3 d)	Reduction in bilirubin levels (larger in Prometheus). Hemodynamic improvement (larger in MARS patients).	Laleman et al[43]
	24	Decompensated cirrhosis Bil >20 mg/dL unresponsive to SMT	MARS + SMT vs SMT Up to 10 sessions	Improved 30-d survival. Decrease in bilirubin. Improvement in renal failure and HE.	Heemann et al[31]
	189	ACLF Bil> 20 mg/dL and/or HE greater than grade II and/or HRS	MARS + SMT vs SMT Up to 10 sessions (6–8 h)	No changes in survival. Improvement in HE. Improvement in HRS. No differences in overall adverse events.	Banares et al[29]
	102	ALF	MARS + SMT (53) vs SMT (49) 8-h session	Six-month survival rate (84.9% vs 75.5%; not significant)	Saliba et al[28]

Device	N	Patient population	Study design	Results	Reference
Prometheus	24	Decompensated cirrhosis	One single 6-h session with Prometheus, MARS, or hemodialysis	No hemodynamic effects. No adverse events. Decrease in platelet count. Reduction in bilirubin levels (larger in Prometheus). Hemodynamic improvement (larger in MARS patients).	Dethloff et al[44]
	18	ACLF in severe AAH	MARS + SMT vs Prometheus + SMT or SMT alone (3 d)		Laleman et al[43]
	145	ACLF	Prometheus + SMT vs SMT Up to 8–11 sessions	No changes in overall survival. Survival benefit in posthoc analysis in type I HRS and MELD score>30.	Kribben et al[32]
Hepat-Assist	171	FHF or SFHF and primary nonfunction after liver transplantation	Hepat-Assist (6 h daily) + SMT vs SMT	Nonsignificant improvement in 30-d survival (71% vs 62%). Posthoc multivariate analysis excluding primary nonfunction. Adjusted hazard ratio, 0.58; $P = .048$.	Demetriou et al[21]
ELAD	24	ALF with potential recoverable lesion or fulfilment of criteria for liver transplantation	ELAD (median period of 72 h) vs SMT	Good biocompatibility. Survival similar to SMT. DIC or hypersensitivity reaction.	Ellis et al[19]

Abbreviations: AAH, acute alcoholic hepatitis; Bil, bilirubin; DIC, disseminated intravascular coagulation; FHF, fulminant hepatic failure; HE, hepatic encephalopathy; SFHF, subfulminant hepatic failure.

The first study evaluated the effect of albumin dialysis in patients with type I hepatorenal syndrome.[33] In this small study, 13 patients were randomly selected to receive either MARS (n = 8) or hemodiafiltration (n = 5). Patients allocated to MARS presented significant decreases in serum bilirubin and creatinine compared with patients allocated to hemodiafiltration. In addition, 7-day survival was significantly better in MARS-treated patients (27.5% vs 0%). Although the results of the study were promising, its small size and the absence of the currently established medical therapy with vasoconstrictors and volume expansion precluded a conclusive evaluation of the efficacy of MARS in this context. In a more recent noncontrolled pilot study performed in patients with hepatorenal syndrome unresponsive to vasoconstrictors, MARS therapy was associated with decreases in nitric oxide plasma concentration and serum creatinine, but without concomitant improvements in glomerular filtration rate.[36]

A second study was performed in 24 patients with ACLF that were randomly allocated to receive MARS or SMT.[31] The primary endpoint was to obtain a 3-day stable reduction of serum bilirubin less than 15 mg/dL. MARS therapy was significantly associated not only with a decrease in serum bilirubin level but also to lower mortality. These results, however, should be cautiously interpreted, because the trial was not designed to detect differences in mortality, and the inclusion criteria were poorly defined.

A third controlled trial evaluated the effects of MARS in patients with cirrhosis and advanced encephalopathy.[30] Albumin dialysis significantly improved the probability of recovery from hepatic encephalopathy compared with SMT, which included conventional hemofiltration when indicated (58% vs 37% at 72 hours; $P = .045$). Interestingly, the survival rate of patients who recovered from encephalopathy was higher than that of patients without improvement of hepatic coma in both treatment arms, indicating the strong influence of hepatic encephalopathy in survival. Even though the methodology for assessing encephalopathy and the lack of effect of MARS therapy on survival have been criticized,[37] it is important to remark that the trial was neither designed nor powered to detect differences in survival.

Despite these encouraging results, 2 large randomized trials of liver support devices in patients with ACLF failed to show a significant impact on survival. One study evaluated the impact of fractionated plasma separation and adsorption (FPSA; the Prometheus device) on the survival of patients with ACLF.[32] In this trial, 145 patients were randomly assigned to receive FPSA plus SMT versus SMT alone. Primary endpoints of the study were the probability of survival at days 28 and 90, irrespective of liver transplantation. Both groups were similar at the baseline. Serum bilirubin level decreased significantly in patients randomly assigned to receive FPSA compared with the group receiving SMT alone. In an intention-to-treat analysis, the probability of 28-day survival was 66% in the FPSA group and 63% in the SMT group ($P = .70$), and the probability of 90-day survival was 47% and 38%, respectively ($P = .35$). Baseline factors independently associated with poor prognosis were a high Sequential Organ Failure Assessment (SOFA) score, bleeding, female sex, spontaneous bacterial peritonitis, intermediate increases in serum creatinine concentration, and the combination of alcoholic and viral etiologies of liver disease. Finally a survival benefit was shown in a predetermined posthoc analysis performed in patients with type I hepatorenal syndrome (HRS) and Model for End-Stage Liver Disease (MELD) score greater than 30 at admission.

The results of the largest randomized trial of the use of artificial liver support systems in patients with ACLF (RELIEF study) have been recently reported.[29] In this study, 189 patients with ACLF from 19 European centers were randomly assigned to receive either MARS plus SMT (n = 95) or SMT alone (n = 94). The main endpoint of the study was 28-day survival. Patients randomly assigned to the MARS arm received up to ten

6- to 8-hour sessions of MARS. Importantly, the first 4 sessions were performed in the first 4 days after randomization. Remarkably, the mean number of MARS sessions was 6.5, and the median time under MARS therapy was just 42 hours, 6.3% of the 28-day study period. Even though both groups were similar at baseline, the proportion of patients with MELD scores greater than 20 points and with spontaneous bacterial peritonitis as the precipitating event was almost significantly higher in the MARS group. At day 4, a greater decrease in serum creatinine level ($P = .02$) and bilirubin level ($P = .001$) was observed in patients treated with MARS. Improvement of hepatic encephalopathy was also more frequent in the MARS arm (from grade II–IV to grade 0–I; 62.5% vs 38.2%; $P = .07$). These beneficial effects on intermediate variables, however, were not translated into an improvement of 28-day survival, which was similar in the 2 groups in intention-to-treat and in per-protocol population (60. 7% vs 58.9%; 60% vs 59.2%, respectively). After adjusting for confounders, a significant beneficial effect of MARS on survival was not observed either (overall risk, 0.87; 95% confidence interval [CI], 0.44–1.72). MELD score and hepatic encephalopathy at admission and the increase in serum bilirubin level at day 4 were independent predictors of mortality. Remarkably, severe adverse events were similar in both groups, a fact that has been observed across the different studies.

COMPARATIVE ANALYSIS OF ARTIFICIAL AND BIOARTIFICIAL LIVER SUPPORT SYSTEMS IN CLINICAL STUDIES

Several systematic reviews and meta-analyses have been published in recent years with heterogeneous results. Kjaergard and colleagues[38] reviewed the experience with artificial and bioartificial liver support systems for both ALF and ACLF from 12 randomized trials (483 patients). Compared with SMT, liver support systems had a significant beneficial effect on hepatic encephalopathy (risk ratio [RR], 0.67; 95% CI, 0.52–0.86), but they had no significant effects on mortality (RR, 0.86; 95% CI, 0.65–1.12) or bridging to liver transplantation (RR, 0.87; 95% CI, 0.73–1.05). Meta-regression analysis indicated that the effect of liver support systems depended on the type of liver failure ($P = .03$). In subgroup analyses, artificial liver support systems seemed to reduce mortality by 33% in ACLF (RR, 0.67; 95% CI, 0.51–0.90) but not in ALF (RR, 0.95; 95% CI, 0.71–1.29). In contrast, the meta-analysis by Stutchfield and colleagues[35] concluded that extracorporeal liver support devices (both artificial and bioartificial) significantly improved survival in ALF (RR, 0.70; $P = .05$) but not in ACLF (RR, 0.87; $P = .37$). Finally, the most recent meta-analysis,[34] which included studies from 1973 to 2012, found a decrease in mortality in patients with ACLF treated with artificial liver support systems (RR, 0.80; 95% CI, 0.66–0.96, $P = .018$) and in patients with ALF treated with bioartificial liver support systems (RR, 0.69; 95% CI, 0.50–0.94; $P = .018$).

These comparative meta-analyses present important limitations, as the observational nature of all meta-analyses expose them to multiple bias or confounders. Furthermore, the heterogeneity of the trials included follow-up periods of variable durations and diverse patient populations regarding the severity and etiology of the liver failure, therefore, precluding definitive conclusions.

REQUIREMENTS OF AN IDEAL LIVER SUPPORT SYSTEM/FUTURE CONSIDERATIONS

Although important advances in liver support systems have been reached in the last decade, it is obvious that current devices are far from ideal. An appropriate liver support system should be clinically effective, provide metabolic and synthetic liver function, and influence the pathophysiologic alterations of liver failure. Importantly, this ideal system should also provide support for end-organ dysfunction. In addition, it should be safe, cost effective, and relatively easy to use. Even if such ideal systems were available, it is important to emphasize the difficulty of performing large well-designed clinical trials in the setting of liver failure to conclusively show their value.

Several issues should be addressed to reach this complex aim. First, it is important to improve current liver support devices. In the case of bioartificial devices, new approaches need to be directed toward identifying functional cell sources (human hepatocytes from stem cells, immortalized human hepatocytes, genetically engineered liver cell lines, humanized pig cells, combination of cell sources). Such cell sources should be expandable in large quantities and should maintain their viability and provide liver functions to the failing liver for prolonged periods. Construction of unique bioreactors that resemble the 3-dimensional liver cell environment with optimum cell-cell interactions and easy scaling from microscopic to clinical size is also critical. The procurement of 3-dimensional, naturally derived scaffolds with an intact vascular tree[39] amenable of grafting with human cells represents a new appealing approach to this problem. The 3-dimensional printing technology combining the potential of engineering and biology to create living human tissues that mimic the shape and functions of native tissues is also promising.

In the case of artificial devices, the production of new prototypes with greater detoxification capacities could result in improved clinical efficacy.

A second important point that needs to be addressed is the optimization of therapy delivery. It is possible that the current limited schedules (in duration and intensity of therapy) are insufficient to provide adequate support.

Finally, it is important to carefully analyze the clinical applicability of liver support systems in terms of definition of target population and disease or condition to be treated. In addition, efficacy should be assessed by adequately defined clinically relevant variables (survival, bridging to liver transplantation), and not by its potential effects on pathophysiologic endpoints or surrogate markers. It is also especially important to consider the impact of liver transplantation in the design of future trials.[40]

REFERENCES

1. Wlodzimirow KA, Eslami S, Abu-Hanna A, et al. A systematic review on prognostic indicators of acute on chronic liver failure and their predictive value for mortality. Liver Int 2013;33:40–52.
2. Bernal W, Auzinger G, Dhawan A, et al. Acute liver failure. Lancet 2010;376: 190–201.
3. Jalan R, Gines P, Olson JC, et al. Acute-on chronic liver failure. J Hepatol 2012; 57:1336–48.
4. Allen JW, Hassanein T, Bhatia SN. Advances in bioartificial liver devices. Hepatology 2001;34:447–55.
5. Carpentier B, Gautier A, Legallais C. Artificial and bioartificial liver devices: present and future. Gut 2009;58:1690–702.
6. Nyberg SL. Bridging the gap: advances in artificial liver support. Liver Transpl 2012;18(Suppl 2):S10–14.
7. Sen S, Williams R. Liver substitution. In: Hakim NS, editor. Artificial Organs: New Techniques in Surgery Series. London: Springer-Verlag; 2009. p. 57–76.
8. Jalan R, Schnurr K, Mookerjee RP, et al. Alterations in the functional capacity of albumin in patients with decompensated cirrhosis is associated with increased mortality. Hepatology 2009;50:555–64.
9. Leckie P, Davenport A, Jalan R. Extracorporeal liver support. Blood Purif 2012;34: 158–63.

10. Tritto G, Davies NA, Jalan R. Liver replacement therapy. Semin Respir Crit Care Med 2012;33:70–9.

11. Nevens F, Laleman W. Artificial liver support devices as treatment option for liver failure. Best Pract Res Clin Gastroenterol 2012;26:17–26.

12. Kapoor D. Molecular adsorbent recirculating system: albumin dialysis-based extracorporeal liver assist device. J Gastroenterol Hepatol 2002;17(Suppl 3):S280–286.

13. Sen S, Davies NA, Mookerjee RP, et al. Pathophysiological effects of albumin dialysis in acute-on-chronic liver failure: a randomized controlled study. Liver Transpl 2004;10:1109–19.

14. Rincon D, Lo Iacono O, Ripoll C, et al. Prognostic value of hepatic venous pressure gradient for in-hospital mortality of patients with severe acute alcoholic hepatitis. Aliment Pharmacol Ther 2007;25:841–8.

15. Mookerjee RP, Malaki M, Davies NA, et al. Increasing dimethylarginine levels are associated with adverse clinical outcome in severe alcoholic hepatitis. Hepatology 2007;45:62–71.

16. Catalina MV, Barrio J, Anaya F, et al. Hepatic and systemic haemodynamic changes after MARS in patients with acute on chronic liver failure. Liver Int 2003;23(Suppl 3):39–43.

17. Lanjuan L, Qian Y, Jianrong H, et al. Severe hepatitis treated with an artificial liver support system. Int J Artif Organs 2001;24:297–303.

18. Sen S, Mookerjee RP, Cheshire LM, et al. Albumin dialysis reduces portal pressure acutely in patients with severe alcoholic hepatitis. J Hepatol 2005;43:142–8.

19. Ellis AJ, Hughes RD, Wendon JA, et al. Pilot-controlled trial of the extracorporeal liver assist device in acute liver failure. Hepatology 1996;24:1446–51.

20. Millis JM, Cronin DC, Johnson R, et al. Initial experience with the modified extracorporeal liver-assist device for patients with fulminant hepatic failure: system modifications and clinical impact. Transplantation 2002;74:1735–46.

21. Demetriou AA, Brown RS, Busuttil RW, et al. Prospective, randomized, multicenter, controlled trial of a bioartificial liver in treating acute liver failure. Ann Surg 2004;239:660–70.

22. Schmidt LE, Wang LP, Hansen BA, et al. Systemic hemodynamic effects of treatment with the molecular adsorbents recirculating system in patients with hyperacute liver failure: a prospective controlled trial. Liver Transpl 2003;9:290–7.

23. Sen S, Rose C, Ytrebo LM, et al. Effect of albumin dialysis on intracranial pressure increase in pigs with acute liver failure: a randomized study. Crit Care Med 2006;34:158–64.

24. Novelli G, Rossi M, Pretagostini R, et al. A 3-year experience with Molecular Adsorbent Recirculating System (MARS): our results on 63 patients with hepatic failure and color Doppler US evaluation of cerebral perfusion. Liver Int 2003;23(Suppl 3):10–5.

25. Novelli G, Rossi M, Pretagostini R, et al. MARS (Molecular Adsorbent Recirculating System): experience in 34 cases of acute liver failure. Liver 2002;22(Suppl 2):43–7.

26. Mitzner S, Loock J, Peszynski P, et al. Improvement in central nervous system functions during treatment of liver failure with albumin dialysis MARS–a review of clinical, biochemical, and electrophysiological data. Metab Brain Dis 2002;17:463–75.

27. Camus C, Lavoue S, Gacouin A, et al. Liver transplantation avoided in patients with fulminant hepatic failure who received albumin dialysis with the molecular adsorbent recirculating system while on the waiting list: impact of the duration of therapy. Ther Apher Dial 2009;13:549–55.

28. Saliba F, Camus C, Durand F, et al. Albumin dialysis with a noncell artificial liver support device in patients with acute liver failure: a randomized, controlled trial. Ann Intern Med 2013;159:522–31.

29. Banares R, Nevens F, Larsen FS, et al. Extracorporeal albumin dialysis with the molecular adsorbent recirculating system in acute-on-chronic liver failure: the RELIEF trial. Hepatology 2013;57:1153–62.

30. Hassanein TI, Tofteng F, Brown RS Jr, et al. Randomized controlled study of extracorporeal albumin dialysis for hepatic encephalopathy in advanced cirrhosis. Hepatology 2007;46:1853–62.

31. Heemann U, Treichel U, Loock J, et al. Albumin dialysis in cirrhosis with superimposed acute liver injury: a prospective, controlled study. Hepatology 2002;36: 949–58.

32. Kribben A, Gerken G, Haag S, et al. Effects of fractionated plasma separation and adsorption on survival in patients with acute-on-chronic liver failure. Gastroenterology 2012;142:782–9.e3.

33. Mitzner SR, Stange J, Klammt S, et al. Improvement of hepatorenal syndrome with extracorporeal albumin dialysis MARS: results of a prospective, randomized, controlled clinical trial. Liver Transpl 2000;6:277–86.

34. Zheng Z, Li X, Li Z, et al. Artificial and bioartificial liver support systems for acute and acute-on-chronic hepatic failure: a meta-analysis and meta-regression. Exp Ther Med 2013;6:929–36.

35. Stutchfield BM, Simpson K, Wigmore SJ. Systematic review and meta-analysis of survival following extracorporeal liver support. Br J Surg 2011;98:623–31.

36. Wong F, Raina N, Richardson R. Molecular adsorbent recirculating system is ineffective in the management of type 1 hepatorenal syndrome in patients with cirrhosis with ascites who have failed vasoconstrictor treatment. Gut 2010;59: 381–6.

37. Ferenci P, Kramer L. MARS and the failing liver-Any help from the outer space? Hepatology 2007;46:1682–4.

38. Kjaergard LL, Liu J, Als-Nielsen B, et al. Artificial and bioartificial support systems for acute and acute-on-chronic liver failure: a systematic review. JAMA 2003;289: 217–22.

39. Baptista PM, Siddiqui MM, Lozier G, et al. The use of whole organ decellularization for the generation of a vascularized liver organoid. Hepatology 2011;53: 604–17.

40. Kantola T, Koivusalo AM, Parmanen S, et al. Survival predictors in patients treated with a molecular adsorbent recirculating system. World J Gastroenterol 2009;15: 3015–24.

41. Ash SR. Hemodiabsorption in treatment of acute hepatic failure and chronic cirrhosis with ascites. Artif Organs 1994;18:355–62.

42. El Banayosy A, Kizner L, Schueler V, et al. First use of the molecular adsorbent recirculating system technique on patients with hypoxic liver failure after cardiogenic shock. ASAIO J 2004;50:332–7.

43. Laleman W, Wilmer A, Evenepoel P, et al. Effect of the molecular adsorbent recirculating system and Prometheus devices on systemic haemodynamics and vasoactive agents in patients with acute-on-chronic alcoholic liver failure. Crit Care 2006;10:R108.

44. Dethloff T, Tofteng F, Frederiksen HJ, et al. Effect of Prometheus liver assist system on systemic hemodynamics in patients with cirrhosis: a randomized controlled study. World J Gastroenterol 2008;14:2065–71.

Intensive Care Unit Management of Patients with Liver Failure

M. Shadab Siddiqui, MD, R. Todd Stravitz, MD*

KEYWORDS

- Cirrhosis • Hepatic encephalopathy • Sepsis • Portal hypertension
- Acute liver failure

KEY POINTS

- Patients with acute liver failure (ALF) have no underlying liver disease and have high mortality without liver transplantation, usually attributable to multiorgan system failure.
- Etiology-specific treatments of the liver insult in patients with ALF are available only for acetaminophen overdose; steroids for autoimmune ALF and nucleos(t)ide analogues for fulminant hepatitis B, and other etiology-specific treatments, remain unproven in efficacy.
- Management of the systemic complications of ALF remains poorly defined, but includes prevention of cerebral edema and infection. Liver transplantation remains the management option of last resort, and its need must be anticipated by frequent assessment of clinical clues.
- Patients with acute-on-chronic liver failure (ACLF) have underlying cirrhosis and portal hypertension, and acutely decompensate after a precipitating event such as infection or gastrointestinal bleeding.
- The primary cause of mortality in ACLF is multiorgan system failure, which optimally should be managed by intensivists with an understanding of liver disease. Liver transplantation in patients with ACLF is contraindicated unless the precipitating event can be contained.

ACUTE LIVER FAILURE
Definition of the Syndrome

Acute liver failure (ALF) is defined as the development of hepatic encephalopathy (HE) and coagulopathy (international normalized ratio [INR] ≥1.5) in a patient with no history of previous liver disease, with the onset of HE within 26 weeks of jaundice. ALF is a

Financial Disclosure: The authors have no conflicts of interest to disclose.
Section of Hepatology, Hume-Lee Transplant Center, Virginia Commonwealth University, 1200 East Broad Street, Richmond, VA 23222, USA
* Corresponding author. Section of Hepatology, Virginia Commonwealth University, 1200 East Broad Street, PO Box 980341, Richmond, VA 23298.
E-mail address: rstravit@vcu.edu

syndrome acquired from at least a dozen causes, and therefore the severity of liver injury, complications, and outcome vary tremendously. Unfortunately, the optimal management of ALF has not been well defined because of the heterogeneity of the syndrome and its relative scarcity (2000–3000 cases per year in the United States). There are 3 possible outcomes after ALF: spontaneous survival without liver transplantation (LT), LT, or death. In the ALF Study Group Registry of more than 2000 enrollees, approximately one-third of patients died, one-quarter underwent orthotopic LT, and the remainder recovered spontaneously.[1] Recent reports have highlighted improvement in survival rates from 17% to 25% in the 1970s to 65% in current series.[2]

Two types of complications lead to death or the need for LT in patients with ALF: those related to hepatocellular failure, and multiorgan system failure (MOSF). The relative frequency of complications leading to death has changed considerably in the last 35 years. Bleeding complications were once a relatively frequent cause of death (27%), but very rarely contribute to death at present (<5% in a recent analysis of the ALF Study Group Registry; R. Todd Stravitz, MD, and colleagues, unpublished data, 2013). The incidence of intracranial hypertension, also once a frequent cause of death, appears to have decreased because of improvements in management.[2]

Etiology and Relative Incidence

In the ALF Study Group (ALFSG) Registry (**Table 1**), acetaminophen (APAP) accounts for approximately 45% of cases,[1] half attributable to ingestion of a single large dose

Table 1
Etiology, prevalence, and evaluation of ALF

Etiology	Prevalence (%)	Evaluation
APAP	45	History; APAP level
HBV	7	Anti-HBc (IgM and total), HBsAg, anti-HBs, HBV DNA, anti-HDV
AIH	5	ANA, ASMA, anti-LKM, immunoglobulins
HAV	4	Anti-HAV (IgM and total)
Shock liver	4	Echocardiogram, brain natriuretic peptide
Wilson disease	3	Serum ceruloplasmin and copper; urine copper; slit-lamp eye examination
BCS	2	Doppler ultrasonography of liver
Malignancy	1	Contrast-enhanced CT; MRI (preferred)
AFLP/HELLP	1	Pregnancy test
HSV	0.5	Anti-HSV 1/2, HSV DNA
Other	4	Anti-HCV/HCV RNA, anti-CMV/CMV DNA, anti-EBV/EBV DNA, toxicology screen
Indeterminate	14	All of above negative
Idiosyncratic drug	13	History; all of above negative

Prevalence of causes are estimates based on the US Acute Liver Failure Study Group Registry (N = ~2000; W.M. Lee, personal communication, 2012).

Abbreviations: AFLP, acute fatty liver of pregnancy; AIH, autoimmune hepatitis; ALF, acute liver failure; ANA, antinuclear antibody; APAP, acetaminophen; ASMA, anti–smooth muscle antibody; BCS, Budd-Chiari syndrome; CMV, cytomegalovirus; CT, computed tomography; EBV, Epstein-Barr virus; HAV, hepatitis A virus; HBc, hepatitis B core antibody; HBs, hepatitis B surface antibody; HBsAg, HBs antigen; HBV, hepatitis B virus; HCV, hepatitis C virus; HDV, hepatitis D virus; HELLP, hemolysis + elevated liver enzymes + low platelet count; HSV, herpes simplex virus; IgM, immunoglobulin M; LKM, liver kidney microsome antibody; MRI, magnetic resonance imaging.

with suicidal intent, and the other half as a "therapeutic misadventure."[3] The second most common cause of ALF remains indeterminate even after extensive evaluation (15% of cases), although many cases may represent unrecognized autoimmune ALF.[4] Idiosyncratic drug-induced liver injury (DILI) represents approximately 13% of ALF cases in the United States, with the most common offenders being antimicrobial agents, neuropsychiatric drugs, and dietary/herbal supplements.[5] The incidence of fulminant hepatitis A and B is decreasing, and now accounts for 4% and 7% of cases, respectively. Autoimmune ALF has been estimated to cause 5% to 7% of cases of ALF, but may be underrecognized because serologies (antinuclear antibodies ± anti–smooth muscle antibodies) are negative in 37% of cases and liver biopsy is infrequently performed. Acute hepatic vein thrombosis (Budd-Chiari syndrome), hypotension ("shock liver"), fulminant Wilson disease, malignant infiltration of the liver, and pregnancy-associated ALF (acute fatty liver of pregnancy and HELLP syndrome [hemolysis + elevated liver enzymes + low platelet count]) comprise fewer than 5% of cases each. It remains controversial whether acute hepatitis C virus infection causes ALF, but case reports exist (3 instances out of 2000 in the ALFSG Registry).

Management of Patients with ALF

Etiology-specific treatment of the liver injury

The first goal when presented with a patient with ALF is to identify the cause, as specific therapies may be applicable (**Table 2**). The diagnosis of APAP overdose in a patient who is unable or unwilling to give an accurate account of the ingestion presents a frequent diagnostic dilemma, because APAP concentrations in blood have a short half-life resulting in false-negative tests, and false-positive APAP levels also occur in patients with severe hyperbilirubinemia (>10 mg/dL).[6] A novel APAP-protein adduct assay has been developed, the results of which remain positive for a week after the ingestion.[7] Intravenous N-acetylcysteine (NAC) should be administered when a patient has HE of grade higher than 1 to 2, or in patients who do not tolerate oral dosing. Because the administration of NAC, even late after ingestion, seems to confer survival benefit, dosing should continue until evidence of severe liver injury resolves (INR <1.5 and resolution of HE), rather by completion of a set number of doses of the drug.[8]

Other medications that may be considered in patients with ALF resulting from non-APAP etiology are outlined in **Table 2**, but are generally unproven. A randomized controlled study of lamivudine in patients with severe acute hepatitis B (many of whom

Table 2	
Etiology-specific therapy for patients with ALF	
Etiology	**Therapy to Be Considered**
APAP	NAC oral: 140 mg/kg load, then 70 mg/kg every 4 h
	NAC IV: 150 mg/kg load, then 12.5 mg/kg/h × 4 h, then 6.25 mg/kg/h
Amanita	Penicillin G: 1 g/kg/d IV and NAC (as in APAP overdose)
HSV	Acyclovir: 30 mg/kg/d IV
AIH	Methylprednisolone 60 mg/d IV
HBV	Lamivudine 100–150 mg/d oral
Wilson disease	Plasmapheresis, ᴅ-penicillamine
AFLP/HELLP	Delivery of fetus

Abbreviations: IV, intravenous; NAC, N-acetylcysteine.

had ALF) showed no benefit.[9] Similarly, the ALFSG recently reported resoundingly negative results in patients with autoimmune ALF treated with corticosteroids.[10] Remedies recommended for other causes are based only on anecdotal experience.

Non–etiology-specific treatment of the liver injury

NAC has been tested with mixed results in ALF of non-APAP etiology. In the ALFSG trial, 173 patients with non-APAP ALF were randomized to receive a 72-hour infusion of NAC or placebo.[11] Although the secondary end point of the trial, transplant-free survival, was more common in NAC-treated than placebo-treated patients (40% vs 27%, respectively; $P = .043$), the primary end point of overall survival was not significantly different between groups. A similarly designed trial in pediatric patients actually suggested that NAC might be harmful.[12] Several smaller, nonrandomized studies have suggested that NAC may improve outcome in non-APAP ALF, but a preponderance of high-quality data leaves its efficacy in question.

Management of specific complications of ALF

General management The optimal management of patients with ALF requires a multi-disciplinary team of experienced physicians. Worsening or exceeding grade 2 HE are indications for admission to the intensive care unit (ICU).

Neurologic complications By definition, patients with ALF have varying degrees of HE, which may portend the development of cerebral edema in 38% to 81% of cases that reach grade 3 or 4.[13] Studies have repeatedly shown that ammonia levels elevated above 150 to 200 μM increase the risk of cerebral edema.[14–16] Conversely, herniation rarely occurs when serum ammonia levels remain lower than 100 μM. In the setting of cerebral edema and intracranial hypertension, cerebral perfusion pressure (CPP = mean arterial pressure [MAP] minus intracranial pressure [ICP]) must be carefully monitored as systemic vascular resistance is often low, and patients are consequently vulnerable to cerebral ischemia.

Considering the central importance of ammonia in the pathogenesis of HE and cerebral edema, lowering serum ammonia levels in patients with ALF seems reasonable. However, data supporting ammonia-lowering therapies in ALF remain elusive. The most commonly used agents in alcoholic chronic liver disease, nonabsorbable disaccharides (eg, lactulose) and oral antibiotics (neomycin, rifaximin, or metronidazole), have not been adequately studied in patients with ALF. A blinded, placebo-controlled study of L-ornithine L-aspartate (LOLA), an ammonia-scavenging agent, showed no benefit on serum ammonia or HE, but may not provide an adequate mechanism of excretion of glutamine to prevent deamidation back into ammonia and glutamate.[17] A similar agent, ornithine phenylacetate (OPA), seems to provide a pathway to renal excretion of glutamine,[18] and is in clinical trials.

The diagnosis and treatment of cerebral edema remains a poorly defined and contentious aspect of managing ALF. Although a head computed tomography (CT) scan may detect cerebral edema, it is poorly sensitive.[19] Because ICP cannot be routinely determined noninvasively and carries important prognostic implications for spontaneous survival and neurologic recovery after LT, many experts advocate ICP monitor placement in LT candidates with stage III or IV HE. However, placement of an ICP monitor has never been shown to improve neurologic outcome or survival in ALF, although it may change management.[20]

The specific management of cerebral edema in patients with ALF resembles that of other causes of intracranial hypertension, with the important caveat that hyperemia plays an important additional pathogenic role in the former. Endotracheal intubation and mechanical ventilation should be performed under deep sedation and neuromuscular blockade to lower the risk of increasing ICP, avoid hypoxemia and hypercapnia, and reduce aspiration risk. Once intubated, patients should receive adequate analgesia and sedation with short-acting agents such as morphine and propofol, and may require paralysis with cisatracurium.[21] Hyperventilation causes cerebral vasoconstriction and a reduction in cerebral blood volume, effects that can be used therapeutically to reduce ICP; therefore, spontaneous hyperventilation and respiratory alkalosis should not be corrected. However, forced hyperventilation may sensitize some regions of the brain to ischemia in ALF, and is generally not advocated.[22]

In a randomized, placebo-controlled study, Murphy and colleagues[23] showed that hypernatremia induced with hypertonic saline (HTS) to a serum sodium level of 145 to 155 mEq/L was more effective in preventing the development of cerebral edema than management at normal serum sodium. Although there are no clinical studies of the use of HTS to treat cerebral edema once established, experience in other disease states such as traumatic brain injury suggest that HTS is a reasonable treatment. Another osmotic agent, mannitol, has been shown to lower ICP in small human case series of ALF, and has appeared to improve survival.[24] A general indication for the administration of mannitol includes persistently (>10 minutes) elevated ICP (>20 mm Hg). The optimal dose of mannitol remains untested, but smaller boluses (eg, 0.25–0.5 g/kg every 4–6 hours) seem to be as effective as larger ones. High-dose barbiturates (pentobarbital or thiopental) can be used as rescue therapy when other interventions have been maximized.

Fever increases ICP in ALF, and should be treated promptly with cooling blankets. Similarly, the induction of mild hypothermia may be considered when the measures discussed here fail to control the ICP. Hypothermia interferes with many aspects of the pathogenesis of cerebral edema.[25] Temperatures of 32°C to 34°C have been induced usually with cooling blankets, and may provide a bridge to LT.[26] However, induced hypothermia has never been shown to bridge a patient to spontaneous recovery of liver function, may interfere with hepatic regeneration, and has many untoward effects, including interference with coagulation and an increased risk of infection. Therefore, therapeutic hypothermia must be considered experimental. However, patients with ALF frequently develop mild (35°–36°C) spontaneous hypothermia, particularly in those on renal replacement therapy, and should not be rewarmed.

Cardiopulmonary complications Hypotension is a frequent complication of ALF and reflects systemic inflammatory response syndrome (SIRS)-associated low systemic vascular resistance. As patients with ALF often arrive intravascularly depleted, hypotension should always first be treated with volume (normal saline, or sodium bicarbonate in half-normal saline in patients with acidemia), in addition to empiric broad-spectrum antibiotics. After normovolemia has been assured, persistent hypotension should be treated with norepinephrine, with vasopressin added in refractory cases. Finally, "relative" adrenal insufficiency should be suspected in refractory hypotension and treated with hydrocortisone (50–100 mg intravenously every 6–8 hours).[27] The goal MAP is generally greater than 60 to 65 mm Hg, and CPP greater than 50 to 60 mm Hg; if an ICP monitor is not placed, clinicians should err on the side of a slightly higher MAP.

As many as 37% of patients with ALF develop acute lung injury (ALI) or acute respiratory distress syndrome (ARDS).[28] Although liver failure may have a direct effect, the etiology may also include neurogenic pulmonary edema, aspiration pneumonitis, nosocomial pneumonia, or extrapulmonary infection. With established ALI or ARDS, tidal volumes should be limited to 6 mL/kg of predicted body weight. Positive end-expiratory pressure settings should be sufficient to achieve adequate oxygenation while concomitantly ensuring that ICP, blood pressure, and cardiac output are not compromised.

Renal failure Acute renal failure complicates ALF in up to 50% of cases, and more frequently in APAP overdose.[29] Two types of renal failure are peculiar to patients with ALF. The first is the result of hepatotoxin-induced nephrotoxicity. Examples include APAP and trimethoprim-sulfamethoxazole, and the clinical picture is one of acute tubular necrosis early after the liver injury. The second is a functional renal failure similar to hepatorenal syndrome in patients with cirrhosis. ALF patients develop functional renal failure as a consequence of intense renal vasoconstriction, and the clinical presentation is one of oliguric renal failure with preserved ability to concentrate the urine at a time period more removed from the liver injury. Early institution of renal replacement therapy (RRT) should be considered, because renal failure per se compounds the problem of hyperammonemia, and electrolyte abnormalities may exacerbate HE and hemodynamic instability. Continuous RRT is preferred over intermittent hemodialysis because of the more stable hemodynamics and greater time-averaged dialysis dose in the former.[30]

Infection ALF patients are relatively immunocompromised because of several mechanisms, and are at high risk (incidence 40%) of nosocomial infections with both bacterial and fungal pathogens.[31] Early diagnosis can be difficult because patients often have subtle manifestations. Daily surveillance cultures and chest radiographs should be considered, as they may improve early diagnosis and guide selection of antimicrobial agents.[32] Although prophylactic antibiotics (enteral and parenteral) decrease the risk of infection in ALF, they have not been shown to improve survival and may promote infection with resistant pathogens.[33] Indications for broad-spectrum antibiotics include significant isolates on surveillance cultures,[31] unexplained progression of HE,[34] or signs of SIRS.[35]

Coagulopathy Despite a deficiency of prohemostatic clotting factors, low fibrinogen, thrombocytopenia, and platelet dysfunction, spontaneous (non–procedure-related) bleeding is infrequent in patients with ALF, approximately 10% based on recent analysis of the ALFSG Registry (R. Todd Stravitz, MD, and colleagues, unpublished data, 2013). Furthermore, increasing evidence suggests that global hemostasis is well preserved in patients with ALF.[36–38] Therefore, the routine use of blood products to correct these abnormalities is not justified because they are unnecessary, ineffective, and interfere with the prognostic utility of the INR. Vitamin K deficiency has been reported to contribute to the coagulopathy of ALF,[39] and should be repleted parenterally (10 mg subcutaneously or slow [over 30 minutes] intravenous infusion). Recombinant factor VIIa (rFVIIa) (40 µg/kg) may be considered in patients with life-threatening bleeding, and before placement of an ICP monitor or performance of a liver biopsy. However, the risk of thrombosis with rFVIIa may be high among patients with ALF.[40] Coagulopathy and mechanical ventilation are well-established indications for gastrointestinal stress ulcer prophylaxis, and deep venous thrombosis prophylaxis should be administered to patients with ALF.

Liver transplantation for ALF

LT remains the treatment of last resort for ALF. Unfortunately, identifying which patients will die without an LT is difficult, despite numerous prognostic schemes (**Table 3**).[41] The single most important clinical feature predicting outcome after ALF is etiology, as some causes are associated with greater than 50% to 60% spontaneous survival rates (APAP, hepatitis A, ischemic ALF, and pregnancy-associated

Table 3
Schemes for predicting poor prognosis and the need for liver transplantation in patients with ALF

Scheme	Etiology of ALF	Criteria for Liver Transplantation	Reference
King's College criteria	APAP	Arterial pH <7.30 or All of the following: 1. PT >100 s, and 2. Creatinine >3.4 mg/dL, and 3. Grade 3/4 encephalopathy	O'Grady et al,[44] 1989
	Non-APAP	PT >100 s (INR >6.5) or Any 3 of the following: 1. NANB/drug/halothane etiology 2. Jaundice to encephalopathy >7 d 3. Age <10 or >40 y 4. PT >50 s 5. Bilirubin >17.4 mg/dL	
Factor V	Viral	Age <30 y: factor V <20% Or Any age: factor V <30% and grade 3/4 encephalopathy	Bernuau et al,[134] 1986
Factor VIII/V ratio	APAP	Factor VIII/V ratio >30	Pereira et al,[135] 1992
Liver biopsy	Mixed	Hepatocyte necrosis >70%	Donaldson et al,[136] 1993
Arterial phosphate	APAP	>1.2 mmol/L	Schmidt and Dalhoff,[46] 2002
Arterial lactate	APAP	>3.5 mmol/L	Bernal et al,[45] 2002
Arterial ammonia	Mixed	>150–200 µmol/L	Clemmesen et al,[14] 1999
APACHE II/III score	APAP	Score >15	Polson et al,[41] 2008
SOFA score	APAP		Cholongitas et al,[137] 2012

Abbreviations: APACHE, Acute Physiology and Chronic Health Evaluation; APAP, acetaminophen; INR, international normalized ratio; Mixed, mixed etiology; NANB, non-A non-B hepatitis; PT, prothrombin time.

ALF), whereas others have dismal spontaneous survival rates (≤25%: indeterminate ALF, autoimmune ALF, hepatitis B, idiosyncratic DILI).[42] The length of time between the onset of symptoms and the onset of HE constitutes another helpful clinical clue about estimating prognosis, with hyperacute cases having much better spontaneous survival rates than subacute cases.[43] The decision to list an ALF patient for LT is thus based on several clinical clues, including etiology, tempo of progression, severity of abnormal chemistries (INR, bilirubin, lactate, and phosphate), and presence of systemic complications, particularly the severity of HE and intracranial hypertension.[44–46]

In the United States, criteria for listing a patient with ALF according to policy of the United Organization for Organ Sharing include a life expectancy without LT of less than 7 days, onset of HE within 8 weeks of the first symptoms of liver disease, and no history of preexisting liver disease. At present, patients with ALF are given priority to receive a cadaveric organ over all patients with chronic liver disease (Status 1). In addition, patients must be in the ICU, and must fulfill 1 of the following 3 criteria: (1) be ventilator-dependent; (2) require dialysis or RRT; or (3) have an INR greater than

2.0. A detailed re-review of the patient's neurologic status must be made just before going to the operating suite so that LT is not performed when the likelihood of neurologic recovery is poor. Severe, sustained intracranial hypertension predicts brainstem herniation during LT or poor neurologic recovery after LT, and patients with an ICP greater than 40 mm Hg or CPP less than 40 mm Hg for more than 2 hours appear to be particularly vulnerable to disastrous outcomes.[47]

ACUTE-ON-CHRONIC LIVER FAILURE

Cirrhotic patients are prone to developing acute hepatic decompensation often resulting from gastrointestinal hemorrhage or bacterial infections.[48–51] Acute-on-chronic liver failure (ACLF) is an acute decompensation of hepatic function in cirrhotic patients, either secondary to superimposed liver injury or caused by systemic precipitating factors culminating in MOSF.[52] ACLF has been recently further defined as a clinically distinct entity consisting of acute hepatic decompensation (inclusion criteria, present in all patients), organ failure (defined by the Chronic Liver Failure-Sequential Organ Failure Assessment or CLIF-SOFA score), and high 28-day mortality.[53] The estimated number of ICU admissions related to cirrhosis in the United States is in excess of 26,000 per year, with an estimated financial burden of more than $3 billion.[54]

Pathophysiology

Although exact pathogenesis of ACLF remains to be elucidated, it usually results from an inciting event and alteration in host-response to injury leading to clinical deterioration. These events could be either liver-related (ie, alcoholic hepatitis, superimposed viral hepatitis, portal vein thrombosis, DILI) or non–liver-related (ie, trauma, surgery, infections). However, a lack of a specific precipitating event can be found in as many as 40% of patients with ACLF. In addition to the precipitating factors, the role of host injury and inflammation is being recognized as a key component in the propagation of ACLF. Multiple proinflammatory and anti-inflammatory cytokines including tumor necrosis factor (TNF)-α, sTNF-αR1, sTNF-αR2, interleukin (IL)-2, IL-2R, IL-6, IL-8, IL-10, and interferon-γ have been implicated in ACLF.[55,56]

Initial Assessment of Prognosis in Patients with ACLF

The initial assessment of prognosis in cirrhotic patients admitted to the ICU is essential to identify patients in whom aggressive treatment is futile. Several prognostic scores in cirrhotic patients in the ICU have been validated and are routinely used to assess outcomes (**Table 4**).[57] Although several liver-specific models for predicting in-hospital mortality exist, those using general organ system assessment appear to be more accurate.[58–60] The in-hospital mortality in cirrhotic patients is closely associated with organ dysfunction, and increases from 33% in patients with single-organ failure to 97% in those with failure in 3 or more organs within 24 hours after ICU admission.[59,60]

Infection

Infection is the most common precipitant of ACLF.[61,62] Bacterial infections occur in 34% of cirrhotic patients admitted to hospital, compared with 5% to 7% observed in patients without cirrhosis.[63,64] The increased risk of infection in patients with cirrhosis is multifactorial, being due to portosystemic shunting of the reticuloendothelial system and impaired monocyte activation, cytokine secretion, and phagocytosis.[65–68] In addition, intestinal bacterial translocation to portal circulation increases the risk for spontaneous bacterial peritonitis and bacteremia.[53,69–72]

Table 4
Prognostic scores in cirrhotic patients admitted to the ICU

Study	Study Period	Mortality	Discrimination Ability of Predictive Scores (ROC AUC)
Das et al,[138] 2010 (N = 138)	2005–2008	ICU: 41% 6 mo: 54%	CTP (0.76) MELD (0.77); MELD Na (0.75) SAPS II (0.78) Modified SOFA (0.84)
Filloux et al,[139] 2010 (N = 86)	2002–2007	ICU: 37%	CTP (0.69) MELD (0.70) SAPS II (0.81) SOFA (0.86)
Juneja et al,[140] 2009 (N = 104)	2007–2008	ICU: 42.3 In hospital: 56.7	APACHE II (0.90) SOFA (0.93)
Levesque et al,[141] 2012 (N = 377)	2005–2007	ICU: 34.7% In hospital: 42.9%	SOFA (0.92) SAPS II (0.89) MELD (0.82); MELD Na (0.79) CTP (0.79)
Olmez et al,[142] 2012 (N = 201)	2007–2010	ICU: 41.8%	APACHE II (0.82) CTP (0.72) MELD (0.79) SOFA (0.85)
Rabe et al,[143] 2004 (N = 76)	1993–2003	ICU: 59% In hospital: 70%	APACHE II (0.66) CTP (0.87)
Tu et al,[144] 2011 (N = 202)	2008–2009	In hospital: 59.9%	CTP (0.71) MELD (0.87) SOFA (0.87)
Wehler et al,[59] 2001 (N = 143)	1993–1998	ICU: 36% In hospital: 46%	APACHE II (0.79) CTP (0.74) SOFA (0.95)

Abbreviations: APACHE, Acute Physiology and Chronic Health Evaluation; CTP, Child-Turcotte-Pugh; MELD, Model for End-Stage Liver Disease; MELD Na, MELD sodium model; ROC AUC, area under the receiver-operating characteristic curve; SAPS, Simplified Acute Physiology Score; SOFA, Sequential Organ Failure Assessment.

Management of hemodynamic instability and septic shock

Because of cirrhosis-associated immune dysfunction, patients with cirrhosis who experience infection are at greater risk of developing sepsis syndromes.[55,61,73] Furthermore, in-hospital mortality is disproportionately higher in cirrhotic patients with severe sepsis or septic shock.[74–76] Historically, gram-negative organisms were the most common bacterial infections in patients admitted to the ICU, but recent series suggest that the prevalence of gram-positive infections is increasing.[77,78] The management of sepsis in cirrhosis parallels the general ICU population, with minor differences. There are no specific studies evaluating early goal-directed therapy (EGDT) or optimal end points for resuscitation in cirrhotic patients per se. However, the general principles of EGDT in the management of septic patients should be applied (**Fig. 1**).[79]

Cirrhotic patients have vascular hyporeactivity and a hyperdynamic circulation characterized by higher cardiac index and lower systemic vascular resistance.[76] Therefore, central venous oxygen saturation of more than 70% may be normal in cirrhotic patients and may not be an ideal end point while providing EGDT. In addition, because lactate metabolism is often impaired in cirrhosis, it is difficult to monitor as a

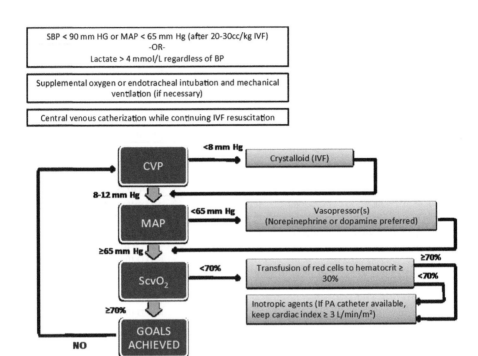

Fig. 1. Early goal-directed therapy (EGDT) in the management of severe sepsis. As defined by EGDT, it is important to meet the following parameters expeditiously to improve ICU-related mortality: (1) central venous pressure (CVP) between 8 and 12 mm Hg; (2) mean arterial pressure (MAP) 65 mm Hg or higher; (3) urine output 0.5 mL/kg/h or higher; and (4) central venous oxygen saturation (ScvO$_2$) 70% or more. These parameters are met through the use of intravenous fluid (IVF) resuscitation, blood transfusions, vasopressors, and inotropes. BP, blood pressure; PA, pulmonary artery; SBP, systolic blood pressure.

marker of tissue hypoperfusion in cirrhotic patients.[80] The optimal choice of intravenous fluid therapy is controversial; because patients with cirrhosis are usually hypoalbuminic but have effective hypervolemia, albumin is often advocated over other volume expanders. Indeed, post hoc analysis of the SAFE study has suggested that albumin use in septic patients with cirrhosis might improve survival.[81] While implementing EGDT, it is imperative to evaluate cirrhotic patients for potential sources of infection. Blood, urine, and sputum cultures should be sent early to help direct antibiotics, with chest radiographs and diagnostic paracentesis if ascites is present. Early empiric institution of antibiotics in patients with components of the SIRS is imperative; in critically ill cirrhotic patients presenting with septic shock, in-hospital mortality was as high as 76%, and delay in antimicrobial therapy was associated with increased mortality (adjusted odds ratio per hour 1.1).[82] Choice of initial empiric antibiotic treatment will depend on several factors including history of known pathogens, institutional antibiotic resistance pattern, and prior antibiotic treatment.

Despite a 20% to 60% prevalence of relative adrenal insufficiency in noncirrhotic patients with sepsis,[83] routine use of stress-dosed steroid is not recommend because of the increased risk of infection.[84] Similarly, adrenal insufficiency in cirrhotics with septic shock is common (51%–77%), and associated with a higher mortality rate (81% vs 37%) in comparison with those without adrenal insufficiency.[74,85] However, the limited data available do not support the use of routine high-dose steroids in cirrhotic patients with septic shock.[86]

At present there are no trials evaluating the efficacy of different vasoactive agents in patients with cirrhosis. Consequently, vasoactive drugs in cirrhotic patients with sepsis should be administered to cirrhotic patients with hypotension refractory to volume, similarly to those of the general population.[79,87] Although positive inotropic agents are often used in septic patients with myocardial dysfunction, their efficacy in cirrhotic patients is not as clear because most cirrhotic patients have high cardiac output resulting from hyperdynamic circulation.[76]

Acute kidney injury

Acute kidney injury (AKI) affects 40% to 60% of cirrhotic patients and is an independent predictor of death after admission to the ICU.[88–92] Although not ideally suited to cirrhotics owing to poor muscle mass, the currently used definition of AKI in cirrhotic patients is a serum creatinine level of greater than 1.5 mg/dL.[93,94] To be able to identify AKI sooner, the Acute Kidney Injury Network (AKIN) and Risk, Injury, Failure, Loss and End-stage kidney disease (RIFLE) definitions have been recommended[95–97] but are not used widely. According to the AKIN criteria, cirrhosis-associated AKI is defined by an increase in serum creatinine by more than 50% from a stable baseline value in less than 3 months, or by 0.3 mg/dL in less than 48 hours.[98] In a cohort of 337 patients with cirrhosis, the newly proposed definition of cirrhosis-associated AKI accurately predicted 30-day mortality, length of hospital stay, and organ failure.[98]

The etiology of AKI in cirrhotic patients is often multifactorial, and includes sepsis, hypovolemia secondary to overdiuresis or shock, drug-induced nephrotoxicity, parenchymal renal disease, and hepatorenal syndrome (HRS). Analysis of urine sediment and sodium can differentiate between acute tubular necrosis (ATN) and other causes of renal failure in cirrhosis. In prerenal azotemia and HRS, the urine sediment is normal and urine sodium is low (<10 mEq/L), whereas in ATN there is renal tubular cell debris and high urine sodium. It is of paramount importance to be able to distinguish between these causes because HRS (particularly type 1) is associated with high mortality.[99,100] Given the close association between HRS and bacterial infections, an infectious workup should be undertaken in any cirrhotic patients admitted to the ICU with renal failure.[94,99,100] The cornerstone of management of HRS continues to be albumin (1 g/kg initially followed by 20–40 g/d) and vasopressor therapy to mitigate splanchnic and systemic vasodilatation (**Fig. 2**). Terlipressin (a vasopressin analogue) and albumin have been shown to reverse type 1 HRS in up to 50% of patients.[101,102] Complete response is defined as a decrease in serum creatinine to less than 1.5 mg/dL, and usually occurs in 7 to 10 days.[101,102] Norepinephrine has also been shown to be effective in the treatment of type 1 HRS in small studies.[103,104] RRT is not considered a treatment option for HRS or cirrhosis-induced AKI, but is often used as a bridge to LT.

Neurologic complications

Altered mentation is practically universal in ACLF. HE is a diagnosis of exclusion, and other causes of altered sensorium should be sought.[105,106] After screening for toxic and metabolic derangements, an obtunded patient should undergo a non–contrast-enhanced head CT scan to rule out intracranial bleed. After common reversible causes of altered mental status have been ruled out, the diagnosis of HE should be considered. Treatment of HE begins by identifying and treating precipitating factors, particularly infection and gastrointestinal hemorrhage (**Table 5**). Because serum ammonia levels do not correlate with clinical outcomes, their routine use in the management of HE is not recommended.[107] Prompt intubation of patients with advanced HE should

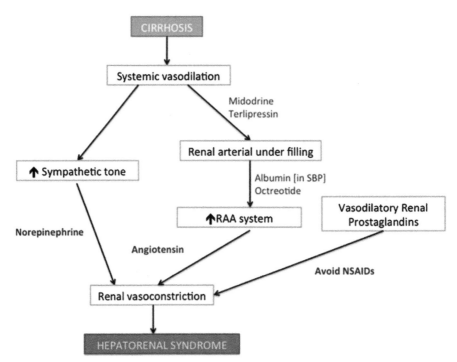

Fig. 2. Pathophysiologic mechanism and management of hepatorenal syndrome. NSAIDs, nonsteroidal anti-inflammatory drugs; RAA, renin-angiotensin-aldosterone; SBP, spontaneous bacterial peritonitis.

be undertaken to protect the airway. Nonabsorbable disaccharides (lactulose and lactilol) are the mainstay of therapy and are administered to achieve 2 to 3 soft stools per day. In addition, oral rifaximin (1100 mg/d), a nonabsorbable derivative of rifamycin, has been shown to be an effective treatment of HE.[108,109] Lactulose in patients with ACLF should be administered cautiously, as aspiration pneumonia, gaseous distention of the bowel, toxic megacolon, poor glycemic control, and electrolyte imbalance may ensue. The benzodiazepine receptor antagonist, flumazenil (1 mg intravenously) may transiently improve HE, particularly for those in whom HE may

Table 5
Precipitating events and mechanisms of hepatic encephalopathy in cirrhosis

Event	Mechanism
Excessive protein ingestion Constipation Gastrointestinal bleed	Gut ammonia production
Portosystemic shunting Fever Infection	Neurotoxin clearance (ammonia, endogenous benzodiazepines)
Dehydration Azotemia Hypokalemia	Renal excretion of ammonia
Sedative (benzodiazepines)	Inhibitory neurotransmission (γ-aminobutyric acid)

be due to overzealous or unintentional benzodiazepine use, but the benefit wanes within 2 hours.[110] Finally, extracorporeal albumin dialysis (MARS system) may also improve HE in refractory cases, but does not improve mortality and cannot yet be considered a bridge to LT.[111,112]

In patients requiring sedation protocol for mechanical ventilation, daily interruption of continuous sedation should be utilized to reassess the need for continued mechanical ventilation.[79] If possible the use of benzodiazepines should be avoided, as they can precipitate or exacerbate HE and may prolong the need for mechanical ventilation.[113] Sedatives with a shorter-acting half-life, such as propofol, are preferred because of the lower risk of precipitating HE.

Gastrointestinal bleeding

Variceal bleeding is related to the degree of underlying portal hypertension, not the presence of coagulopathy. Poor prognostic factors associated with high mortality include active bleeding at the time of endoscopy, decompensated cirrhosis (Child-Turcotte-Pugh [CTP] grade C or Model for End-Stage Liver Disease score > 20), portosystemic gradient greater than 20 mm Hg, and MOSF.[50] Advances in medical and endoscopic therapy for variceal bleeding has improved survival, but mortality remains high in patients with CTP grade C cirrhosis.[114] The optimal care of cirrhotic patients with acute variceal hemorrhage is a multipronged approach optimizing fluid resuscitation, replacement of blood products, vasoactive therapy, antibiotic prophylaxis, and endoscopy. Blood volume should be resuscitated urgently with the goals of maintaining hemodynamic stability and a hemoglobin level of approximately 8 g/dL[115]; transfusion to a higher hemoglobin level increases portal pressure to levels higher than baseline,[116] and increases the risk of rebleeding and mortality.[117] Overzealous resuscitation with crystalloids should also be avoided because, in addition to increasing the risk of rebleeding, it exacerbates fluid accumulation in extravascular sites. Although plasma and platelet transfusions are commonly used in volume resuscitation, a large, multicenter, placebo-controlled trial of rFVIIa in cirrhotic patients with gastrointestinal hemorrhage failed to show a beneficial effect of rFVIIa over standard therapy.[118]

Pharmacologic therapy with vasoactive agents (ie, terlipressin, somatostatin, or octreotide) should be initiated as soon as the diagnosis of variceal hemorrhage is suspected, even before endoscopy, and should be continued for up to 5 days. Somatostatin and its analogues such as octreotide can also improve bleeding control by increasing splanchnic vasoconstriction. Although these agents have a better safety profile and may improve bleeding control, they have not been shown to improve mortality.[119,120] Terlipressin, a synthetic analogue of vasopressin that is not yet approved in the United States, has a more favorable safety profile than vasopressin, is effective in bleeding control, and improves mortality.[121,122]

After the initial assessment and initiation of medical therapy, an endoscopy should be performed within 6 to 12 hours. Owing to the risk of aspiration, endotracheal intubation before endoscopy should be considered. Endoscopic variceal ligation (EVL) and sclerotherapy are both effective means of controlling bleeding. However, compared with sclerotherapy, EVL is more effective in the control of bleeding, with fewer complications (esophageal ulcers, stricture, rupture),[115] and has replaced sclerotherapy as the endoscopic treatment of choice.[123] In patients with acute variceal bleeding from gastric varices, cyanoacrylate injection into the gastric varix can be considered,[124] or placement of a transjugular portosystemic shunt (TIPS).

Cirrhotic patients with gastrointestinal bleeding have a high risk of bacterial infection ranging from 22% to 66%.[125] Patients who develop infections are not only at a higher risk for developing sepsis and sepsis-related complications but also at higher risk of variceal bleeding and mortality.[126,127] The use of short-term prophylactic antibiotics in patients with cirrhosis and gastrointestinal hemorrhage has been shown to not only reduce the risk of bacterial infections and rebleeding but also improve survival.[125,128] Cephalosporins (relative risk [RR] 0.16; 95% confidence interval [CI] 0.05–0.48) may be more effective in reducing the risk of infection in comparison with fluoroquinolones (RR 0.27; 95% CI 0.18–0.30).[129]

In 10% to 20% of patients with variceal hemorrhage, endoscopic and pharmacologic therapy will fail to achieve hemostasis. TIPS insertion controls bleeding in 90% of refractory cases, with a 52% 1-year survival rate.[130] In a randomized controlled trial comparing the use of TIPS performed within 24 to 48 hours of admission with vasoactive drugs and endoscopic therapy, early TIPS was associated with lower rebleeding rates and mortality.[131]

Pulmonary complications

Respiratory failure accounts for up to 40% of ICU admissions in patients with cirrhosis.[60] Complications of cirrhosis including ascites and hepatic hydrothorax (HH) can impair pulmonary physiology and lead to respiratory failure. HH, the accumulation of ascitic fluid within the pleural space, may occur in the absence of ascites and results from negative intrathoracic pressure generated during inspiration. Treatment options include diuretics and therapeutic thoracentesis. TIPS can be considered in refractory HH, although relapse-free 1-year survival is only 35%.[132,133] Chest tube placement and pleurodesis should be avoided because they increase the risk of infections and procedural complications, and are associated with increased mortality.

SUMMARY

ALF and ACLF are distinct clinical syndromes with high mortality. The optimal management of ALF is particularly poorly defined because of its rarity and heterogeneity, and continues to be based on local institutional experience. Although the management of ACLF has been more systematically studied, the definition of the syndrome remains controversial and has only recently received attention from researchers. Future studies on the management of patients with ALF and ACLF in the ICU should be designed by specialists from multiple disciplines, particularly intensivists with an understanding of liver disease.

REFERENCES

1. Lee WM. Acute liver failure in the United States. Semin Liver Dis 2003;23(3):217–26.
2. Bernal W, Hyyrylainen A, Gera A, et al. Lessons from look-back in acute liver failure? A single centre experience of 3300 patients. J Hepatol 2013;59(1):74–80.
3. Zimmerman HJ, Maddrey WC. Acetaminophen (paracetamol) hepatotoxicity with regular intake of alcohol: analysis of instances of therapeutic misadventure. Hepatology 1995;22(3):767–73.
4. Stravitz RT, Leftkowitch JH, Sterling RK, et al. Autoimmune hepatitis presenting as acute liver failure: distinguishing clinical and histological features [abstract]. Am J Transplant 2008;8:195.
5. Reuben A, Koch DG, Lee WM, Acute Liver Failure Study Group. Drug-induced acute liver failure: results of a U.S. multicenter, prospective study. Hepatology 2010;52(6):2065–76.
6. Polson J, Wians FH Jr, Orsulak P, et al. False positive acetaminophen concentrations in patients with liver injury. Clin Chim Acta 2008;391(1–2):24–30.

7. Davern TJ 2nd, James LP, Hinson JA, et al. Measurement of serum acetaminophen-protein adducts in patients with acute liver failure. Gastroenterology 2006;130(3):687–94.

8. Harrison PM, Keays R, Bray GP, et al. Improved outcome of paracetamol-induced fulminant hepatic failure by late administration of acetylcysteine. Lancet 1990;335(8705):1572–3.

9. Kumar M, Satapathy S, Monga R, et al. A randomized controlled trial of lamivudine to treat acute hepatitis B. Hepatology 2007;45(1):97–101.

10. Karkhanis J, Verna EC, Chang MS, et al. Steroid use in acute liver failure. Hepatology 2014;59(2):612–21.

11. Lee WM, Hynan LS, Rossaro L, et al. Intravenous N-acetylcysteine improves transplant-free survival in early stage non-acetaminophen acute liver failure. Gastroenterology 2009;137(3):856–64, 864.e1.

12. Squires RH, Dhawan A, Alonso E, et al. Intravenous N-acetylcysteine in pediatric patients with nonacetaminophen acute liver failure: a placebo-controlled clinical trial. Hepatology 2013;57(4):1542–9.

13. Butterworth RF. Molecular neurobiology of acute liver failure. Semin Liver Dis 2003;23(3):251–8.

14. Clemmesen JO, Larsen FS, Kondrup J, et al. Cerebral herniation in patients with acute liver failure is correlated with arterial ammonia concentration. Hepatology 1999;29(3):648–53.

15. Bernal W, Hall C, Karvellas CJ, et al. Arterial ammonia and clinical risk factors for encephalopathy and intracranial hypertension in acute liver failure. Hepatology 2007;46(6):1844–52.

16. Himmelseher S. Hypertonic saline solutions for treatment of intracranial hypertension. Curr Opin Anaesthesiol 2007;20(5):414–26.

17. Jalan R, Lee WM. Treatment of hyperammonemia in liver failure: a tale of two enzymes. Gastroenterology 2009;136(7):2048–51.

18. Jalan R, Wright G, Davies NA, et al. L-ornithine phenylacetate (OP): a novel treatment for hyperammonemia and hepatic encephalopathy. Med Hypotheses 2007;69(5):1064–9.

19. Wijdicks EF, Plevak DJ, Rakela J, et al. Clinical and radiologic features of cerebral edema in fulminant hepatic failure. Mayo Clin Proc 1995;70(2):119–24.

20. Vaquero J, Fontana RJ, Larson AM, et al. Complications and use of intracranial pressure monitoring in patients with acute liver failure and severe encephalopathy. Liver Transpl 2005;11(12):1581–9.

21. Wijdicks EF, Nyberg SL. Propofol to control intracranial pressure in fulminant hepatic failure. Transplant Proc 2002;34(4):1220–2.

22. Strauss GI, Hogh P, Moller K, et al. Regional cerebral blood flow during mechanical hyperventilation in patients with fulminant hepatic failure. Hepatology 1999;30(6):1368–73.

23. Murphy N, Auzinger G, Bernel W, et al. The effect of hypertonic sodium chloride on intracranial pressure in patients with acute liver failure. Hepatology 2004;39(2):464–70.

24. Canalese J, Gimson AE, Davis C, et al. Controlled trial of dexamethasone and mannitol for the cerebral oedema of fulminant hepatic failure. Gut 1982;23(7):625–9.

25. Stravitz RT, Larsen FS. Therapeutic hypothermia for acute liver failure. Crit Care Med 2009;37(7 Suppl):S258–64.

26. Jalan R, Olde Daminink SW, Deutz NE, et al. Moderate hypothermia in patients with acute liver failure and uncontrolled intracranial hypertension. Gastroenterology 2004;127(5):1338–46.

27. Harry R, Auzinger G, Wendon J. The clinical importance of adrenal insufficiency in acute hepatic dysfunction. Hepatology 2002;36(2):395–402.
28. Trewby PN, Warren R, Contini S, et al. Incidence and pathophysiology of pulmonary edema in fulminant hepatic failure. Gastroenterology 1978;74(5 Pt 1):859–65.
29. Moore K. Renal failure in acute liver failure. Eur J Gastroenterol Hepatol 1999; 11(9):967–75.
30. Davenport A, Will EJ, Davison AM, et al. Changes in intracranial pressure during machine and continuous haemofiltration. Int J Artif Organs 1989;12(7):439–44.
31. Rolando N, Philpott-Howard J, Williams R. Bacterial and fungal infection in acute liver failure. Semin Liver Dis 1996;16(4):389–402.
32. Rolando N, Harvey F, Brahm J, et al. Prospective study of bacterial infection in acute liver failure: an analysis of fifty patients. Hepatology 1990;11(1):49–53.
33. Rolando N, Gimson A, Wade J, et al. Prospective controlled trial of selective parenteral and enteral antimicrobial regimen in fulminant liver failure. Hepatology 1993;17(2):196–201.
34. Vaquero J, Polson J, Chung C, et al. Infection and the progression of hepatic encephalopathy in acute liver failure. Gastroenterology 2003;125(3):755–64.
35. Rolando N, Wade J, Davalos M, et al. The systemic inflammatory response syndrome in acute liver failure. Hepatology 2000;32(4 Pt 1):734–9.
36. Stravitz RT, Lisman T, Luketic VA, et al. Minimal effects of acute liver injury/acute liver failure on hemostasis as assessed by thromboelastography. J Hepatol 2012;56(1):129–36.
37. Lisman T, Bakhtiari K, Adelmeijer J, et al. Intact thrombin generation and decreased fibrinolytic capacity in patients with acute liver injury or acute liver failure. J Thromb Haemost 2012;10(7):1312–9.
38. Hugenholtz GC, Adelmeijer J, Meijers JC, et al. An unbalance between von Willebrand factor and ADAMTS13 in acute liver failure: Implications for hemostasis and clinical outcome. Hepatology 2013;58(2):752–61.
39. Pereira SP, Rowbotham D, Fitt S, et al. Pharmacokinetics and efficacy of oral versus intravenous mixed-micellar phylloquinone (vitamin K1) in severe acute liver disease. J Hepatol 2005;42(3):365–70.
40. Pavese P, Bonadona A, Beaubien J, et al. FVIIa corrects the coagulopathy of fulminant hepatic failure but may be associated with thrombosis: a report of four cases. Can J Anaesth 2005;52(1):26–9.
41. Polson J. Assessment of prognosis in acute liver failure. Semin Liver Dis 2008; 28(2):218–25.
42. Lee WM. Etiologies of acute liver failure. Semin Liver Dis 2008;28(2):142–52.
43. Gimson AE, O'Grady J, Ede RJ, et al. Late onset hepatic failure: clinical, serological and histological features. Hepatology 1986;6(2):288–94.
44. O'Grady JG, Alexander GJ, Hayllar KM, et al. Early indicators of prognosis in fulminant hepatic failure. Gastroenterology 1989;97(2):439–45.
45. Bernal W, Donaldson N, Wyncoll D, et al. Blood lactate as an early predictor of outcome in paracetamol-induced acute liver failure: a cohort study. Lancet 2002;359(9306):558–63.
46. Schmidt LE, Dalhoff K. Serum phosphate is an early predictor of outcome in severe acetaminophen-induced hepatotoxicity. Hepatology 2002;36(3):659–65.
47. Lidofsky SD, Bass NM, Prager MC, et al. Intracranial pressure monitoring and liver transplantation for fulminant hepatic failure. Hepatology 1992;16(1):1–7.
48. Moore KP, Wong F, Gines P, et al. The management of ascites in cirrhosis: report on the consensus conference of the international ascites club. Hepatology 2003; 38(1):258–66.

49. Khungar V, Poordad F. Management of overt hepatic encephalopathy. Clin Liver Dis 2012;16(1):73–89.
50. Garcia-Tsao G, Bosch J. Management of varices and variceal hemorrhage in cirrhosis. N Engl J Med 2010;362(9):823–32.
51. Arvaniti V, D'Amico G, Fede G, et al. Infections in patients with cirrhosis increase mortality four-fold and should be used in determining prognosis. Gastroenterology 2010;139(4):1246–56.e5.
52. Jalan R, Gines P, Olson JC, et al. Acute-on chronic liver failure. J Hepatol 2012; 57(6):1336–48.
53. Moreau R, Jalan R, Gines P, et al. Acute-on-chronic liver failure is a distinct syndrome that develops in patients with acute decompensation of cirrhosis. Gastroenterology 2013;144(7):1426–37, 1437.e1–9.
54. Olson JC, Kamath PS. Acute-on-chronic liver failure: concept, natural history, and prognosis. Curr Opin Crit Care 2011;17(2):165–9.
55. Gustot T, Durand F, Lebrec D, et al. Severe sepsis in cirrhosis. Hepatology 2009; 50(6):2022–33.
56. Sen S, Davies NA, Mookerjee RP, et al. Pathophysiological effects of albumin dialysis in acute-on-chronic liver failure: a randomized controlled study. Liver Transpl 2004;10(9):1109–19.
57. Vincent JL, Moreno R. Clinical review: scoring systems in the critically ill. Crit Care 2010;14(2):207.
58. Ho YP, Chen YC, Yang C, et al. Outcome prediction for critically ill cirrhotic patients: a comparison of APACHE II and Child-Pugh scoring systems. J Intensive Care Med 2004;19(2):105–10.
59. Wehler M, Kokoska J, Reulbach U, et al. Short-term prognosis in critically ill patients with cirrhosis assessed by prognostic scoring systems. Hepatology 2001;34(2):255–61.
60. Cholongitas E, Senzolo M, Patch D, et al. Risk factors, sequential organ failure assessment and model for end-stage liver disease scores for predicting short term mortality in cirrhotic patients admitted to intensive care unit. Aliment Pharmacol Ther 2006;23(7):883–93.
61. Tandon P, Garcia-Tsao G. Bacterial infections, sepsis, and multiorgan failure in cirrhosis. Semin Liver Dis 2008;28(1):26–42.
62. Caly WR, Strauss E. A prospective study of bacterial infections in patients with cirrhosis. J Hepatol 1993;18(3):353–8.
63. Fernandez J, Navasa M, Gomez J, et al. Bacterial infections in cirrhosis: epidemiological changes with invasive procedures and norfloxacin prophylaxis. Hepatology 2002;35(1):140–8.
64. Borzio M, Salerno F, Piantoni L, et al. Bacterial infection in patients with advanced cirrhosis: a multicentre prospective study. Dig Liver Dis 2001;33(1): 41–8.
65. Ghassemi S, Garcia-Tsao G. Prevention and treatment of infections in patients with cirrhosis. Best Pract Res Clin Gastroenterol 2007;21(1):77–93.
66. Katz S, Jimenez MA, Lehmkuhler WE, et al. Liver bacterial clearance following hepatic artery ligation and portacaval shunt. J Surg Res 1991;51(3):267–70.
67. Wasmuth HE, Kunz D, Yagmur E, et al. Patients with acute on chronic liver failure display "sepsis-like" immune paralysis. J Hepatol 2005;42(2):195–201.
68. Shawcross DL, Wright GA, Stadlbauer V, et al. Ammonia impairs neutrophil phagocytic function in liver disease. Hepatology 2008;48(4):1202–12.
69. Bajaj JS. Defining acute-on-chronic liver failure: will east and west ever meet? Gastroenterology 2013;144(7):1337–9.

70. Chang CS, Chen GH, Lien HC, et al. Small intestine dysmotility and bacterial overgrowth in cirrhotic patients with spontaneous bacterial peritonitis. Hepatology 1998;28(5):1187–90.

71. Garcia-Tsao G, Wiest R. Gut microflora in the pathogenesis of the complications of cirrhosis. Best Pract Res Clin Gastroenterol 2004;18(2):353–72.

72. Runyon BA, Squier S, Borzio M. Translocation of gut bacteria in rats with cirrhosis to mesenteric lymph nodes partially explains the pathogenesis of spontaneous bacterial peritonitis. J Hepatol 1994;21(5):792–6.

73. Foreman MG, Mannino DM, Moss M. Cirrhosis as a risk factor for sepsis and death: analysis of the national hospital discharge survey. Chest 2003;124(3):1016–20.

74. Tsai MH, Peng YS, Chen YC, et al. Adrenal insufficiency in patients with cirrhosis, severe sepsis and septic shock. Hepatology 2006;43(4):673–81.

75. Tsai M, Peng Y, Chen Y, et al. Low serum concentration of apolipoprotein A-I is an indicator of poor prognosis in cirrhotic patients with severe sepsis. J Hepatol 2009;50(5):906–15.

76. Moreau R, Hadengue A, Soupison T, et al. Septic shock in patients with cirrhosis: hemodynamic and metabolic characteristics and intensive care unit outcome. Crit Care Med 1992;20(6):746–50.

77. Gines P, Rimola A, Planas R, et al. Norfloxacin prevents spontaneous bacterial peritonitis recurrence in cirrhosis: results of a double-blind, placebo-controlled trial. Hepatology 1990;12(4 Pt 1):716–24.

78. European Association for the Study of the Liver. EASL clinical practice guidelines on the management of ascites, spontaneous bacterial peritonitis, and hepatorenal syndrome in cirrhosis. J Hepatol 2010;53(3):397–417.

79. Dellinger RP, Levy MM, Rhodes A, et al. Surviving sepsis campaign: international guidelines for management of severe sepsis and septic shock, 2012. Intensive Care Med 2013;39(2):165–228.

80. Rivers E, Nguyen B, Havstad S, et al. Early goal-directed therapy in the treatment of severe sepsis and septic shock. N Engl J Med 2001;345(19):1368–77.

81. Finfer S, Bellomo R, Boyce N, et al, SAFE Study Investigators. A comparison of albumin and saline for fluid resuscitation in the intensive care unit. N Engl J Med 2004;350(22):2247–56.

82. Arabi YM, Dara SI, Memish Z, et al. Antimicrobial therapeutic determinants of outcomes from septic shock among patients with cirrhosis. Hepatology 2012;56(6):2305–15.

83. Marik PE, Pastores SM, Annane D, et al. Recommendations for the diagnosis and management of corticosteroid insufficiency in critically ill adult patients: consensus statements from an international task force by the American College of Critical Care Medicine. Crit Care Med 2008;36(6):1937–49.

84. Sprung CL, Annane D, Keh D, et al. Hydrocortisone therapy for patients with septic shock. N Engl J Med 2008;358(2):111–24.

85. Fernandez J, Escorsell A, Zabalza M, et al. Adrenal insufficiency in patients with cirrhosis and septic shock: effect of treatment with hydrocortisone on survival. Hepatology 2006;44(5):1288–95.

86. Arabi YM, Aljumah A, Dabbagh O, et al. Low-dose hydrocortisone in patients with cirrhosis and septic shock: a randomized controlled trial. CMAJ 2010;182(18):1971–7.

87. De Backer D, Biston P, Devriendt J, et al. Comparison of dopamine and norepinephrine in the treatment of shock. N Engl J Med 2010;362(9):779–89.

88. Cholongitas E, Calvaruso V, Senzolo M, et al. RIFLE classification as predictive factor of mortality in patients with cirrhosis admitted to intensive care unit. J Gastroenterol Hepatol 2009;24(10):1639–47.

89. du Cheyron D, Bouchet B, Parienti JJ, et al. The attributable mortality of acute renal failure in critically ill patients with liver cirrhosis. Intensive Care Med 2005;31(12):1693–9.

90. Terra C, Guevara M, Torre A, et al. Renal failure in patients with cirrhosis and sepsis unrelated to spontaneous bacterial peritonitis: value of MELD score. Gastroenterology 2005;129(6):1944–53.

91. Cardenas A, Gines P, Uriz J, et al. Renal failure after upper gastrointestinal bleeding in cirrhosis: incidence, clinical course, predictive factors, and short-term prognosis. Hepatology 2001;34(4 Pt 1):671–6.

92. Gines A, Escorsell A, Gines P, et al. Incidence, predictive factors, and prognosis of the hepatorenal syndrome in cirrhosis with ascites. Gastroenterology 1993; 105(1):229–36.

93. Arroyo V, Gines P, Gerbes AL, et al. Definition and diagnostic criteria of refractory ascites and hepatorenal syndrome in cirrhosis. International ascites club. Hepatology 1996;23(1):164–76.

94. Gines P, Schrier RW. Renal failure in cirrhosis. N Engl J Med 2009;361(13): 1279–90.

95. Bellomo R, Ronco C, Kellum JA, et al, Acute Dialysis Quality Initiative Workgroup. Acute renal failure - definition, outcome measures, animal models, fluid therapy and information technology needs: the second International Consensus Conference of the Acute Dialysis Quality Initiative (ADQI) group. Crit Care 2004; 8(4):R204–12.

96. Joannidis M, Druml W, Forni LG, et al. Prevention of acute kidney injury and protection of renal function in the intensive care unit. Expert opinion of the working group for nephrology, ESICM. Intensive Care Med 2010;36(3):392–411.

97. Wong F, Nadim MK, Kellum JA, et al. Working party proposal for a revised classification system of renal dysfunction in patients with cirrhosis. Gut 2011;60(5): 702–9.

98. Wong F, O'Leary JG, Reddy KR, et al. New consensus definition of acute kidney injury accurately predicts 30-day mortality in patients with cirrhosis and infection. Gastroenterology 2013;145(6):1280–8.e1.

99. Arroyo V, Fernandez J, Gines P. Pathogenesis and treatment of hepatorenal syndrome. Semin Liver Dis 2008;28(1):81–95.

100. Bagshaw SM, George C, Dinu I, et al. A multi-centre evaluation of the RIFLE criteria for early acute kidney injury in critically ill patients. Nephrol Dial Transplant 2008;23(4):1203–10.

101. Sanyal AJ, Boyer T, Garcia-Tsao G, et al. A randomized, prospective, double-blind, placebo-controlled trial of terlipressin for type 1 hepatorenal syndrome. Gastroenterology 2008;134(5):1360–8.

102. Martin-Llahi M, Pepin MN, Guevara M, et al. Terlipressin and albumin vs albumin in patients with cirrhosis and hepatorenal syndrome: a randomized study. Gastroenterology 2008;134(5):1352–9.

103. Sharma P, Kumar A, Shrama BC, et al. An open label, pilot, randomized controlled trial of noradrenaline versus terlipressin in the treatment of type 1 hepatorenal syndrome and predictors of response. Am J Gastroenterol 2008;103(7):1689–97.

104. Alessandria C, Ottobrelli A, Debernardi-Venon W, et al. Noradrenalin vs terlipressin in patients with hepatorenal syndrome: a prospective, randomized, unblinded, pilot study. J Hepatol 2007;47(4):499–505.

105. Bismuth M, Funakoshi N, Cadranel JF, et al. Hepatic encephalopathy: from pathophysiology to therapeutic management. Eur J Gastroenterol Hepatol 2011;23(1):8–22.

106. Blei AT, Cordoba J, Practice Parameters Committee of the American College of Gastroenterology. Hepatic encephalopathy. Am J Gastroenterol 2001;96(7): 1968–76.

107. Bajaj JS. Review article: the modern management of hepatic encephalopathy. Aliment Pharmacol Ther 2010;31(5):537–47.

108. Mas A, Rodes J, Sunyer L, et al. Comparison of rifaximin and lactitol in the treatment of acute hepatic encephalopathy: results of a randomized, double-blind, double-dummy, controlled clinical trial. J Hepatol 2003;38(1):51–8.

109. Bass NM, Mullen KD, Sanyal A, et al. Rifaximin treatment in hepatic encephalopathy. N Engl J Med 2010;362(12):1071–81.

110. Barbaro G, Di Lorenzo G, Soldini M, et al. Flumazenil for hepatic encephalopathy grade III and IVa in patients with cirrhosis: an Italian multicenter double-blind, placebo-controlled, cross-over study. Hepatology 1998;28(2):374–8.

111. Hassanein TI, Tofteng F, Brown RS Jr, et al. Randomized controlled study of extracorporeal albumin dialysis for hepatic encephalopathy in advanced cirrhosis. Hepatology 2007;46(6):1853–62.

112. Heemann U, Treichel U, Loock J, et al. Albumin dialysis in cirrhosis with superimposed acute liver injury: a prospective, controlled study. Hepatology 2002; 36(4 Pt 1):949–58.

113. Khamaysi I, William N, Olga A, et al. Sub-clinical hepatic encephalopathy in cirrhotic patients is not aggravated by sedation with propofol compared to midazolam: a randomized controlled study. J Hepatol 2011;54(1):72–7.

114. Carbonell N, Pauwels A, Serfaty L, et al. Improved survival after variceal bleeding in patients with cirrhosis over the past two decades. Hepatology 2004;40(3):652–9.

115. de Franchis R. Revising consensus in portal hypertension: report of the Baveno V consensus workshop on methodology of diagnosis and therapy in portal hypertension. J Hepatol 2010;53(4):762–8.

116. Kravetz D, Sikuler E, Groszmann RJ. Splanchnic and systemic hemodynamics in portal hypertensive rats during hemorrhage and blood volume restitution. Gastroenterology 1986;90(5 Pt 1):1232–40.

117. Castaneda B, Morales J, Lionetti R, et al. Effects of blood volume restitution following a portal hypertensive-related bleeding in anesthetized cirrhotic rats. Hepatology 2001;33(4):821–5.

118. Bosch J, Thabut D, Bendtsen F, et al. Recombinant factor VIIa for upper gastrointestinal bleeding in patients with cirrhosis: a randomized, double-blind trial. Gastroenterology 2004;127(4):1123–30.

119. Ioannou GN, Doust J, Rockey DC. Systematic review: terlipressin in acute oesophageal variceal haemorrhage. Aliment Pharmacol Ther 2003;17(1): 53–64.

120. D'Amico G, Pagliaro L, Bosch J. Pharmacological treatment of portal hypertension: an evidence-based approach. Semin Liver Dis 1999;19(4):475–505.

121. Teran JC, Imperiale TF, Mullen KD, et al. Primary prophylaxis of variceal bleeding in cirrhosis: a cost-effectiveness analysis. Gastroenterology 1997; 112(2):473–82.

122. Levacher S, Letoumelin P, Pateron D, et al. Early administration of terlipressin plus glyceryl trinitrate to control active upper gastrointestinal bleeding in cirrhotic patients. Lancet 1995;346(8979):865–8.

123. Garcia-Pagan JC, Bosch J. Endoscopic band ligation in the treatment of portal hypertension. Nat Clin Pract Gastroenterol Hepatol 2005;2(11):526–35.
124. Lo GH, Lai KH, Cheng JS, et al. A prospective, randomized trial of butyl cyano-acrylate injection versus band ligation in the management of bleeding gastric varices. Hepatology 2001;33(5):1060–4.
125. Bernard B, Grange JD, Khac EN, et al. Antibiotic prophylaxis for the prevention of bacterial infections in cirrhotic patients with gastrointestinal bleeding: a meta-analysis. Hepatology 1999;29(6):1655–61.
126. Bernard B, Cadranel JF, Valla D, et al. Prognostic significance of bacterial infection in bleeding cirrhotic patients: a prospective study. Gastroenterology 1995; 108(6):1828–34.
127. Goulis J, Armonis A, Patch D, et al. Bacterial infection is independently associated with failure to control bleeding in cirrhotic patients with gastrointestinal hemorrhage. Hepatology 1998;27(5):1207–12.
128. Soares-Weiser K, Brezis M, Tur-Kaspa R, et al. Antibiotic prophylaxis for cirrhotic patients with gastrointestinal bleeding. Cochrane Database Syst Rev 2002;(2): CD002907.
129. Chavez-Tapia NC, Barrientos-Gutierrez T, Tellez-Avila FI, et al. Antibiotic prophylaxis for cirrhotic patients with upper gastrointestinal bleeding. Cochrane Database Syst Rev 2010;(9):CD002907.
130. Azoulay D, Castaing D, Majno P, et al. Salvage transjugular intrahepatic porto-systemic shunt for uncontrolled variceal bleeding in patients with decompensated cirrhosis. J Hepatol 2001;35(5):590–7.
131. Garcia-Pagán JC, Di Pascoli M, Caca K, et al. Use of early-TIPS for high-risk variceal bleeding: results of a post-RCT surveillance study. J Hepatol 2013;58(1):45–50.
132. Siegerstetter V, Deibert P, Ochs A, et al. Treatment of refractory hepatic hydro-thorax with transjugular intrahepatic portosystemic shunt: long-term results in 40 patients. Eur J Gastroenterol Hepatol 2001;13(5):529–34.
133. Rossle M, Gerbes AL. TIPS for the treatment of refractory ascites, hepatorenal syndrome and hepatic hydrothorax: a critical update. Gut 2010;59(7):988–1000.
134. Bernuau J, Rueff B, Benhamou JP. Fulminant and subfulminant liver failure: definitions and causes. Semin Liver Dis 1986;6(2):97–106.
135. Pereira LM, Langley PG, Hayllar KM, et al. Coagulation factor V and VIII/V ratio as predictors of outcome in paracetamol induced fulminant hepatic failure: relation to other prognostic indicators. Gut 1992;33(1):98–102.
136. Donaldson BW, Gopinath R, Wanless IR, et al. The role of transjugular liver biopsy in fulminant liver failure: relation to other prognostic indicators. Hepatology 1993;18(6):1370–6.
137. Cholongitas E, Theocharidou E, Vasianopoulou P, et al. Comparison of the sequential organ failure assessment score with the king's college hospital criteria and the model for end-stage liver disease score for the prognosis of acetaminophen-induced acute liver failure. Liver Transpl 2012;18(4):405–12.
138. Das V, Boelle PY, Galbois A, et al. Cirrhotic patients in the medical intensive care unit: early prognosis and long-term survival. Crit Care Med 2010;38(11): 2108–16.
139. Filloux B, Chagneau-Derrode C, Ragot S, et al. Short-term and long-term vital outcomes of cirrhotic patients admitted to an intensive care unit. Eur J Gastroenterol Hepatol 2010;22(12):1474–80.
140. Juneja D, Gopal PB, Kapoor D, et al. Outcome of patients with liver cirrhosis admitted to a specialty liver intensive care unit in India. J Crit Care 2009; 24(3):387–93.

141. Levesque E, Hoti E, Azoulay D, et al. Prospective evaluation of the prognostic scores for cirrhotic patients admitted to an intensive care unit. J Hepatol 2012;56(1):95–102.

142. Olmez S, Gumurdulu Y, Tas A, et al. Prognostic markers in cirrhotic patients requiring intensive care: a comparative prospective study. Ann Hepatol 2012; 11(4):513–8.

143. Rabe C, Schmitz V, Paashaus M, et al. Does intubation really equal death in cirrhotic patients? Factors influencing outcome in patients with liver cirrhosis requiring mechanical ventilation. Intensive Care Med 2004;30(8):1564–71.

144. Tu KH, Jenq CC, Tsai MH, et al. Outcome scoring systems for short-term prognosis in critically ill cirrhotic patients. Shock 2011;36(5):445–50.

Index

Note: Page numbers of article titles are in **boldface** type.

A

ACLF. *See* Acute-on-chronic liver failure (ACLF)
Acute kidney injury (AKI)
  in ACLF patients, 967
Acute liver failure (ALF), 957–964
  causes of, 958–959
  defined, 957–958
  incidence of, 958–959
  management of, 959–964
    bioartificial liver support systems in
      clinical efficacy of, 948–949
    cause-specific, 959–960
    complications-related, 960–962
    liver transplantation in, 962–964
    non-cause-specific, 960
Acute-on-chronic liver failure (ACLF)
  described, 964
  management of
    artificial liver support systems in
      clinical efficacy of, 949–953
    ICU, 964–970
  pathophysiology of, 964
  prognosis of
    initial assessment of, 964–970
Acute variceal bleeding (AVB), **793–808**
  described, 793–794
  management of
    esophageal stents in, 800–803
    general, 795
    hemostatic therapies in, 795–800
      EBL, 796–800
      endoscopic therapy, 796
      splanchnic vasoconstrictors, 795–796
    TIPS in, 855
  natural history/diagnosis of, 794–795
  refractory
    TIPS for, 855–857
AKI. *See* Acute kidney injury (AKI)
Alcoholic hepatitis
  HVPG measurement in, 785
ALF. *See* Acute liver failure (ALF)

Clin Liver Dis 18 (2014) 979–989
http://dx.doi.org/10.1016/S1089-3261(14)00078-6
1089-3261/14/$ – see front matter © 2014 Elsevier Inc. All rights reserved.

liver.theclinics.com

Ascites
   refractory
      TIPS for, 857
AVB. *See* Acute variceal bleeding (AVB)

B

Balloon-occluded retrograde transvenous obliteration (BRTO) procedure
   in gastric varices management, 819, 833–847
      outcomes in American institutions, 844–846
      outcomes in Asian institutions, 837–844
      TIPS with
         outcomes of, 846–847
Balloon tamponade
   in gastric varices management, 814
Bile duct stones
   cholangioscopy for
   outcomes of, 932–934
Biliary anastomotic strictures
   after liver transplantation
      cholangioscopy for, 921
      diagnostic approach to, 915–916
      ERCP for, **913–926**. *See also* Endoscopic retrograde cholangiopancreatography
         (ERCP), for biliary anastomotic strictures after liver transplantation
      recurrence of, 920
      risk factors for, 915
      treatment of, 916–920
Biliary malignancies
   suspected
      cholangioscopy for
         outcomes of, 934–937
Biliary strictures
   anastomotic. *See* Biliary anastomotic strictures
   LDLT and, 920–921
   types of, 914–915
Bleeding
   acute variceal, **793–808**. *See also* Acute variceal bleeding (AVB)
   gastrointestinal
      in ACLF patients, 969–970
   refractory
      gastric varices and portal hypertensive gastropathy and, 857
   variceal. *See* Variceal bleeding
BRTO procedure. *See* Balloon-occluded retrograde transvenous obliteration (BRTO)
   procedure
Budd-Chiari syndrome
   TIPS for, 859

C

Cancer(s). *See also* Carcinoma(s)
   liver

radioembolization for, 882–883

TACE for, **877–890**. *See also* Transarterial chemoembolization (TACE), for liver
cancer

Carcinoma(s). *See also* Cancer(s)

hepatocellular. *See* Hepatocellular carcinoma (HCC)

Chemoembolization

transarterial

for liver cancer. *See also* Transarterial chemoembolization (TACE)

Cholangiocarcinoma

benign stenosis *vs.*

in PSC patients, 906–907

described, 891

ERCP for, **891–897**. *See also* Endoscopic retrograde cholangiopancreatography
(ERCP)

Cholangioscopy

in liver disease, **927–944**

approach to, 929–930

for bile duct stones

outcomes of, 932–934

for biliary anastomotic strictures after liver transplantation, 921

clinical implications of, 938

complications/management of, 938

current controversies/future considerations in, 938–939

follow-up care, 938

indications/contraindications to, 928

introduction, 927–928

outcomes of, 931–937

postprocedure care, 938

preparation for, 928–929

for PSC, 907

outcomes of, 937

reporting of, 938

for suspected biliary malignancies

outcomes of, 934–937

technique for, 930–931

Cholangitis

primary sclerosing

ERCP for, **899–911**. *See also* Endoscopic retrograde cholangiopancreatography
(ERCP), for PSC; Primary sclerosing cholangitis (PSC)

Chronic liver disease (CLD)

described, 768

Cirrhosis

prognosis of

HVPG measurement in, 784–785

severity of

HVPG measurement in, 784–785

CLD. *See* Chronic liver disease (CLD)

Conventional TACE (cTACE)

for liver cancer

technique/procedure for, 879–881

D

Drug-eluting bead TACE
    for liver cancer
        technique/procedure for, 882

E

EBL. *See* Endoscopic band ligation (EBL)
Endoscopic band ligation (EBL)
    in AVB management, 796–800
    in gastric varices management, 816
Endoscopic retrograde cholangiopancreatography (ERCP)
    for biliary anastomotic strictures after liver transplantation, **913–926**
        complications of, 921
        dilation and plastic stent placement, 917
        introduction, 913–914
        limitations of, 918–920
        self-expandable metal stents, 917–918
    for cholangiocarcinoma, **891–897**
        complications/management of, 894–895
        current controversies/future considerations in, 896
        indications/contraindications to, 891–892
        outcomes of, 895–896
        postoperative care, 895
        technique/procedure for, 892–894
    introduction, 891
    for PSC, **899–911**. *See also* Primary sclerosing cholangitis (PSC)
        complications of, 905–907
        introduction, 899–900
Endoscopic sphincterotomy
    for PSC, 902
Endoscopic stent placement
    for PSC, 903–904
Endoscopic stricture dilation
    for PSC, 902–903
Endoscopic therapies
    in AVB management, 796
    combined
        in gastric varices management, 818
    in gastric varices management, 814
    in gastric varices prevention, 820
Endoscopic ultrasound (EUS)–guided therapy
    in gastric varices management, 818–819
Endovascular procedures
    in gastric varices management, **829–851**. *See also specific methods and* Gastric
        varices, management of, endovascular
ERCP. *See* Endoscopic retrograde cholangiopancreatography (ERCP)
Esophageal stents
    in AVB management, 800–803
EUS. *See* Endoscopic ultrasound (EUS)

G

Gastric varices
    acute
        management of, 813
    anatomy related to, 830–833
        vascular, 811–812
    classification of, 810, 830–833
    hemodynamic features of, 811–812
    introduction, 809–810
    management of, **809–851**
        balloon tamponade in, 814
        band ligation in, 816
        BRTO procedure in, 819, 833–847
        endoscopic therapies in, 814
            combined, 818
        endovascular, **829–851**
            BRTO procedure, 833–837
                outcomes in American institutions, 844–846
                outcomes in Asian institutions, 837–844
            introduction, 829–830
            TIPS only in
                outcomes of, 846
        EUS–guided treatment in, 818–819
        medical, 813–814
        obturation in, 815–816
        primary prophylaxis in, 812–813
        radiologic interventions in, 819
        risk factors associated with, 813
        sclerotherapy in, 814–815
        secondary prophylaxis in, 820–821
        thrombin in, 817–818
        TIPS in, 819
    refractory bleeding from
        TIPS for, 857
    terminology related to, 830–833
Gastroesophageal varices. See also Gastric varices
    introduction, 809–810
Gastrointestinal bleeding
    in ACLF patients, 969–970
Gastropathy
    portal hypertensive
        refractory bleeding from
            TIPS for, 857

H

HCC. See Hepatocellular carcinoma (HCC)
Hemodynamic instability
    in ACLF patients
        management of, 965–967

Hemostatic therapies
    in AVB management, 795–800. *See also* Acute variceal bleeding (AVB), management
        of, hemostatic therapies in
Hepatic venoocclusive disease
    TIPS for, 859
Hepatic venous pressure gradient (HVPG) measurement, 780–782
    applications of, 783–788
        alcoholic hepatitis, 785
        assessment of new therapeutic agents, 788
        assessment of response to pharmacologic therapy to decrease portal pressure,
          786–788
        cirrhosis prognosis, 784–785
        cirrhosis severity, 784–785
        hepatocellular carcinoma, 786
        liver transplantation, 785–786
        portal hypertension classification, 784
        portal hypertension diagnosis, 783–784
        viral hepatitis, 785
Hepatitis
    alcoholic
        HVPG measurement in, 785
    viral
        HVPG measurement in, 785
Hepatocellular carcinoma (HCC)
    HVPG measurement in, 786
    introduction, 877–879
Hepatopulmonary syndrome (HPS)
    TIPS for, 858–859
Hepatorenal syndrome (HRS)
    TIPS for, 859
HPS. *See* Hepatopulmonary syndrome (HPS)
HRS. *See* Hepatorenal syndrome (HRS)
HVPG. *See* Hepatic venous pressure gradient (HVPG)
Hydrothorax
    refractory hepatic
        TIPS for, 858
Hypertension
    portal. *See* Portal hypertension

    I

ICU. *See* Intensive care unit (ICU)
Infection(s)
    in ACLF patients, 964
Intensive care unit (ICU)
    liver failure patients in
        management of, **957–978**. *See also* Liver failure, ICU management of patients with
Interventional radiologic approach
    in gastric varices prevention, 820

L

LDLT. *See* Living donor liver transplantation (LDLT)
Liver biopsy
  transjugular, **767–778**. *See also* Transjugular liver biopsy (TJLB)
Liver cancer
  radioembolization for, 882–883
  TACE for, **877–890**. *See also* Transarterial chemoembolization (TACE), for liver
    cancer
Liver disease
  cholangioscopy in, **927–944**. *See also* Cholangioscopy, in liver disease
Liver failure
  acute. *See* Acute liver failure (ALF)
  acute-on-chronic. *See* Acute-on-chronic liver failure (ACLF)
  ICU management of patients with, **957–978**
    ACL patients, 957–964. *See also* Acute liver failure (ALF)
    ACLF patients, 964–970
  liver support systems in, **945–956**. *See also* Liver support systems
Liver support systems
  bioartificial
    in ALF, 948–949
  extracorporeal
    technical characteristics of, 946
  in liver failure, **945–956**
    artificial *vs.* bioartificial systems analysis
      clinical studies, 953
    clinical efficacy of, 948–953
      in ACLF, 949–953
      in ALF, 949
      bioartificial liver support systems in ALF, 948–949
    future considerations, 953–954
    ideal
      requirements for, 953–954
    in improving liver regeneration, 948
    in improving portal and systemic hemodynamics, 947–948
    rationale for, 946–948
    in toxins elimination, 946–947
  necessity of, 945–946
Liver transplantation
  for ALF, 962–964
  biliary anastomotic strictures after. *See also* Biliary anastomotic strictures, after liver
    transplantation
    ERCP for, **913–926**. *See also* Biliary anastomotic strictures; Endoscopic retrograde
      cholangiopancreatography (ERCP), for biliary anastomotic strictures after liver
      transplantation
  HVPG measurement and, 785–786
  living donor
    biliary strictures and, 920–921
Living donor liver transplantation (LDLT)
  biliary strictures and, 920–921

M

Malignancy(ies)
 biliary
  suspected
   cholangioscopy for, 934–937
Medical therapies
 in gastric varices prevention, 820

N

Neurologic complications
 in ACLF patients, 967–969

O

Obturation
 in gastric varices management, 815–816

P

Partial splenic embolization (PSE)
 in gastric varices prevention, 820
Portal hypertension
 classification of
  HVPG measurement in, 784
 described, 779–780
 diagnosis of
  HVPG measurement in, 783–784
Portal hypertensive gastropathy
 refractory bleeding from
  TIPS for, 857
Portal pressure
 decrease in
  HVPG measurement in assessment of response to pharmacologic therapy for,
   786–788
 introduction, 779–780
 measurement of, **779–792**
  HVPG–related, 780–782
Primary sclerosing cholangitis (PSC)
 cholangioscopy for
  outcomes of, 937
 cholangioscopy in
  role of, 907
 described, 899–900
 diagnosis of, 900
 dominant stricture in, 900–901
  management of
   endoscopic, 902–904
   medical, 901
   nonendoscopic, 901–902
   percutaneous, 901
   surgical, 902

endoscopic management of
    efficacy of, 904
ERCP for, **899–911**. *See also* Endoscopic retrograde cholangiopancreatography
    (ERCP), for PSC
PSC. *See* Primary sclerosing cholangitis (PSC)
PSE. *See* Partial splenic embolization (PSE)
Pulmonary complications
    in ACLF patients, 970

R

Radioembolization
    for liver cancer, 882–883
Radiologic procedures
    in gastric varices management, 819
Refractory acute variceal bleeding
    TIPS for, 855–857
Refractory ascites
    TIPS for, 857
Refractory bleeding
    gastric varices and portal hypertensive gastropathy and
        TIPS for, 857
Refractory hepatic hydrothorax
    TIPS for, 858

S

Sclerotherapy
    in gastric varices management, 814–815
Septic shock
    in ACLF patients
        management of, 965–967
Sphincterotomy
    endoscopic
        for PSC, 902
Splanchnic vasoconstrictors
    in AVB management, 795–796
Stent(s)
    esophageal
        in AVB management, 800–803
Suspected biliary malignancies
    cholangioscopy for
        outcomes of, 934–937

T

TACE. *See* Transarterial chemoembolization (TACE)
Thrombin
    in gastric varices management, 817–818
TIPS. *See* Transjugular intrahepatic portosystemic shunts (TIPS)
TJLB. *See* Transjugular liver biopsy (TJLB)

Toxin(s)
    liver failure–related
        elimination of
            liver support systems in, 946–947
Transarterial chemoembolization (TACE)
    for liver cancer, **877–890**
        clinical implications of, 884–885
        complications/management of, 883
        cTACE
            technique/procedure for, 879–881
        current controversies/future considerations in, 886–888
        drug-eluting bead–type
            technique/procedure for, 882
        follow-up care, 884–885
        indications/contraindications for, 879
        introduction, 877–879
        outcomes of, 885–886
        postprocedure care, 883–884
        reporting related to, 884–885
        technique/procedure for, 879–883
Transjugular intrahepatic portosystemic shunts (TIPS), **853–876**
    advanced/alternative techniques for, 864
    complications of, 864–867
    conventional technique for, 860–864
    evaluation prior to, 859–860
    follow-up care, 867
    future considerations in, 867
    in gastric varices management, 819
        with BRTO procedure
            outcomes of, 846–847
        outcomes of, 846
    indications for, 854–859
        AVB, 855
            refractory, 855–857
        Budd-Chiari syndrome, 859
        hepatic venoocclusive disease, 859
        HPS, 858–859
        HRS, 859
        refractory ascites, 857
        refractory bleeding from gastric varices and portal hypertensive gastropathy, 857
        refractory hepatic hydrothorax, 858
        variceal hemorrhage prevention, 854–855
    introduction, 853–854
    maintenance care, 867
    patient selection for, 859–860
Transjugular liver biopsy (TJLB), **767–778**
    complications/management of, 774
    current controversies/future considerations in, 776
    indications/contraindications to, 768
    sample quality and clinical implications in, 774–776
    technique/procedure for, 768–774

Transplantation(s)
  liver. *See* Liver transplantation

V

Variceal bleeding
  acute
    refractory
      TIPS for, 855–857
    TIPS for, 855
  prevention of
    TIPS in, 854–855
Varices
  gastric. *See* Gastric varices
Vasoconstrictor(s)
  splanchnic
    in AVB management, 795–796
Venoocclusive disease
  hepatic
    TIPS for, 859
Viral hepatitis
  HVPG measurement in, 785

United States Postal Service

Statement of Ownership, Management, and Circulation
(All Periodicals Publications Except Requestor Publications)

1. Publication Title	2. Publication Number	3. Filing Date
Clinics in Liver Disease	0 1 6 - 7 5 4	9/14/14

4. Issue Frequency	5. Number of Issues Published Annually	6. Annual Subscription Price
Feb, May, Aug, Nov	4	$295.00

7. Complete Mailing Address of Known Office of Publication (Not printer) (Street, city, county, state, and ZIP+4®)

Elsevier Inc.
360 Park Avenue South
New York, NY 10010-1710

Contact Person
Stephen R. Bushing

Telephone (Include area code)
215-239-3688

8. Complete Mailing Address of Headquarters or General Business Office of Publisher (Not printer)

Elsevier Inc., 360 Park Avenue South, New York, NY 10010-1710

9. Full Names and Complete Mailing Addresses of Publisher, Editor, and Managing Editor (Do not leave blank)

Publisher (Name and complete mailing address)

Linda Belfus, Elsevier Inc., 1600 John F. Kennedy Blvd., Suite 1800, Philadelphia, PA 19103-2899

Editor (Name and complete mailing address)

Kerry Holland, Elsevier Inc., 1600 John F. Kennedy Blvd., Suite 1800, Philadelphia, PA 19103-2899

Managing Editor (Name and complete mailing address)

Adrianne Brigido, Elsevier Inc., 1600 John F. Kennedy Blvd., Suite 1800, Philadelphia, PA 19103-2899

10. Owner (Do not leave blank. If the publication is owned by a corporation, give the name and address of the corporation immediately followed by the names and addresses of all stockholders owning or holding 1 percent or more of the total amount of stock. If not owned by a corporation, give the names and addresses of the individual owners. If owned by a partnership or other unincorporated firm, give its name and address as well as those of each individual owner. If the publication is published by a nonprofit organization, give its name and address.)

Full Name	Complete Mailing Address
Wholly owned subsidiary of	1600 John F. Kennedy Blvd, Ste. 1800
Reed/Elsevier, US holdings	Philadelphia, PA 19103-2899

11. Known Bondholders, Mortgagees, and Other Security Holders Owning or Holding 1 Percent or More of Total Amount of Bonds, Mortgages, or Other Securities. If none, check box ☐ None

Full Name	Complete Mailing Address
N/A	

12. Tax Status (For completion by nonprofit organizations authorized to mail at nonprofit rates) (Check one)
The purpose, function, and nonprofit status of this organization and the exempt status for federal income tax purposes:
☐ Has Not Changed During Preceding 12 Months
☐ Has Changed During Preceding 12 Months (Publisher must submit explanation of change with this statement)

13. Publication Title	14. Issue Date for Circulation Data Below
Clinics in Liver Disease	August 2014

15. Extent and Nature of Circulation		Average No. Copies Each Issue During Preceding 12 Months	No. Copies of Single Issue Published Nearest to Filing Date
a. Total Number of Copies (Net press run)		406	442
b. Paid Circulation (By Mail and Outside the Mail)	(1) Mailed Outside-County Paid Subscriptions Stated on PS Form 3541. (Include paid distribution above nominal rate, advertiser's proof copies, and exchange copies)	151	132
	(2) Mailed In-County Paid Subscriptions Stated on PS Form 3541 (Include paid distribution above nominal rate, advertiser's proof copies, and exchange copies)		
	(3) Paid Distribution Outside the Mails Including Sales Through Dealers and Carriers, Street Vendors, Counter Sales, and Other Paid Distribution Outside USPS®	71	87
	(4) Paid Distribution by Other Classes Mailed Through the USPS (e.g. First-Class Mail®)		
c. Total Paid Distribution (Sum of 15b (1), (2), (3), and (4))	▶	222	219
d. Free or Nominal Rate Distribution (By Mail and Outside the Mail)	(1) Free or Nominal Rate Outside-County Copies Included on PS Form 3541	85	103
	(2) Free or Nominal Rate In-County Copies Included on PS Form 3541		
	(3) Free or Nominal Rate Copies Mailed at Other Classes Through the USPS (e.g. First-Class Mail)		
	(4) Free or Nominal Rate Distribution Outside the Mail (Carriers or other means)		
e. Total Free or Nominal Rate Distribution (Sum of 15d (1), (2), (3) and (4))	▶	85	103
f. Total Distribution (Sum of 15c and 15e)	▶	307	322
g. Copies not Distributed (See instructions to publishers #4 (page #3))	▶	99	120
h. Total (Sum of 15f and g)	▶	406	442
i. Percent Paid (15c divided by 15f times 100)		72.31%	68.01%

16. Total circulation includes electronic copies. Report circulation on PS Form 3526-X worksheet.

17. Publication of Statement of Ownership
If the publication is a general publication, publication of this statement is required. Will be printed in the November 2014 issue of this publication.

18. Signature and Title of Editor, Publisher, Business Manager, or Owner

Stephen R. Bushing – Inventory Distribution Coordinator

Date: September 14, 2014

I certify that all information furnished on this form is true and complete. I understand that anyone who furnishes false or misleading information on this form or who omits material or information requested on the form may be subject to criminal sanctions (including fines and imprisonment) and/or civil sanctions (including civil penalties).

PS Form 3526, August 2012 (Page 1 of 3 (Instructions Page 3)) PSN 7530-01-000-9931 PRIVACY NOTICE: See our Privacy policy in www.usps.com

PS Form 3526, August 2012 (Page 2 of 3)

Printed and bound by CPI Group (UK) Ltd, Croydon, CR0 4YY

03/10/2024

01040485-0003